The IMA Volumes in Mathematics and its Applications

Volume 116

Series Editor
Willard Miller, Jr.

Springer
New York
Berlin
Heidelberg
Barcelona
Hong Kong
London
Milan
Paris
Singapore
Tokyo

Institute for Mathematics and its Applications IMA

The **Institute for Mathematics and its Applications** was established by a grant from the National Science Foundation to the University of Minnesota in 1982. The IMA seeks to encourage the development and study of fresh mathematical concepts and questions of concern to the other sciences by bringing together mathematicians and scientists from diverse fields in an atmosphere that will stimulate discussion and collaboration.

The IMA Volumes are intended to involve the broader scientific community in this process.

Willard Miller, Jr., Professor and Director

* * * * * * * * * *

IMA ANNUAL PROGRAMS

1982–1983	Statistical and Continuum Approaches to Phase Transition
1983–1984	Mathematical Models for the Economics of Decentralized Resource Allocation
1984–1985	Continuum Physics and Partial Differential Equations
1985–1986	Stochastic Differential Equations and Their Applications
1986–1987	Scientific Computation
1987–1988	Applied Combinatorics
1988–1989	Nonlinear Waves
1989–1990	Dynamical Systems and Their Applications
1990–1991	Phase Transitions and Free Boundaries
1991–1992	Applied Linear Algebra
1992–1993	Control Theory and its Applications
1993–1994	Emerging Applications of Probability
1994–1995	Waves and Scattering
1995–1996	Mathematical Methods in Material Science
1996–1997	Mathematics of High Performance Computing
1997–1998	Emerging Applications of Dynamical Systems
1998–1999	Mathematics in Biology
1999–2000	Reactive Flows and Transport Phenomena
2000–2001	Mathematics in Multimedia
2001–2002	Mathematics in the Geosciences

Continued at the back

M. Elizabeth Halloran   Donald Berry
Editors

Statistical Models in Epidemiology, the Environment, and Clinical Trials

With 32 Illustrations

Springer

M. Elizabeth Halloran
Department of Biostatistics
Rollins School of Public Health
Emory University
1518 Clifton Road, NE
Atlanta, GA 30322, USA
betz@bear.sph.emory.edu

Donald Berry
Institute of Statistics and Decision Sciences
and Cancer Center Biostatistics
Box 90251
223 Old Chemistry Bldg., Main Campus
Duke University
Durham, NC 27708-0251, USA

Series Editor:
Willard Miller, Jr.
Institute for Mathematics and its Applications
University of Minnesota
Minneapolis, MN 55455, USA

Mathematics Subject Classification (1991): 62-06, 62-07, 62A10, 62A15, 65D05, 65D15, 65D30

Library of Congress Cataloging-in-Publication Data
Statistical models in epidemiology, the environment, and clinical trials / editors, M. Elizabeth Halloran, Donald Berry.
p. cm. — (The IMA volumes in mathematics and its applications : v. 116)
Includes bibliographical references.
ISBN 0-387-98924-2 (hc. : alk. paper)
1. Epidemiology—Statistical methods Congresses. I. Halloran, M. Elizabeth. II. Berry, Donald A. III. Series: IMA volumes in mathematics and its applications ; v. 116.
RA652.2.M3S735 1999
614.4′07′27—dc21 99-43260

Printed on acid-free paper.

Production managed by A. Orrantia; manufacturing supervised by Joe Quatela.
Camera-ready copy prepared by the IMA.
Printed and bound by Sheridan Books, Inc., Ann Arbor, MI.
Printed in the United States of America.

9 8 7 6 5 4 3 2 1

ISBN 0-387-98924-2 Springer-Verlag New York Berlin Heidelberg SPIN 10743210

FOREWORD

This IMA Volume in Mathematics and its Applications

STATISTICAL MODELS IN EPIDEMIOLOGY, THE ENVIRONMENT, AND CLINICAL TRIALS

is a combined proceedings on "Design and Analysis of Clinical Trials" and "Statistics and Epidemiology: Environment and Health." This volume is the third series based on the proceedings of a very successful 1997 IMA Summer Program on "Statistics in the Health Sciences."

I would like to thank the organizers: M. Elizabeth Halloran of Emory University (Biostatistics) and Donald A. Berry of Duke University (Institute of Statistics and Decision Sciences and Cancer Center Biostatistics) for their excellent work as organizers of the meeting and for editing the proceedings. I am grateful to Seymour Geisser of University of Minnesota (Statistics), Patricia Grambsch, University of Minnesota (Biostatistics); Joel Greenhouse, Carnegie Mellon University (Statistics); Nicholas Lange, Harvard Medical School (Brain Imaging Center, McLean Hospital); Barry Margolin, University of North Carolina-Chapel Hill (Biostatistics); Sandy Weisberg, University of Minnesota (Statistics); Scott Zeger, Johns Hopkins University (Biostatistics); and Marvin Zelen, Harvard School of Public Health (Biostatistics) for organizing the six weeks summer program.

I also take this opportunity to thank the National Science Foundation (NSF) and the Army Research Office (ARO), whose financial support made the workshop possible.

Willard Miller, Jr., Professor and Director

PREFACE

This volume contains refereed papers by participants in the two weeks on Clinical Trials and one week on Epidemiology and the Environment held as part of the six weeks workshop on Statistics in the Health Sciences Applications at the Institute for Mathematics and its Application (IMA) in the summer 1997. The clinical trials weeks had a few dozen participants. The week on Epidemiology and the Environment had about 20 participants. Donald Berry was in charge of the weeks on clinical trials, and Elizabeth Halloran organized the week on epidemiology and the environment. Not all participants actually contributed papers since the IMA publications can include only papers that were not published elsewhere. Given the similarity of the themes of clinical trials and epidemiology, we chose to publish the papers together as one volume.

The focus of the two weeks on clinical trials was innovation in design and analysis. Clinical trials are essential for evaluating the safety and efficacy of therapeutic agents and vaccines. Issues addressed at the workshop included early stopping, censoring, handling missing data, multiple comparisons, synthesis of information across trials, screening and prevention trials, ethical considerations, and using surrogate markers. Both frequentist and Bayesian perspectives were presented, contrasted, and discussed.

The idea in the week on epidemiology and the environment was to bring together people that do not often talk with one another. Spatial mapping and analysis of disease data, including the use of geographic information systems (GIS), remote sensing, and various sources of publicly collected are increasingly being used in epidemiologic and etiologic studies. Hierarchical and Bayesian models are often used in the analysis of such data. The studies of spatial correlations and environmental factors present new challenges for epidemiologic methods. These include the use of case-control methods, analysis of missing data in observational studies, exposure assessment and errors-in-variables, and causal inference. Participants were invited who represented these various fields. The first talks were on mapping and examples of spatial analysis. This laid the groundwork then for discussion of the different methodologies in observational studies. Particularly fun was an afternoon devoted to discussing the semiparametric efficient approach to missing data that was led by Jamie Robins and Mark van der Laan.

We are pleased to include a major contribution from Jamie Robins, Andrea Rotnitzky, and Daniel Scharfstein on sensitivity analysis for selection bias and unmeasured confounding in missing data and causal inference models. In this paper, they present a new class of non-parametric (just) identified models. These models are used to conduct a sensitivity analysis in observational studies about how uncertain the inference is and how biased the results might be. The authors show the relation to the understanding of confounding in usual methods of analysis. In another paper, Jamie Robins presents a new class of causal models called marginal structural models. Alan Hubbard, Mark van der Laan, and Jamie Robins present a methodology for consistent and efficient estimation of treatment-specific survival functions in observational settings where not all subjects receive the treatment of interest. All three of these papers show the similarity in the paradigm for clinical, or randomized trials and how they can become similar to observational studies through choices in changing treatment regimes.

From the spatial and environmental arena, Brian Leroux, Xingye Lei, and Norman Breslow present a new mixed model for spatial dependence for estimating disease rates in small areas. Andrew Lawson and Allan Clark demonstrate the use of Markov Chain Monte Carlo methods for clustering in spatial epidemiology. The approach is based on point process models. Colin Chen, David Chock, and Sandra Winkler present a simulation study examining confounding in estimation of the epidemiologic effect of air pollution.

In the clinical trials area, Dalene Stangl discusses some fundamental issues related to the use of reference priors and Bayes factors in analyzing clinical trials. Stephen George discusses the role of surrogate endpoints in cancer clinical trials, including prevention, screening, and therapeutic trials.

We thank Patricia V. Brick of the IMA for her infinite patience in getting this volume finished. We also thank Robert Gulliver for his energy in helping us organize the six weeks workshop. We thank all of our colleagues who contributed with great vigor to the stimulating discussions. We are especially grateful to Avner Friedman, the Director of the IMA up through the summer of 1997, for inviting us to be on the organizing group of the workshop on Statistics in the Health Sciences at the IMA.

M. Elizabeth Halloran
Department of Biostatistics
Emory University

Donald Berry
Institute of Statistics and Decision Sciences and Cancer Center
Biostatistics Duke University

April, 1999

CONTENTS

SENSITIVITY ANALYSIS FOR SELECTION BIAS AND UNMEASURED CONFOUNDING IN MISSING DATA AND CAUSAL INFERENCE MODELS

JAMES M. ROBINS*, ANDREA ROTNITZKY†, AND DANIEL O. SCHARFSTEIN‡

Table of Contents

Sections 1–5 by *J.M. Robins, A. Rotnitzky, and D.O. Scharfstein*

Sections 6–11 by *J.M. Robins*

*Departments of Epidemiology and Biostatistics, Harvard School of Public Health, 677 Huntington Avenue, Boston, MA 02115; robins@hsph.harvard.edu.

†Department of Biostatistics, Harvard School of Public Health, Boston, MA 02115.

‡Department of Biostatistics, Johns Hopkins School of Hygiene and Public Health, Baltimore, MD 21205.

1. Introduction. In both observational and randomized studies, subjects commonly drop out of the study (i.e., become censored) before end of follow-up. If, conditional on the history of the observed data up to t, the hazard of dropping out of the study (i.e., censoring) at time t does not depend on the possibly unobserved data subsequent to t, we say drop-out is ignorable or explainable (Rubin, 1976). On the other hand, if the hazard of drop-out depends on the possibly unobserved future, we say drop-out is non-ignorable or, equivalently, that there is selection bias on unobservables. Neither the existence of selection bias on unobservables nor its magnitude is identifiable from the joint distribution of the observables. In view of this fact, we argue that the data analyst should conduct a "sensitivity analysis" to quantify how one's inference concerning an outcome of interest varies as a function of the magnitude of non-identifiable selection bias.

In Sections 2 and 3, we present a new class of non-parametric (just) identified (NPI) models that are useful for this purpose. These models are non-parametric (i.e., saturated) in the sense that each model in the class places no restrictions on the joint distribution of the observed data. Hence, each model in the class fits the observed data perfectly and cannot be rejected by any statistical test. Each model is (just) identified in the sense that the model identifies the distribution of the underlying full data (i.e., the distribution of the data that would have been observed in the absence of drop-out). Each NPI model in the class is indexed by a selection bias function that quantifies the magnitude of selection bias due to unobservables. Since each model is non-parametric, this selection bias function is not identified from the distribution of the observed data. However, we show that one can perform a sensitivity analysis that examines how inferences concerning functionals of the full data change as the non-identified selection bias function is varied over a plausible range. A nice feature of our approach is that, as discussed in Section 4, for each choice of the non-identified selection bias function, the full data functionals of interest can be estimated at $n^{\frac{1}{2}}$-rates using the modern theory of estimation in semiparametric models with missing data (Robins and Rotnitzky, 1992; Bickel et al., 1993; van der Vaart, 1991; Robins and Ritov, 1997). The results in Sec. 4 draw in part on as yet unpublished work by the authors (Scharfstein, Rotnitzky, and Robins, 1999).

In Sec. 5, we study in further detail a particular NPI model — the selection odds NPI model. This model is the unique NPI model that has both a "pattern mixture" (Little, 1993) and a selection model interpretation. Under this model, we derive an explicit formula, the selection bias g-computation algorithm formula, for the distribution of the full (i.e., complete) data. This formula generalizes the g-computation algorithm formula of Robins (1986) to the setting in which drop-out is non-ignorable.

There is a close connection between selection bias due to unobserved factors in follow-up studies with drop-out and selection bias due to unmeasured confounding factors in causal inference models. In Secs. 6 and 7, we use this connection to generalize our NPI selection bias models to NPI causal inference models. Unfortunately, we show in Sec. 7.2 that there is major difficulty with trying to construct semiparametric estimators of the parameters of a NPI selection odds causal inference model. One solution to this difficulty is to give up the attempt to construct simple semiparametric estimators and, instead, use fully parametric likelihood-based inference. This approach is briefly discussed in the last remark of Sec. 8.6.1. A second and better approach is to develop alternative NPI causal inference models that simultaneously allow for unmeasured confounding and admit simple semiparametric estimators. This latter approach is considered in Sec. 8. In that section, we generalize both the structural nested models of Robins (1989, 1997b) and the marginal structural models of Robins (1998ab) to allow for selection bias due to unmeasured confounding.

In Secs. 9 and 10, we return to the subject of missing data models. The NPI missing data models discussed in Sections 2, 3 assume a monotone missing data pattern. In Section 10, we construct NPI models, the selection bias permutation missingness models, for non-monotone missing data with positive probability of complete observations. These models generalize the permutation missingness models of Robins (1997a).

In Section 11, we consider a Bayesian, as opposed to a sensitivity analysis, approach to summarizing our uncertainty.

Other work on NPI models with non-ignorable missing data includes the papers by Baker et al. (1992), Robins (1997a), Rotnitzky, Robins, and Scharfstein (1998), Zheng and Klein (1994, 1995), Slud and Rubenstein (1983), Klein and Moeschberger (1988), Nordheim (1984), Little (1994), and Moeschberger and Klein (1995). In contrast with our approach, except for Robins (1997a) and Rotnitzky, Robins, and Scharfstein (1998), the NPI models described in these papers do not allow for the incorporation of data on high-dimensional time-dependent covariate processes. The availability of such data has become very frequent in both longitudinal randomized and non-randomized studies.

Rosenbaum (1995) has published a considerable body of work on sensitivity analysis for selection bias and unmeasured confounding. However, Rosenbaum's approach differs from ours in that his approach is not based on a class of NPI models indexed by selection bias functions. Thus, in Rosenbaum's approach, causal contrasts of interest are not consistently estimated as a function of the non-identified strength of residual unmeasured confounding.

A large body of previous work, originating with Cornfield (1959), on sensitivity analysis in causal inference models has assumed the existence of an unmeasured confounder of U. In a sensitivity analysis, one varies the association of U with the outcome Y (within levels of treatment and measured confounders) and the association of U with the treatment (within levels of measured confounders) (Schlesselman, 1978; Rosenbaum and Rubin, 1983; Lin et al., 1998). In contrast, in our approach, we simply model the association of the counterfactual outcome variable with the treatment (within levels of measured confounders). The advantage of our approach is that *(i)* there are many fewer sensitivity parameters to vary, and *(ii)* the (essentially impossible) decision as to whether to view U as univariate or multivariate, continuous or discrete is done away with. A link between the two approaches is that the counterfactual variable can be considered the ultimate unmeasured confounder U. This reflects the fact that, given the counterfactual and treatment, other unmeasured covariates U fail to predict the observed outcome (and thus are superfluous and can be dispensed with), since the observed outcome variable is a deterministic function of the treatment and the counterfactual outcome.

In our opinion, the unmeasured confounder U approach should be preferred to our counterfactual approach only in circumstances, where *(i)* U represents a known confounder (e.g., cigarette smoking) that for logistical reasons was not measured in a particular study, and furthermore, *(ii)* there exists reasonable historical knowledge about the magnitude of association of U with both the outcome (conditional on treatment and measured confounders) and the treatment (conditional on measured confounders). In contrast, when U is to represent all possible unmeasured factors, we believe that it is substantively easier for subject-matter experts to give their opinions about the plausible magnitude of the association of the counterfactual outcome with treatment than about the question of whether any unmeasured confounders U are continuous or discrete, single or multidimensional, and the associations of such confounders with treatment and the outcome.

In the setting of a single time-independent treatment, our counterfactual approach leads to extremely simple computations that can be carried out with standard software. Specifically, as described in Remark 8.14 of Sec. 8.5, when the outcome Y is dichotomous, it is possible to use a standard logistic regression program equipped with an offset option that allows the analyst to fix coefficients of certain regressors to known values. In contrast, as discussed by Lin et al. (1998), there can be formidable computational difficulties associated with the approach based on positing an unmeasured covariate U. Even in the presence of time-varying treatments and covariates, the counterfactual approach to sensitivity analysis can remain computationally simple provided one uses the semiparametric estimation methods described in Sec. 8.

2. Identification in monotone missing data problems.

2.1. Single occasion. Consider a study designed such that a vector or scalar variable L_i is to be measured on each of n units $i, i = 1, \ldots, n$. The entire vector L_i is missing on a subset of the units. We therefore observe n i.i.d. copies of

$$O = (\Delta, \Delta L) \tag{2.1}$$

where $\Delta = 1$ if L is observed and $\Delta = 0$ otherwise. Throughout we refer to L_i as the *full data* on unit i. Thus, under our assumptions, (L_i, Δ_i) and $O_i, i = 1, \ldots, n$ are n i.i.d. copies of random variables (L, Δ) and O with cumulative distribution functions denoted by $F_{L,\Delta}$ and F_O respectively. In what follows, F_L is used to denote the cumulative distribution function of L. Here and henceforth we suppress the i subscript denoting unit. Little and Rubin (1987) refer to the product variable ΔL as L_{obs}. We assume that

$$pr\,(\Delta = 1) \neq 0. \tag{2.2}$$

The simple paradigmatic theorem underlying many of the results of this paper is the following.

In the following theorem and until Sec. 8, $\Phi\,(x)$ will denote a known, continuous, monotone increasing distribution function [i.e., $\Phi\,(x)$ is strictly increasing in x and $\Phi\,(x) \to 0$ as $x \to -\infty$ and $\Phi\,(x) \to 1$ as $x \to \infty$].

THEOREM 2.1. *Given (i) a law F_O of O satisfying (2.2), (ii) a continuous, monotone increasing, distribution function $\Phi\,(x)$, and (iii) a function $q\,(L)$, there exists a unique joint law $F_{L,\Delta}$ for (L, Δ) with marginal F_O for O satisfying*

$$pr\,[\Delta = 1 \mid L] = \Phi\,[h + q\,(L)] \tag{2.3}$$

for some $h \in (-\infty, \infty]$. Specifically, the constant h is the unique solution to

$$E_O\,[\Delta / \Phi\,\{h + q\,(L)\}] = 1 \tag{2.4}$$

and the marginal F_L of L under $F_{L,\Delta}$ is

$$F_L\,(\ell) = E_O\,[\Delta I\,(L \leq \ell) / \Phi\,\{h + q\,(L)\}] \tag{2.5}$$

where $E_O\,[\cdot]$ denotes expectation w.r.t. F_O, and, for multivariate L and ℓ, $L \leq \ell$ means that each component of L is less than or equal to the corresponding component of ℓ.

REMARK 2.1. If $q\,(L)$ is a constant not depending on L, then (2.3) says that, under $F_{L,\Delta}$, the data are missing at random in the sense defined by Rubin (1976). A choice $q\,(L)$ that is a non-constant function of L corresponds to Rubin's (1976) definition of a non-ignorable non-response process. Note that in the preceding Theorem, h can take the value $+\infty$. Indeed, h is equal to $+\infty$ if and only if $pr\,(\Delta = 1) = 1$. Eq. (2.2) guarantees h will always exceed $-\infty$.

REMARK 2.2. **Semiparametric model a:** Consider the semiparametric model **a** for the law of (Δ, L) defined by the following conditions:

$$F_L \text{ is unrestricted,} \tag{2.6}$$

$pr(\Delta = 1 \mid L) = \Phi\{h + q(L)\}$ where $q(\cdot)$ is a fixed and known function, $\Phi(\cdot)$ is a known, strictly increasing, distribution function, and h is unknown and ranges over $(-\infty, +\infty]$. By Theorem 2.1, this model places no restrictions on the law F_O of the observables and it is therefore non-parametric for the law F_O of the observed data. That is, Theorem 2.1 establishes that every F_O is the marginal of a law $F_{L,\Delta}$ allowed by the model, and thus for each choice of $q(L)$ the model fits the data perfectly and cannot be rejected by any statistical test. Second, the model is identified in the sense that the unknowns F_L and h in the model, and thus the joint distribution $F_{L,\Delta}$ are uniquely determined by the law F_O of the observed data. We refer to model **a** as a non-parametric (just) identified (NPI) model for (Δ, L). Robins (1997b) referred to NPI models as non-parametric saturated.

The NPI model **a** is useful for conducting sensitivity analysis as the following example illustrates.

REMARK 2.3. In Theorem 2.1 and Remark 2.2, we implicitly assume that the law F_O lay in some large set $\mathcal{F}$ of possible laws for O. In Theorem 2.1, as well as in similar remarks in Theorems to follow, we assume that the non-ignorable selection bias function q belongs to a set of functions $\mathcal{Q}$ satisfying the restriction that for all $F_O \in \mathcal{F}$ and $q \in \mathcal{Q}$, all expectations and integrals occurring in the statement of the theorem are finite. For example, if $\mathcal{F} = \{F_O; F_{L|\Delta=1}$ *is absolutely continuous with respect to Lebesgue measure*$\}$, i.e., L is a continuous random variable with potentially unbounded support, then $\mathcal{Q} = \{q(\ell); |q(\ell)|$ *is bounded by a constant* $c\}$ is a suitable choice for $\mathcal{Q}$. In contrast, if $\mathcal{F} = \left\{F_O; F_{L|\Delta=1}\ \textit{has support on}\ \{0,1\}\right\}$ (i.e., L is dichotomous), the set $\mathcal{Q}$ would be unrestricted. If we included laws in $\mathcal{F}$ for which the aforementioned integrals and expectations did not exist then model **a** would not be a nonparametric model since there would exist laws F_O in $\mathcal{F}$ which would not be the marginal of any law for (L, Δ) satisfying (2.3).

REMARK 2.4. Consider the following example.

EXAMPLE 2.1. Consider the special case of semiparametric model **a** in which $\Phi(x) = e^x/(1+e^x)$, L is scalar, and $q(L) = \alpha_1 L$. Then α_1 "quantifies" the magnitude of selection bias on a logistic scale with $\alpha_1 = 0$ denoting no selection bias, i.e., missing at random data. Now suppose the parameter of interest is $F_L(10)$, the marginal probability that L is less than 10 (were there no missing data). Then, given a law F_O for the observed data, by (2.4) and (2.5) we obtain $F_L(10)$ as a function of α_1 as shown in the schematic graph below. Figure 1 demonstrates that our inferences about $F_L(10)$ based on F_O depend on our choice of α_1. Note that α_1 is not identified by F_O since, by Theorem 2.1, F_O is perfectly compatible with any choice of α_1. Thus, in Figure 1, we have specified a range of values for α_1 and used these together with F_O to identify $F_L(10)$ as a function of the chosen α_1.

In practice, the law F_O of O is unknown but can be estimated at the usual $n^{\frac{1}{2}}$-rate by the empirical law F_n of the data that puts mass

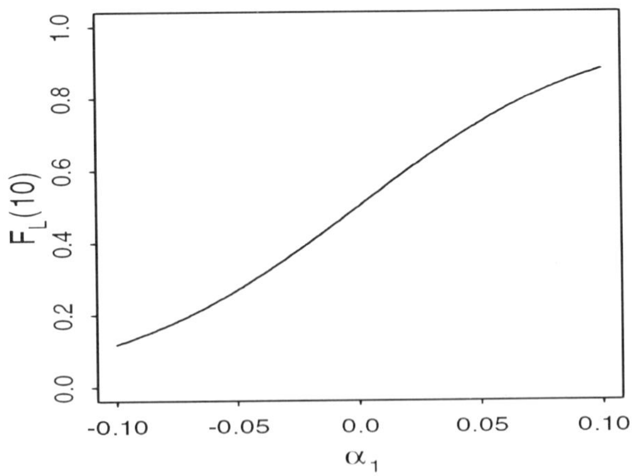

FIG. 1. $F_L(10)$ *as a function of* α_1.

$1/n$ on each of the n observations $(\Delta_i, \Delta_i L_i)$. Thus, in practice we would replace Figure 1 by Figure 2 where the solid line is the estimate $\widehat{F}_L(10)$ of $F_L(10)$ computed under F_n and the vertical bars between the dashed curves represent a 95 percent confidence interval for $F_L(10)$. $\widehat{F}_L(10)$ is obtained by the empirical versions of (2.4) and (2.5) in which $E_O[\cdot]$ is replaced by $\widetilde{E}_n[\cdot]$ where, for any random variable, $H_i, \widetilde{E}_n[H] = n^{-1}\sum_{i=1}^{n} H_i$. We delay to Section 4 describing how confidence intervals for $F_L(10)$ can be computed.

Since Theorem 2.1 implies that there will never be any data evidence that can determine either the magnitude of α_1 or that the function $q(\ell)$ is a linear function of ℓ, it follows that we might wish to repeat the preceding sensitivity analysis for other functions $q(\ell)$ such as $\alpha_1 e^{\ell}$. Note that this substantive meaning of the magnitude of α_1 depends on whether we choose $q(L)$ to be linear in L or exponential in L.

Two functions $q_1(L)$ and $q_2(L)$ that differ by a constant K result in the same semiparametric model (a) for the law of (Δ, L) because $\Phi(h + q_1(L)) = \Phi(h^* + q_2(L))$ where $h^* = h + K$ and the constant h is allowed to vary over the entire extended interval $(-\infty, \infty]$. It is therefore desirable to restrict the class of functions $q(L)$ over which a sensitivity analysis is to be conducted to a class of functions where different functions yield different models for the law of (Δ, L). One way to accomplish this is to restrict attention to functions $q(L)$ such that $q(0) = 0$. With this restriction, the

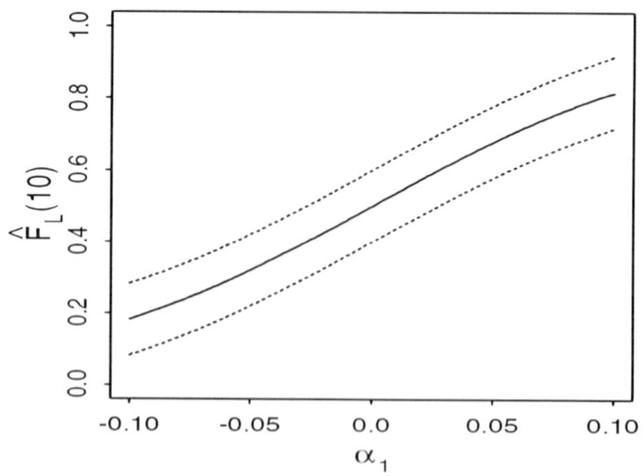

FIG. 2. $\widehat{F}_L(10)$ *as a function of* α_1*, with 95% confidence intervals.*

function $q(L) = 0$ is the unique function that corresponds to the data being missing at random.

Bounds – It would be advantageous to use, in a sensitivity analysis, parameterized functions $q(L) \equiv q(L;\alpha)$ such that in the limit as the parameter $\alpha \to -\infty$ and $\alpha \to \infty$, the implied laws for $F_L(\ell)$ based on the selection bias function $q(L;\alpha)$ converges to the bounds on $F_L(\ell)$ imposed by the law F_O of O. See Sec. 7 of Scharfstein, Rotnitzky, and Robins (1999) for additional discussion.

The reader may feel discouraged that we have only obtained a "sensitivity analysis" for the parameter of interest $F_L(10)$ and that we have been unable to jointly identify this parameter and the selection bias parameter α_1. However, we feel quite the opposite. Since the parameter α_1 represents the magnitude of selection bias due to unmeasured factors, it would not be desirable or scientifically reasonable for α_1 to be identified from the data in the absence of further knowledge of these factors. We would hope it would *not* be identifiable from the data without further well-supported substantive knowledge. Our semi-parametric model a for (L, Δ) operationalizes this desiderata; we cannot identify the magnitude of selection bias, but we can identify the law F_L as a function of the selection bias parameter.

To clarify this point, consider the parametric submodel of our semiparametric model **a** in which we assume that L is normally distributed with unknown mean μ and variance σ^2, and again $\Phi(x)$ is logistic, $q(L;\alpha_1) =$

$\alpha_1 L$, and the "intercept" h in (2.3) is unknown. This parametric model is a special case of the "selection model" proposed by Heckman (1976). The parametric likelihood function for this model is

$$f\left(\Delta, \Delta L; \mu, \sigma^2, h, \alpha_1\right) = \left[\Phi\left(h + \alpha_1 L\right) f\left(L; \mu, \sigma^2\right)\right]^{\Delta} \times \left[\int_{-\infty}^{\infty} \left\{1 - \Phi\left(h + \alpha_1 L\right)\right\} f\left(L; \mu, \sigma^2\right) dL\right]^{1-\Delta}. \tag{2.7}$$

Even if α_1 is unknown, $\left(\mu, \sigma^2, h, \alpha_1\right)$ are all identified when $f\left(L; \mu, \sigma^2\right)$ is a normal density function (Heckman, 1976; Rotnitzky and Robins, 1997). However, our ability to identify both the law of L and the selection parameter α_1 comes solely from the assumption of normality. For example, as noted by Little and Rubin (1987), we can determine whether $\alpha_1 = 0$ (i.e., whether the data are MAR) by checking whether the observed conditional distribution of L given $\Delta = 1$ is skew. This follows because if $\alpha_1 = 0$ and L is normal, $f\left(L \mid \Delta = 1\right)$ is normal and thus is not skew; however, for all $\alpha_1 \neq 0$, $f\left(L \mid \Delta = 1\right)$ is skew. Thus, unless we know *a priori* with certainty that $f\left(L\right)$ is not skew, we should not use such a parametric model to test for selection bias because identification of α_1 comes entirely from the assumed distributional shape. As noted by Little and Rubin (1987), it is rare, if ever, that we would have such prior knowledge. In contrast, the likelihood in our semi-parametric model a in which $F_L\left(\cdot\right)$ is left unspecified is except for being dominated by Lesbesgue measure,

$$f\left(\Delta, \Delta L; \theta, h, \alpha_1\right) = \left[\Phi\left(h + \alpha_1 L\right) f\left(L; \theta\right)\right]^{\Delta} \times \left[\int_{-\infty}^{\infty} \left\{1 - \Phi\left(h + \alpha_1 L\right)\right\} f\left(L; \theta\right) dL\right]^{1-\Delta} \tag{2.8}$$

where θ is an infinite dimensional parameter indexing the laws of L that are dominated by a Lesbesgue measure and $\left(\theta, h, \alpha_1\right)$ are not jointly identified. However, given α_1 known, the NPMLE of h and $F_L\left(\ell\right)$ is given precisely by (2.4) and (2.5) with E_O replaced by $\widetilde{E}_n$ (where, as is usual in defining the NPMLE, when maximizing (2.8) we allow $f\left(L; \theta\right)$ to be any distribution, including discrete distributions). The NPMLE of F_L is a discrete distribution which jumps only at the observed values of L among subjects with $\Delta = 1$.

REMARK 2.5. Although the NPMLE can be used for sensitivity analysis in the simple "toy" selection model of this subsection, it will fail in the more realistic models discussed in the next two subsections due to the curse of dimensionality (Robins and Ritov, 1997). Estimation of more realistic semiparametric models uses estimating equations derived from the theory of semiparametric models (Bickel et al., 1993; Rotnitzky and Robins, 1997; Rotnitzky, Robins, and Scharfstein, 1998).

2.2. Longitudinal monotone missing data in discrete time. We now generalize our results to a longitudinal study in which the full data is $\overline{L}_{K+1} = (L_0, \ldots, L_{K+1})$ where L_k is a scalar or vector variable measured at occasion $k, k = 0, \ldots, K+1$, and we adopt the notation that, for any time-dependent variable Z_k, $\overline{Z}_k = (Z_0, Z_1, \ldots, Z_k)$ is the history of the variable through time k. By convention, we set $Z_{-1} = \overline{Z}_{-1}$ equal to zero with probability 1. We assume some subjects drop out of the study so that the observed data is $O = \left(C, \overline{L}_C\right)$ where the censoring time C denotes the last occasion on which L_k is observed. We assume that missingness is monotone so that if L_k is not observed, then L_{k+1} is also not observed. Note $C = K+1$ for a subject whose full data $\bar{L}_{K+1}$ are observed. We use $F_{C,L}$ to denote the joint distribution of C and L and $\lambda_k(L)$ to denote the conditional discretized hazard of censoring at time k given L, i.e., $\lambda_k(L) = pr(C = k \mid C \geq k, L)$. For notational convenience, we will often use Λ_k to denote the random variable $\lambda_k(L)$. Note we are not using Λ_k to denote a cumulative hazard function. Then let $\Delta = I(C = K+1)$ be the indicator for observing full data and denote $\overline{L}_{K+1}$ by L. We assume that (2.2) holds. Then in analogy to Theorem 2.1, we have the following Theorem 2.2. Its proof is given in Rotnitzky, Robins, and Scharfstein (1998). Theorem 2.1 above is a special case of Theorem 2.2.

THEOREM 2.2. *Given (i) a law F_O of O satisfying $pr[C \neq k \mid C \geq k, \overline{L}_k] \geq \sigma > 0$ w.p.1, $k = 0, \ldots, K$, (ii) a continuous, monotone increasing, distribution function $\Phi(x)$, and (iii) known functions $q_k(L), k = 0, \ldots, K$, there exists a unique joint law $F_{C,L}$ for (C, L) with marginal F_O for O satisfying the condition that, for $k = 0, \ldots, K$, one minus the discrete hazard $\Lambda_k = \lambda_k(L)$ of becoming censored at k given L is*

$$1 - \Lambda_k \equiv pr\left[C \neq k \mid C \geq k, L\right] = \Phi\left[h_k\left(\overline{L}_k\right) + q_k(L)\right] \tag{2.9}$$

for some functions $h_k\left(\overline{\ell}_k\right)$ taking values in $(-\infty, \infty]$. Specifically, $h_K(\cdot)$ is the unique solution to

$$E_O\left\{\Delta / \Phi\left[h_K\left(\overline{L}_K\right) + q_K(L)\right] \mid \overline{L}_K, C \geq K\right\} = 1\ ; \tag{2.10}$$

$h_m(\cdot)$, $m = K-1, \ldots, 0$ is recursively obtained as the unique solution to

$$E_O\left[\Delta \Big/ \left\{\prod_{j=m+1}^{K} (1 - \Lambda_j)\, \Phi\left[h_m\left(\overline{L}_m\right) + q_m(L)\right]\right\} \mid \overline{L}_m, C \geq m\right] = 1, \tag{2.11}$$

(where the $\Lambda_j, j = m+1, \ldots, K$ have been previously obtained), and the marginal F_L of L is

$$F_L(\ell) = E_O\left[\Delta I(L \leq \ell) \Big/ \prod_{j=0}^{K} (1 - \Lambda_j)\right]. \tag{2.12}$$

REMARK 2.6. **Semiparametric model a**: In analogy to Section 2.1, consider the semiparametric model **a** for the law of (C, L) defined by the following conditions:

F_L is unrestricted

$1-\lambda_k(L) = \Phi\left\{h_k\left(\overline{L}_k\right) + q_k(L)\right\}$ *where $q_k(\cdot)$ is an arbitrary fixed and known function $k = 0, \ldots, K$,*

$\Phi(\cdot)$ is a known, strictly increasing, distribution function, and $h_k(\cdot)$ is unknown and ranges over $[-\infty, \infty]$.

Theorem 2.2 implies that model **a** places no restrictions on the law F_O of O and, furthermore, that the unknowns F_L and $h_k(\cdot)$ are identified. That is, model **a** is non-parametric (just) identified. In particular, the functions $q_k(\cdot)$ are not amendable to empirical verification, i.e., cannot be rejected by any statistical test, because all choices of $q_k(\cdot)$ are compatible with the observed data. As in Section 2.1, in order to avoid the possibility that different functions $q_k(\cdot)$ yield the same semiparametric model for $F_{C,L}$, we shall restrict attention to functions $q_k(\cdot)$ such that $q_k(L) = 0$ if $\underline{L}_{k+1} \equiv (L_{k+1}, \ldots, L_{K+1}) = 0$. Note if the restriction on the law F_O in *(i)* of Theorem (2.2) did not hold then, in general, identification will fail.

REMARK 2.7. If all the L_m are discrete with only a few levels, the NPMLEs of $h_k\left(\overline{\ell}_k\right)$ and $F_L(\ell)$ are obtained by substituting the population expectation E_O by its sample version in (2.10)–(2.12). In general, however, if the L_m has continuous components or many discrete components (L_m may be a random vector), then, due to the curse of dimensionality, the NPMLE will be undefined. As discussed in Section 4, in practice, inference in such settings requires placing additional restrictions on the functions $h_k(\cdot)$. One such approach would be to impose only smoothness conditions on the functions $h_k(\cdot)$ and to conduct inference about any functional $\beta(F_L)$ of interest (e.g., the mean of L_{K+1}) using smoothing methods to estimate the unknowns $h_k(\cdot)$. However, when the L_m have multiple continuous components, the use of multivariate smoothing techniques for estimating $h_k(\cdot)$ requires impractically large samples. Thus, in practice, more restrictive models are required on the functions $h_k(\cdot)$. Formally, we assume that $h_k\left(\overline{\ell}_k\right)$ lies in a class of functions $h_k\left(\overline{\ell}_k;\gamma\right)$ indexed by a parameter $\gamma \in \Gamma$ where the parameter space Γ may be finite dimensional or infinite dimensional. Therefore, let the semiparametric model $\mathbf{a}_r$ be semiparametric model **a** modified in that $h_k\left(\overline{\ell}_k\right)$ is subject to the restriction that it lies in $\mathcal{H}_k \equiv \left\{h_k\left(\overline{\ell}_k;\gamma\right); \gamma \in \Gamma\right\}$. When $\mathcal{H}_k$ does not contain all possible functions $h_k\left(\overline{\ell}_k\right)$, Theorem 2.2 implies that then there will exist laws F_O that are not the marginal of any law of (L, C) that lies in model $\mathbf{a}_r$ (i.e., $\mathbf{a}_r$ is not a non-parametric model for F_O). Thus, in principle, model $\mathbf{a}_r$ can be subjected to an empirical goodness-of-fit test. Our informal suggestion for conducting sensitivity analysis in this setting is first to *(i)* choose the model for the $h_k(\overline{\ell}_k)$ large enough that nearly any goodness-of-fit test will have little power to reject the model $\mathbf{a}_r$ but *(ii)* choose it small enough so that the estimators described in Sec. 4 below of functionals $\beta(F_L)$ of interest have a nearly normal sampling distribution with the variance small enough to be substantively useful to subject matter experts. It is not clear that both criteria *(i)* and *(ii)* can always be met. Clearly the choice of the size of the model will depend on the size of the data set, the complexity of the functional $\beta(F_L)$, and the precision required by the subject matter experts. Furthermore, since different models $\mathbf{a}_r$ associated with different model choices for the $h_k(\overline{\ell}_k)$ cannot be easily distinguished by goodness-of-fit tests when the advice in *(i)* is followed, we suggest using a large number of different models for $h_k(\overline{\ell}_k)$. Then, for each model for the $h_k(\overline{\ell}_k)$, estimate F_L under many choices for the selection bias functions $q_k(L)$ (still treated as known in the analysis) so that sensitivity both to the choice of the $q_k(L)$ and to the choice of model for $h_k(\overline{\ell}_k)$ can be assessed.

2.3. Longitudinal monotone missing data in continuous time. In this section, we generalize the results of Section 2.2 to allow for drop-out (censoring) in continuous time. The full data are n i.i.d. copies of a, possibly multivariate, continuous time stopped stochastic process, $L \equiv \overline{L}(\tau)$, where for any stochastic process $Z(u), \overline{Z}(t) = \{Z(u); 0 \leq u \leq t\}$ is the history of the process up to t, and the stopping time τ is the (possibly random) administrative end-of-follow-up time. Since τ is the administrative end-of-follow-up time, it is assumed known for each subject at time 0 and thus τ is a component of $L(0)$.

The observed data are now n i.i.d. copies of $O = (C, \overline{L}(C))$ where C is time to drop-out and, by convention, $C \equiv \tau$ if the subject is uncensored (does not drop out) by administrative end-to-follow-up. In analogy to Sec. 2, let $\Delta = I(C = \tau)$ be the indicator that the full data $L = \overline{L}(\tau)$ are observed and we continue to assume (2.2) holds. Furthermore, we let F_O and $F_{C,L}$ denote the CDF of O and (C, L) respectively, and we use $\lambda(u \mid A)$ to denote the conditional hazard of C at u given A, that is, $\lambda(u \mid A) = \lim_{t \to 0} t^{-1} pr(u < C < u + t \mid C \geq u, A)$. Further, we write $\Lambda(u)$ to denote the random variable $\lambda(u \mid L)$. Note $\Lambda(u)$ is not a cumulative hazard function. We then have the following theorem whose proof is given in Appendix 1 of Scharfstein, Rotnitzky, and Robins (1999) in the special case in which the process $\overline{L}(u)$ only jumps at a finite number of fixed non-random times. Richard Gill has proved this theorem for more general processes. His proof will be reported elsewhere.

THEOREM 2.3. *Given (i) a law F_O of $O = (C, \overline{L}(C))$ such that the hazard of C at u given $\overline{L}(u)$ is bounded by a constant c w.p.1 and (ii) a function $q(u, L), u \in [0, \tau)$, there exists a unique joint law $F_{C,L}$ with marginal F_O satisfying, for some function $h(u, \overline{L}(u))$*

$$\lambda(u \mid L) = exp\left[h\left(u, \overline{L}(u)\right) + q(u, L)\right] . \tag{2.13}$$

Specifically, $h\left(u, \overline{L}(u)\right)$ *is the unique function taking values in* $(-\infty, \infty]$ *satisfying*

$$E_O\left[\Delta / \, exp\left[-\int_u^\tau \lambda\left(x \mid L\right) dx\right] \mid \overline{L}\left(u\right), C \geq u\right] = 1 \tag{2.14}$$

and the marginal F_L *of* L *is*

$$F_L\left(\ell\right) = E_O\left[\Delta I\left(L \leq \ell\right) / S\right] \tag{2.15}$$

where

$$S = exp\left[-\int_0^\tau \lambda\left(x \mid L\right) dx\right] \tag{2.16}$$

and $L \leq \ell$ *means each component of the vector* $L(u)$ *is less than or equal to the corresponding component* $\ell(u)$ *for all* $u \in [0, \tau]$.

REMARK 2.8. **Semiparametric model a:** As in Section 2.2, consider the semiparametric model a for the law of (C, L) defined by the conditions *(i)* F_L is unrestricted and *(ii)* $\lambda(u \mid L)$ is given by (2.13) with the selection bias function $q(u, L)$ known and $h\left(u, \overline{L}(u)\right)$ completely unrestricted.

REMARK 2.9. It follows from Theorem 2.3 that model **a** is nonparametric (just) identified. In analogy to Section 2.2, we will restrict attention to a class of functions $q(u, L)$ for which each member results in a different semiparametric model for the law of (C, L). Specifically, we will consider functions $q(u, L)$ satisfying $q(u, L) = 0$ if $\underline{L}(u) \equiv \{L(t); u < t \leq \tau\}$ is equal to 0. This choice ensures that when the drop-out process is ignorable, then $q(u, L) = 0$ and, thus, $h\left\{u, \overline{L}(u)\right\}$ can be directly interpreted as giving the dependence of drop-out process on the recorded past. Here we have used the fact that the data are MAR if and only if $q(u, L) = q\left(u, \overline{L}(u)\right)$.

REMARK 2.10. Consider a study in which one wants to make inferences about time to death. However, we do not observe each subject's death time because of censoring by administrative end of follow-up or drop-out. In order to use the above methods to estimate the time to death distribution, we cannot treat death as a censoring event but rather must include it in the full data. Formally, we can write $L(u) = (D(u), D(u) V(u))$ where $D(u) = 1$ if the subject is alive, $D(u) = 0$ if the subject has died, and $D(u) V(u)$ denotes other characteristics recorded at u in living persons. Let T be time to death, i.e., $D(T) = 0$ and $D(T^-) = 1$. Let Q be time to drop-out (censoring). Theorem 2.3 assumes that censoring time C is always observed. However, in studies with death as the survival time, the censoring time Q is often not known (observed) for deaths. However, such studies can be easily accommodated in our set-up by setting the censoring time to infinity for deaths. That is, we set $C = Q$ if $Q < \min(\tau, T)$ and set $C = \infty$ otherwise. The observed data are now in the required form $\left(C, \overline{L}(C)\right)$. This renaming trick so that the censoring time C is always observed is quite generally applicable (Robins, 1996; Gill, van der Laan, and Robins, 1998). A similar renaming trick will be necessary in Sec. 2.2 when we are interested in mortality as an endpoint. If we are interested in only a single cause of death, we let T be the time to death from that cause and count deaths from other causes as censoring events.

3. Identification of a subcomponent distribution in monotone missing data problems.

3.1. Single occasion. Suppose that in the scenario of Section 2.1, $L = (Y, V)$. However, suppose that interest lies in making inference about some component of the law of Y. That is, in our analysis Y is the sole outcome of interest despite the fact that the study also collects data on a secondary outcome V. Suppose that we are interested in performing a sensitivity analysis only over the magnitude of Y's influence on selection. The following generalization of Theorem 2.1 provides the mathematical justification for the discussion that follows.

THEOREM 3.1. *Given (i), a law F_O of $O = (\Delta, \Delta L)$ satisfying*

$$pr\,(\Delta = 1) \neq 0\,, \tag{3.1}$$

(ii) a continuous, monotone increasing, distribution function $\Phi\,(x)$, and (iii) a known function $q\,(Y)$, there exists joint laws $F_{\Delta,L}$ for (Δ, L) with marginal F_O for O satisfying

$$pr\,[\Delta = 1 \mid Y] = \Phi\,[h + q\,(Y)] \tag{3.2}$$

for some $h \in (-\infty, \infty]$. Specifically, h is the unique solution to

$$E_O\,[\Delta/\Phi\,(h + q\,(Y))] = 1 \tag{3.3}$$

and each law $F_{\Delta,L}$ has the same marginal F_Y for Y given by

$$F_Y\,(y) = E_O\,[\Delta I\,(Y \leq y)\,/\Phi\,\{h + q\,(Y)\}]\ . \tag{3.4}$$

Consider the semiparametric model **b** for the law of (Δ, L) defined by the following conditions: *(i)* the law of F_Y is unrestricted, *(ii)* the law of Δ given Y is given by (3.2) with h unknown, but $\Phi\,(x)$ and $q\,(Y)$ known and *(iii)* the law of V given (Y, Δ) is unrestricted. This model is a non-parametric model for the observed data O in which the constant h and the marginal distribution of Y are just identified. Note, that for a given law F_O and $\Phi\,(x)$, F_Y based on model **b** will generally differ from that based on model **a** of Sec. 2.1 unless the function $q\,(L) = q\,(Y, V)$ chosen in specifying model **a** equals the function $q\,(Y)$ chosen in specifying model **b**. From the point of view of model **a**, choosing $q\,(Y, V)$ to be a function of Y only is equivalent to specifying that Δ and V are conditionally independent given Y, an assumption that cannot be checked from the data since any choice of $q(Y,V)$ is perfectly compatible with the distribution F_O of the observed data.

We now provide a generalization of Theorem 3.1 to the longitudinal monotone missing data setting of Section 2.2. Suppose that $L_k = (Y_k, V_k), k = 0, \ldots, K+1$, and we are interested in making inference about some component of the law F_Y of an outcome of interest $Y = (Y_0, \ldots, Y_{K+1})$. In particular, we want to conduct a sensitivity analysis over the influence of the magnitude of the unobserved parts of Y on the conditional probability of selection at each occasion $k+1$ given the observed past $\overline{L}_k \equiv (L_0, \ldots, L_k)$ and the current and future outcomes $\underline{Y}_{k+1} \equiv (Y_{k+1}, \ldots, Y_{K+1})$. Let $\lambda_k\left(\overline{L}_k, \underline{Y}_{k+1}\right)$ denote $pr\left(C = k \mid C \geq k, \overline{L}_k, \underline{Y}_{k+1}\right)$. On occasions, we write Λ_k for $\lambda_k\left(\overline{L}_k, \underline{Y}_{k+1}\right)$. Note that Λ_k is defined as a conditional probability given $\overline{L}_k$ and $\underline{Y}_{k+1}$, i.e., the observed past and the future outcomes of interest Y. In contrast, in Section 2.2, Λ_k was a conditional probability given the entire vector $(L_0, \ldots, L_{K+1})$. Theorem 3.1 has the following generalization formulated here directly in terms of a semiparametric model **b** to avoid redundancy. A proof follows along the lines of Lemma A.1 of Scharfstein, Rotnitzky, and Robins (1999).

THEOREM 3.2. *Consider the semiparametric model* ***b*** *for* (C, L) *characterized by the sole restrictions*

$$1-\Lambda_k \equiv pr\left[C \neq k \mid C \geq k, \overline{L}_k, \underline{Y}_{k+1}\right] = \Phi\left[h_k\left(\overline{L}_k\right) + q_k\left(\overline{L}_k, \underline{Y}_{k+1}\right)\right] \tag{3.5}$$

$\Phi(\cdot)$ *a continuous, monotone increasing, distribution function,* $q_k(\cdot,\cdot)$ *a known function, and* $h_k(\cdot)$ *an unknown function taking values in* $(-\infty, \infty]$. *Suppose*

$$pr\left(C = k \mid C \geq k, \overline{L}_k\right) \neq 1 \ w.p.1\ . \tag{3.6}$$

Then model ***b*** *is a non-parametric model for the law* F_O *of the observed data* $O = \left(C, \overline{L}_C\right)$. *Furthermore,* F_Y *and the* $h_k\left(\overline{L}_k\right)$ *are identified from data on* O. *Specifically,* $h_m(\cdot), m = K, \ldots, 0$, *are obtained as the unique solutions to the recursive set of equations*

$$E_O\left[\Delta \Big/ \left\{ \prod_{j=m+1}^{K} (1-\Lambda_j)\, \Phi\left[h_m\left(\overline{L}_m\right) + q_m\left(\overline{L}_m, \underline{Y}_{m+1}\right)\right]\right\} \,\Bigg|\, \overline{L}_m, C \geq m\right] = 1 \tag{3.7a}$$

for $m = K, \ldots, 0$, *where* $\prod_{j=a}^{b} V_j \equiv 1$ *if* $a > b$, *and*

$$F_Y(y) = E_O\left[\Delta I(Y \leq y) \Big/ \prod_{j=0}^{K} (1-\Lambda_j)\right]. \tag{3.7b}$$

Furthermore,

$$F_{\underline{Y}_{m+1}}\left(\underline{y}_{m+1}\overline{L}_m, C \geq m\right) = E_O\left[\Delta I\left(\underline{Y}_{m+1} \leq \underline{y}_{m+1}\right) / \prod_{j=m}^{K}(1-\Lambda_j)\,|\overline{L}_m, C \geq m\right]. \tag{3.7c}$$

$$F_{\underline{Y}_{m+1}}\left(\underline{y}_{m+1} \mid \overline{L}_m, C > m\right) = E_O\left[\Delta I\left(\underline{Y}_{m+1} \leq \underline{y}_{m+1}\right) / \prod_{j=m+1}^{K}(1-\Lambda_j)\,|\overline{L}_m, C > m\right]. \tag{3.7d}$$

The key difference between model **a** of Section 2.2 and model **b** of this section is that model **b** imposes a restriction on the conditional probability of response at occasion $k+1$ given $\left(\overline{L}_k, \underline{Y}_{k+1}\right)$ while model **a** imposes a restriction on the conditional probability of response at $k+1$ given $\left(\overline{L}_k, \underline{L}_{k+1}\right)$. Inference about functionals of the law of F_Y under these two models will, quite generally, differ. To see this, notice that with $\Lambda_k \equiv pr\left(C = k \mid C \geq k, \overline{L}_k, \underline{Y}_{k+1}\right)$, as in this section, the density of the observed data $\left(C, \overline{L}_C\right)$ satisfies

$$f\left(C, \overline{L}_C\right) = \int f(Y) \prod_{m=0}^{C} f\left(V_m \mid Y, \overline{V}_m, C \geq m\right)\left\{\prod_{m=0}^{C-1}(1-\Lambda_m)\right\}\Lambda_C^{I(C\neq K+1)}d\mu\left(\underline{Y}_{C+1}\right) \tag{3.8}$$

while with $\Lambda_k \equiv pr\left(C = k \mid C \geq k, \overline{L}_k, \underline{L}_{k+1}\right)$, as in Sec. 2.2, the density of the observed data satisfies

$$f\left(C, \overline{L}_C\right) = \int f(Y) \prod_{m=0}^{C} f\left(V_m \mid Y, \overline{V}_m\right)\left\{\prod_{m=0}^{C-1}(1-\Lambda_m)\right\}\Lambda_C^{I(C\neq K+1)}d\mu\left(\underline{Y}_{C+1}\right) \tag{3.9}$$

where by convention we set $\underline{L}_{K+2} = 0$ and $\overline{V}_{-1} = 0$. Then, given an observed data law $f\left(C, \overline{L}_C\right)$, we conclude that $pr\left(C = k \mid C \geq k, \overline{L}_k, \underline{Y}_{k+1}\right) \neq pr\left(C = k \mid C \geq k, \overline{L}_k, \underline{L}_{k+1}\right)$ for some k (i.e., Λ_k defined in this section differs from Λ_k of Sec. 2.2) if and only if the unique density $f(Y)$ that solves the integral equation (3.8) under model **b** will not be the same as the unique density $f(Y)$ that solves the integral equation (3.9) under model **a**. The two versions of Λ_k will be equal if in model **a** we choose functions $q_k(L)$ that: *(i)* do not depend on $\underline{V}_{k+1} = (V_{k+1}, \ldots, V_{K+1})$, and *(ii)* are identically equal to the function $q_k\left(\overline{L}_k, \underline{Y}_{k+1}\right)$ that we choose in model **b**.

We now proceed to generalize those results to the case in which censoring is measured in continuous time. Henceforth, suppose that in the scenario of Sec. 2.3, $L(u) = (Y(u), V(u))$. Define $\underline{Y}(u) \equiv \{Y(t);\ u \le t \le \tau\}$ and let $\lambda\left(u \mid \underline{Y}(u), \overline{L}(u^-)\right)$ be the conditional hazard of censoring at time u given $\underline{Y}(u)$ and $\overline{L}(u^-)$. On occasions, we write $\Lambda(u)$ for $\lambda\left(u \mid \underline{Y}(u), \overline{L}(u^-)\right)$.

We obtain an analogous result with censoring in continuous time.

THEOREM 3.3. *Consider the semiparametric model* $\boldsymbol{b}$ *for* (C, L) *characterized by the sole restriction on the conditional hazard of* C *given* $(\overline{L}(u^-), \underline{Y}(u) = \{Y(t);u \ge t \ge \tau\})$

$$\begin{aligned} \Lambda(u) &\equiv \lambda\left(u \mid \underline{Y}(u), \overline{L}(u^-)\right) \\ &= \exp\left[h\left(u, \overline{L}(u^-)\right) + q\left(u, \underline{Y}(u), \overline{L}(u^-)\right)\right] \end{aligned} \tag{3.10}$$

with $h\left(u, \overline{L}(u^-)\right)$ *unknown, and* $q\left(u, \underline{Y}(u), \overline{L}(u^-)\right)$ *known. Suppose* $\lambda\left(u \mid \overline{L}(u^-)\right)$ *is bounded w.p.1. Then model* $\boldsymbol{b}$ *is a non-parametric model for the law* F_O *of* $O = \left(C, \overline{L}(C)\right)$ *and* $h\left(u, \overline{L}(u)\right)$ *and* F_Y *are identified from data on* O. *Specifically,* $h\left(u, \overline{L}(u)\right)$ *is the unique function satisfying (2.14) with* $\Lambda(x)$ *redefined as in (3.10) and*

$$F_Y(y) = E_O\left[\Delta I(Y \le y)/S\right] \tag{3.11}$$

where S *is as in (2.16) except with* $\Lambda(x)$ *as redefined in (3.10).*

Theorem 3.3 is proved in Lemma A.1 of Scharfstein, Rotnitzky, and Robins (1999) in the special case where the $\overline{L}(u)$ process jumps only at a finite number of fixed non-random times.

4. Estimation in monotone missing data problems.

4.1. Estimation — Simple example. For brevity, we will consider only the most difficult case, that of longitudinal monotone missing data in continuous time.

We consider estimation of functionals $\beta = \beta(F_L)$ of the distribution F_L from n i.i.d. copies of data $O = \left(C, \overline{L}(C)\right)$. We limit, for the moment, consideration to functionals β that admit unbiased estimating functions $U \equiv U(\beta) = u(L, \beta)$ for β in a semiparametric model in which F_L is unrestricted (non-parametric) but L is always fully observed. When F_L is unrestricted, $U(\beta)$ is unique up to multiplicative constants. For example, if $\beta = E[Y(10)]$, the mean at $t = 10$ of a variable $Y(t)$ that is a component of $L(t)$, then $U(\beta) = Y(10) - \beta$. The functionals β we are considering are those with positive semiparametric information bound when F_L is unrestricted and data on L is available.

If L was always observed, we would estimate β by $\widetilde{\beta}$ solving $\widetilde{E}_n[U(\beta)] = 0$ where $\widetilde{E}_n(H) = n^{-1}\sum_{i=1}^{n} H_i$ is the sample average over the n observations. For example, if $\beta = E[Y(10)]$, $\widetilde{\beta}$ is the sample average $\widetilde{E}_n[Y(10)]$.

We shall now consider estimation of β from data $O = \left(C, \overline{L}(C)\right)$ both in the semiparametric model **a** of Remark (2.8) and the more *restrictive* semiparametric model $\mathbf{a}_r$ in which we assume the unknown function $h\left(u, \overline{L}(u)\right)$ satisfies

$$\exp\left\{h\left(u,\overline{L}\left(u^{-}\right)\right)\right\}=\exp\left[h\left(u\right)+\nu\left(u,\overline{L}\left(u\right);\gamma_{0}\right)\right] \tag{4.1}$$

where $h(u)$ is an unknown function of time, $\nu(\cdot,\cdot,\cdot)$ is a known function, and γ_0 is the finite dimensional parameter to be estimated.

REMARK 4.1. In view of the discussion following Theorem 3.2, the results obtained in this section for estimation of model **a** apply equally to model **b**. Similarly, the results we obtained for estimation of $\mathbf{a_r}$ apply to model $\mathbf{b_r}$ where model $\mathbf{b_r}$ is model **b** with the additional restriction (4.1). This reflects the fact that for the purposes of semiparametric statistical inference, we can consider model **b** to be the special case of model **a** in which the known selection bias function $q(u,L)$ depends on L only through $\left(\underline{Y}(u),\overline{L}(u^{-})\right)$.

As described previously, we need to consider the submodel $\mathbf{a}_r$ of our model **a** because of the curse of dimensionality. Specifically, in general, $\sqrt{n}-$ estimation of β under model **a** requires that we construct an estimate $\widehat{h}\left(u,\overline{L}\left(u^{-}\right)\right)$ that converges to $h\left(u,\overline{L}\left(u^{-}\right)\right)$ at rate $n^{\frac{1}{4}}$ or more, which is not practically possible (even with multivariate non-parametric smoothing techniques) in moderate size samples when $\overline{L}(u)$ is a high-dimensional stochastic process (Robins and Ritov, 1997).

To describe how we estimate β from data $O=\left(C,\overline{L}(C)\right)$ under semiparametric model **a** (when $\overline{L}(u)$ is not high-dimensional) or under model $\mathbf{a}_r$, we need for the moment to consider, as a pedagogic tool, a semiparametric model $\mathbf{a}_p$ (p for pedagogic) in which data *(i)* O is observed, *(ii)* F_L is unrestricted, and *(iii)* $\Lambda(u)\equiv\lambda(u\mid L)$ is completely known. Robins and Rotnitzky (1992) show that under model $\mathbf{a}_p$, the set of all unbiased estimating functions for β is

$$\mathcal{N}_1^{O,\perp}=\left\{N_1^{O,\perp}(\beta)\equiv\Delta U(\beta)/S+N_{car}\ ;\ N_{car}\in\mathcal{N}_{car}\right\} \tag{4.2}$$

where S is given by (2.16) and

$$\begin{aligned}\mathcal{N}_{car}=e\ \{&N_{car}\equiv N_{car}(a)\equiv(1-\Delta)A-\Delta E\left[(1-\Delta)A\mid L\right]/S\ ;\\ &A=a(O)\ \textit{has finite variance}\}\ .\end{aligned} \tag{4.3}$$

The reason for the notation we have chosen will become clear in the next subsection. $\mathcal{N}_{car}$ constitute exactly all functions of the observed data O with mean zero given the full data L. Since $E\left[\Delta U(\beta)/S\mid L\right]=U(\beta)$ and, at the true value β_0 of β, $E\left[U(\beta_0)\right]=0$, it is clear that $E\left[N_1^{O,\perp}(\beta_0)\right]=0$.

In semiparametric model **a** and $\mathbf{a}_r$, $\Lambda(u)$ and thus S are unknown, so the unbiased estimating function $N_1^{O,\perp}(\beta)$ cannot be computed. In this subsection we consider model **a** and assume $\tau_i=\tau$ for all i. To obtain estimates $\widehat{h}\left(u,\overline{L}(u)\right)$ and thus $\widehat{\Lambda}(u)\equiv\widehat{\lambda}(u\mid L)$ of (2.13), we first renumber the subjects $i, i=1,\ldots,n$, such that if $C_i<C_j$, then $i<j$. Next set $\exp\left\{\widehat{h}\left(u,\overline{L}(u)\right)\right\}=0$ unless $u=C_i<\tau_i$ for some $i=1,\ldots,n$. For

$C_i < \tau_i$, recursively define $\exp\left\{\widehat{h}\left(C_i, \overline{L}_i\left(C_i\right)\right)\right\}$ starting from the largest C_i as

$$\left[\sum_{j=1}^{n} \Delta_j I\left[\overline{L}_j\left(C_i\right) = \overline{L}_i\left(C_i\right)\right] \exp\left[q\left(C_i, L_j\right)\right] \Big/ \left\{\prod_{k=i+1}^{n} \left[1 - \widehat{\Lambda}_j\left(C_k\right)\right] I\left(C_k \neq \tau_k\right)\right\}\right]^{-1}. \tag{4.4}$$

Letting $\widehat{N}_1^{O,\perp}(\beta)$ be $N_1^{O,\perp}(\beta)$ with $\widehat{\Lambda}$ substituted for Λ, the estimator $\widehat{\beta}$ solving $0 = \sum_i \widehat{N}_{1i}^{O,\perp}(\beta)$ will be $\sqrt{n}$ -consistent for β in model **a** only if $\sum_{j=1}^{n} I\left(\overline{L}_j\left(C_i\right) = \overline{L}_i\left(C_i\right)\right) \to \infty$ as $n \to \infty$ with probability 1, which is an unreasonable asymptotics in high-dimensional problems due to the curse of dimensionality. In practice we would use model $\mathbf{a}_r$ whose estimation we will consider in Sec. 4.2.

However, for pedagogic purposes, in this subsection, we shall unrealistically continue to assume here that $\overline{L}(u)$ is discrete with only a moderate number of levels for each u so that the estimator $\widehat{\beta}$ is a regular asymptotically linear (RAL) estimator of β in model **a**. Our goal now is to derive a consistent estimator for the asymptotic variance of $n^{\frac{1}{2}}\left(\widehat{\beta} - \beta_0\right)$ so we can construct Wald confidence intervals for β. Recall that an estimator $\widetilde{\beta}$ is RAL with influence function IF if $n^{\frac{1}{2}}\left(\widetilde{\beta} - \beta_0\right) = n^{\frac{1}{2}} \sum_i IF_i + o_p(1)$, the IF_i are i.i.d. with mean zero and finite variance and the convergence of $\widetilde{\beta}$ to β_0 is locally uniform. Here $o_p(1)$ denotes a random variable converging in probability to zero. Thus, a RAL estimator is asymptotically equivalent to a sum of i.i.d. random variables IF_i and the asymptotic variance of $n^{\frac{1}{2}}\left(\widetilde{\beta} - \beta_0\right)$ is $E\left[IF^{\otimes 2}\right]$. Thus, the goal is to find the influence function of the estimator $\widehat{\beta}$ solving $\sum_i \widehat{N}_{1i}^{O,\perp}(\beta) = 0$ and then estimate $E\left[IF^{\otimes 2}\right]$ by $\tilde{E}_n\left[\widehat{IF}^{\otimes 2}\right]$ where $\widehat{IF}^{\otimes 2}$ is a consistent estimator of IF. Since we have seen that the semiparametric model **a** is a non-parametric model for the observed data O, it follows from Bickel et al. (1993) that all RAL estimators of β will have the same influence function. Hence all the $\widehat{\beta}$ will have the identical influence function irrespective of the choice of $A = a(O)$.

In any semiparametric model, the influence function IF of any RAL estimator *(i)* lies in the orthogonal complement to the nuisance tangent space of the model and *(ii)* satisfies $E\left[IFS_{\beta}^{T}\right] = Id$ where Id is the identity matrix, T denotes matrix transposition, and S_β is the score for β evaluated at the true distribution generating the data (Bickel et al., 1993). As just mentioned, in model **a**, there is a unique random variable satisfying both *(i)* and *(ii)*.

Our goal is thus to determine the orthogonal complement to the nuisance tangent space in model **a** which we do in the course of developing the general theory given in the following subsection.

4.2. General theory of estimation. Let $(C, L \equiv \overline{L}(\tau))$ denote the complete data. Suppose we only observe $O = (C, \overline{L}(C))$. Furthermore, we assume that *(i)* L follows an arbitrary semiparametric model, F_L, indexed by a px1 parameter β and an infinite dimensional parameter θ, and *(ii)* C given L follows an arbitrary semiparametric model, $F_{C|L}$, indexed by a qx1 parameter γ and an infinite dimensional parameter η. If the model $F_{C|L}$ is completely non-parametric, then there will be no parameter γ. We assume that the parameters in model F_L are (locally) variation independent of those in the model for $F_{C|L}$. We let β_0, γ_0, θ_0, and η_0 denote the true values of β, γ, θ, and η, respectively. We are interested in estimating $\psi_0 = (\beta_0', \gamma_0')'$. We observe n independent identically distributed copies of O_i.

We shall assume that the probability of complete observations is bounded away from zero. This condition is somewhat stronger than we actually need to obtain the results below, as discussed in Rotnitzky and Robins (1997). Specifically, we assume

$$S \equiv pr[\Delta = 1 \mid L] > \sigma > 0 \ \ w.p.1 \ for\ some\ constant\ \sigma.$$

Let $\mathcal{N}_1 = \mathcal{N}(F_L)$ and $\mathcal{N}_2 = \mathcal{N}(F_{C|L})$ denote the (nuisance) tangent spaces for θ and η, respectively had we observed (C, L). Throughout, all spaces are sub-spaces of the Hilbert space of $q+p$-dimensional mean zero random vectors with the covariance inner product computed under the truth. Note that $\mathcal{N}_1$ and $\mathcal{N}_2$ are orthogonal. For the "observed data", there is an induced semiparametric model which we denote by *Obs*. In model *Obs*, the observed data nuisance tangent space is $\mathcal{N}^O = \overline{\mathcal{N}_1^O + \mathcal{N}_2^O}$, where $\mathcal{N}_1^O$ is the observed data nuisance tangent space for θ and $\mathcal{N}_2^O$ is the observed data nuisance tangent space for η. Specifically, $\mathcal{N}_j^O = \overline{R(g \circ \Pi_j)}$, where $R(\cdot)$ is the range of an operator, $g : \Omega^{(C,L)} \to \Omega^{(O)}$ is the conditional expectation operator $g(\cdot) = E[\cdot|O]$, $\Omega^{(C,L)}$ and $\Omega^{(O)}$ are the spaces of all $p+q$ dimensional random functions of (C, L) and O respectively, Π_j is the Hilbert space projection operator from $\Omega^{(C,L)}$ onto $\mathcal{N}_j$ and $\overline{\mathcal{S}}$ denotes the close linear span of the set $\mathcal{S}$ (Bickel et al., 1993). A space superscripted by $\perp$ denotes the orthogonal complement of that space. We are interested in finding $\mathcal{N}^{O,\perp}$ because, in sufficiently smooth models, the set of influence functions of all asymptotically linear (RAL) estimators of ψ_0 is the set $\left\{E\left[\mathcal{A}S_\psi'\right]^{-1}\mathcal{A}; \mathcal{A} \in \mathcal{N}^{O,\perp}\right\}$ where S_ψ is the score for ψ evaluated at the truth. Another motivation for our interest in this space is as follows. An element in $\mathcal{N}^{O,\perp}$ is a $(p+q)$ dimensional function of the observed data and of the true values of the parameters, ψ_0, θ_0, and η_0. Denote this function by $N^{O,\perp} \equiv N^{O,\perp}(\psi_0, \theta_0, \eta_0)$. Suppose we estimate ψ_0 by $\widehat{\psi}$ solving $\sum_i N_i^{O,\perp}\left(\psi, \widehat{\theta}(\psi), \widehat{\eta}(\psi)\right) = 0$ where $\widehat{\theta}(\psi_0)$ and $\widehat{\eta}(\psi_0)$ converge to θ_0 and η_0, respectively. Then Bickel et al. (1993), van der Vaart (1991), and Newey (1990) show that under suitable regularity conditions $\widehat{\psi}$ is a RAL estimator with influence function $\rho^{-1} N^{O,\perp}$ where $\rho = E\left[N^{O,\perp} S'_{\psi}\right] = -\partial E\left[N^{O,\perp}(\psi, \theta_0, \eta_0)\right] / \partial\psi \mid_{\psi=\psi_0}$. But this is the same influence function as would have been obtained by solving the estimating equation $\sum_i N_i^{O,\perp}(\psi, \theta_0, \eta_0) = 0$ in which the infinite dimensional components (θ_0, η_0) are known rather than estimated. It is precisely the orthogonality of $N^{O,\perp}$ to $\mathcal{N}^O$ which obviates the need to adjust the asymptotic variance for estimation of the nuisance parameters (θ_0, η_0).

Taking orthogonal complements, we can express $\mathcal{N}^{O,\perp}$ as $\mathcal{N}_1^{O,\perp} \cap \mathcal{N}_2^{O,\perp}$. Let $a(L)$ and $b(O)$ be $p+q$ dimensional functions of L and O, respectively. $\mathcal{N}_1^{O,\perp}$ has the interpretation as the orthogonal complement to the nuisance tangent space $\mathcal{N}_1^O$ in the semiparametric model in which $\lambda[u \mid L]$ (i.e., the law of $C \mid L$) is known.

Rotnitzky and Robins (1997) showed how to compute $\mathcal{N}_1^{O,\perp}$. Specifically,

$$(4.5)\quad \mathcal{N}_1^{O,\perp} = \left\{N_1^{O,\perp} = \Delta m(L)/S + N_{car} : m(L) \in \mathcal{N}_1^{\perp} \text{ and } N_{car} \in \mathcal{N}_{car}\right\}.$$

REMARK 4.2. Recall that N_{car} was defined in Eq. (4.3). $\mathcal{N}_{car}$ is exactly the nuisance tangent space (i.e., mean square closure of nuisance scores) corresponding to $\lambda(u \mid L)$ when $\lambda(u \mid L)$ is unrestricted except for the fact that the data are CAR, i.e., $q(u, L) = q\left(u, \overline{L}(u^-)\right)$.

By the relationship between range and null spaces, $\mathcal{N}_2^{O,\perp} = Null\left(\Pi_2^T \circ g^T\right)$, where $Null(\cdot)$ is the null space of an operator, and superscript T denotes the adjoint of an operator. As projection operators $\Pi_j^T = \Pi_j, j = 1, 2$, and $g^T : \Omega^O \rightarrow \Omega^{(C,L)}$ is the identity operator. So,

$$(4.6)\qquad \mathcal{N}_2^{O,\perp} = \{b(O) : \Pi_2[b(O)|\mathcal{N}_2] = 0\} = \{b(O) : b(O) \in \mathcal{N}_2^{\perp}\}.$$

Model a: Our next goal is to determine the orthogonal complement to the nuisance tangent space in semiparametric model **a** of Remark 2.8, except we no longer require that F_L be unrestricted. Rather, we allow F_L to follow a semiparametric model indexed by finite dimensional parameter β and infinite dimensional parameter θ. Under model **a**, $F_{C|L}$ is given by (2.13) with $h\left(u, \overline{L}(u)\right)$ unrestricted and $q(u, L)$ known. In model **a**, there is no parameter γ so that $\psi = \beta$.

If we had observed (C, L), then the nuisance scores corresponding to parametric submodels for the unknown $h\left(u, \overline{L}(u)\right)$ is the set

$$(4.7)\qquad \mathcal{N}_2 = \left\{N_2 = N_2(a) = \int_0^{\tau} d\mathcal{M}(u)\, a\left(u, \overline{L}(u)\right)\right\}$$

where $a\left(u, \overline{L}(u)\right)$ is an arbitrary function of dimension equal to that of β, $\mathcal{M}(u) = I[C \leq u, C < \tau] - \int_0^u \lambda(x \mid L)\, I(C \geq x)\, dx$ is the martingale for censoring conditional on L. Note if $C = \tau$, $I(C \leq u, C < \tau) = 0$ since we do not regard a subject successfully reaching end of follow-up as having been censored.

REMARK 4.3. Note that the N_2 are not necessarily functions of the observed data $O = \left(C, \overline{L}\left(C\right)\right)$. However, if the selection function $q\left(u, L\right) = q\left(u, \overline{L}\left(u\right)\right)$ w.p.1 so that the data are CAR, then $\mathcal{N}_2 = \mathcal{N}_{car}$ and the N_2 are functions of O.

The orthogonal complement to $\mathcal{N}_2$ of (4.7) is

$$\mathcal{N}_2^{\perp} = \left\{ N_2^{\perp} = \int_0^{\tau} d\mathcal{M}\left(u\right) b\left(u, L\right) + m\left(L\right); E\left[m\left(L\right)\right] = 0 \quad and \right. \\ \left. E\left[b\left(u, L\right) S\left(u\right) \exp\left[q\left(u, L\right)\right] \mid \overline{L}\left(u\right)\right] = 0 \quad for\ u \in \left[0, \tau\right] \right\} \tag{4.8}$$

by Ritov and Wellner (1988) and Robins and Rotnitzky (1992). Here

$$S\left(u\right) \equiv \exp\left[-\int_0^u \lambda\left(s \mid L\right) ds\right]. \tag{4.9}$$

Given $\mathcal{N}_2^{\perp}$, we obtain $\mathcal{N}_2^{O,\perp}$ from (4.6).

For concreteness, we shall consider the semiparametric model for F_L in which the conditional mean of $Y \equiv Y\left(10\right)$ given a vector $X \in L\left(0\right)$ follows the parametric regression model

$$E\left[Y \mid X\right] = g\left(X, \beta_0\right) \tag{4.10}$$

where $g\left(X, \beta\right)$ is a known function. Note the non-parametric model for the mean of Y discussed in the previous subsection is a special case of model (4.10) in which X is constant with probability 1 and $g\left(X, \beta_0\right) = \beta_0$. That is,

$$E\left(Y\right) = \beta_0. \tag{4.11}$$

Let $\varepsilon \equiv Y - g\left(X, \beta_0\right)$. In the semiparametric model for F_L given by the sole restriction (4.10), Robins et al. (1994) showed that the orthogonal complement $\mathcal{N}_1^{\perp}$ to the nuisance tangent space $\mathcal{N}_1$ is

$$\mathcal{N}_1^{\perp} = \left\{U = d\left(X\right) \varepsilon\ ;\ d\left(X\right)\ \ arbitrary\right\}. \tag{4.12}$$

In the non-parametric model (4.11),

$$\mathcal{N}_1^{\perp} = \left\{U = c\left(Y - \beta_0\right);\ c\ is\ an\ arbitrary\ constant\right\}. \tag{4.13}$$

For each $m\left(L\right) \in \mathcal{N}_1^{\perp}$, let $a_m\left(u, \overline{L}\left(u\right)\right)$ be the unique solution on $0 \le u < \tau$ to the Volterra integral equation

$$a\left(u, \overline{L}\left(u\right)\right) = J_m\left(u\right) - \int_0^u ds\ a\left(s, \overline{L}\left(s\right)\right) \kappa\left(s, u, \overline{L}\left(u\right)\right) \tag{4.14}$$

where

$$J_m(u) \equiv E\left[m(L)\exp\{q(u,L)\} \mid \overline{L}(u)\right] \Big/ E\left[S(u)\exp\{q(u,L)\} \mid \overline{L}(u)\right], \tag{4.15}$$

with $S(u)$ as defined in (4.9) and

$$\kappa\left(s,u,\overline{L}(u)\right) \equiv E\left[\Lambda(s)\,S(s)\,e^{q(u,L)} \mid \overline{L}(u)\right] \Big/ E\left[S(u)\exp\{q(u,L)\} \mid \overline{L}(u)\right]. \tag{4.16}$$

THEOREM 4.1. *In the semiparametric model* **a** *with* $\mathcal{N}_1^{\perp} = \{m(L)\}$

$$\mathcal{N}^{O,\perp} = \left\{N^{O,\perp} = N^{O,\perp}(m) = \Delta m(L)/S + N_{car}(a_m);\ m(L) \in \mathcal{N}_1^{\perp}\right\} \tag{4.17}$$

Proof. To prove the theorem, we use the following lemma, which we prove following the proof of Theorem 4.1.

LEMMA 4.1. *For any* $m(L)$ *and any* $A = a(O) \equiv a\left(C,\overline{L}(C)\right)$,

$$\Delta m(L)/S + (1-\Delta)A - \Delta\, E[(1-\Delta)A \mid L]/S = m(L) + \int d\mathcal{M}(u)\, b(u,L) \tag{4.18}$$

where

$$b(u,L) \equiv a\left(u,\overline{L}(u)\right) + E\left[a\left(C,\overline{L}(C)\right) I(C<u) \mid L\right]/S(u) - m(L)/S(u). \tag{4.19}$$

Proof of Theorem 4.1. Theorem 4.1 follows by noting that it follows from the characterization of $\mathcal{N}_2^{\perp}$ in (4.8) that the LHS of (4.18) is in $\mathcal{N}_2^{\perp}$ if and only if for $b(u,L)$ given by (4.19), $E\left[b(u,L)\,S(u)\,e^{q(u,L)} \mid \overline{L}(u)\right] = 0$ which implies that

$$a(u,\overline{L}(u))E\left[S(u)\exp q(u,L) \mid \overline{L}(u)\right] - E\left[m(L)\exp\{q(u,L)\} \mid \overline{L}(u)\right] + E\left[E\{a(C,\overline{L}(C))I(C<u) \mid L\}\exp\left\{q(u,L) \mid \overline{L}(u)\right\}\right] = 0. \tag{4.20}$$

The last term on the LHS of (4.20) is $\int_0^u ds\, a\left(s,\overline{L}(s)\right) E\left[\Lambda(s)\,S(s)\exp\{q(u,L)\} \mid \overline{L}(u)\right]$, which completes the proof.

Proof of Lemma 4.1.

$$\Delta m(L)/S = m(L) - \int_0^{\tau} m(L)\, d\mathcal{M}(u)/S(u) \tag{4.21}$$

by Eq. (3.10d) of Robins and Rotnitzky (1992). Furthermore,

$$\int_0^\tau \{dN^*(u) - \Delta S(u) S^{-1} \lambda(u \mid L) I(C \geq u)\, du\}\, a\left(u, \overline{L}(u)\right) = (1-\Delta) A - \Delta E\left[(1-\Delta) A \mid L\right]/S \tag{4.22}$$

where $N^*(u) = I[C \leq u, C < \tau]$ since subjects with $\Delta = 0$ contribute $(1-\Delta)A$ to the LHS of (4.22), and the LHS of (4.22) has mean zero given L, since $E[\Delta S(u)/S \mid L, I(C \geq u)] = I(C \geq u)$ and $E\big[dN^*(u) \mid L, I(C \geq u)\big] = \lambda(u \mid L) I(C \geq u)\, du$. However, by (3.10c) of Robins and Rotnitzky (1992), $\{\Delta S(u)/S\} \lambda(u \mid L) I(C \geq u) = \lambda(u \mid L) I(C \geq u) - S(u) \lambda(u \mid L) \int_u^\tau d\mathcal{M}(x)/S(x)$. So the LHS of (4.22) is $\int_0^\tau d\mathcal{M}(u)\, a(u, \overline{L}(u)) + \int_0^\tau du S(u) \lambda(u \mid L)\, a\left(u, \overline{L}(u)\right) \int_u^\tau d\mathcal{M}(x)/S(x)$.

However, by Fubini's theorem, $\int_0^\tau du S(u) \Lambda(u)\, a\left(u, \overline{L}(u)\right) \int_u^\tau d\mathcal{M}(x)/S(x) = \int_0^\tau d\mathcal{M}(x) \{S(x)\}^{-1} \int_0^x du \left(S(u) \Lambda(u)\, a\left(u, \overline{L}(u)\right)\right) = \int_0^\tau d\mathcal{M}(x)\, E\left[I(C < x)\, a\left[C, \overline{L}(C)\right] \mid L\right]/S(x)$ which proves the lemma. □

REMARK 4.4. In model **a**, with $\beta_0 = E[Y(10)]$ and F_L unrestricted, $\mathcal{N}_1^\perp$ is given by Eq. (4.13). It then follows from Theorem 4.1 that $\mathcal{N}^{O,\perp}$ is comprised of multiples of a single random variable. Hence all RAL estimators of β_0 must have the same influence function.

In model **a** in which F_L follows the semiparametric model characterized by (4.10), there is more than one influence function, and the question arises as to which influence function is optimal. Now the influence function $IF(m)$ associated with an element $N^{O,\perp}(m)$ in $\mathcal{N}^{O,\perp}$ is

$$IF(m) = E\left[N^{O,\perp}(m) S_\beta^T\right]^{-1} N^{O,\perp}(m) \tag{4.23}$$

where S_β is the score for β evaluated at the truth. However, Robins, Rotnitzky, and Zhao (1994) show that

$$E\left[N^{O,\perp}(m) S_\beta^T\right]^{-1} = E\left[m(L) S_{eff}^{F,T}\right]^{-1} \tag{4.24}$$

where $S_{eff}^F = \Pi\left[S_\beta^F \mid \mathcal{N}_1^\perp\right]$ is the efficient score for $\beta_0 = \psi_0$ were the full data (C, L) always observed. Here, and throughout: $\Pi(A \mid \mathcal{A})$ denotes the Hilbert space projection of the random variable A on the space $\mathcal{A}$, and S_β^F is the score for β when data on (C, L) are available.

The efficient influence function, $EIF \equiv IF(m_{eff})$ has minimum variance among all members of the set of influence functions $\{IF(m)\}$. $Var[IF(m_{eff})]$ is the semiparametric variance bound for model **a**. The following lemma is an immediate consequence of (4.23), (4.24), and Theorem 5.3 in Newey and McFadden (1993).

LEMMA 4.2. *$m_{eff}(L)$ is the unique member of $\mathcal{N}_1^\perp$ that satisfies*

$$E\left[m(L) S_{eff}^{FT}\right] = E\left[N^{O,\perp}(m) N^{O,\perp}(m_{eff})^T\right] \tag{4.25}$$

for all $m(L) \in \mathcal{N}_1^\perp$.

COROLLARY 4.1. *$m_{eff}(L)$ is the unique member of $\mathcal{N}_1^{\perp}$ satisfying*

$$S_{eff}^F = \Pi\left[\mathbf{O}^{\dagger}\mathbf{O}\left[m_{eff}(L)\right] \mid \mathcal{N}_1^{\perp}\right]$$

where the operator $\mathbf{O}: \Omega^{(L)} \to \Omega^{(O)}$ maps $m(L)$ into $\mathcal{N}^{O,\perp}(m)$ and $\mathbf{O}^{\dagger}: \Omega^{(O)} \to \Omega^{(L)}$ is the adjoint of $\mathbf{O}$.

Consider model **a** with F_L restricted by (4.10). Chamberlain (1987) shows that $S_{eff}^F = \{\partial g(X,\beta_0)/\partial\beta\} \, var(\varepsilon \mid X)^{-1} \varepsilon$. Further, by (4.12), $m(L) \in \mathcal{N}_1^{\perp} \Leftrightarrow m(L) = d(X)\varepsilon$. Thus the left hand side of (4.25) becomes $E\left[d(X)\{\partial g(X,\beta_0)/\partial\beta\}^T\right]$. The RHS of (4.25) becomes $E\left[d(X)\, d_{eff}(X)\, \kappa^*(X)\right]$ where $\kappa^*(X) = E\left[\{\Delta\varepsilon/S + N_{car}(a_{eff})\}^2 \mid X\right]$, $m_{eff}(X) \equiv d_{eff}(X)\varepsilon$, $a_{eff}\left(u, \overline{L}(u)\right)$ is the solution $a_m\left(u, \overline{L}(u)\right)$ to (4.14) with $m(L) \equiv \varepsilon \equiv Y - g(x,\beta_0)$. [We have used the fact that, for $m(L) = d(X)\varepsilon$, $a_m\left(u, \overline{L}(u)\right) = d(X)\, a_{eff}\left(u, \overline{L}(u)\right)$.] The LHS and RHS of (4.25) must be equal for all $d(X)$. This implies that

$$d_{eff}(X) = \{\partial g(X,\beta_0)/\partial\beta\}/\kappa^*(X) \; . \tag{4.26}$$

4.3. Further details of estimation in model a. We continue to consider semiparametric model **a** with F_L following the semiparametric model (4.10). In practice we will estimate β_0 by $\widehat{\beta}(d)$ solving $0 = \sum_i \widehat{N}_{1i}^{O,\perp}(\beta, d) = 0$ where

$$\widehat{N}_1^{O,\perp}(\beta, d) = \Delta d(X)\,\varepsilon(\beta)/\widehat{S} + \widehat{N}_{car} \; , \tag{4.27}$$

$\widehat{N}_{car} \equiv \widehat{N}_{car}(a) = (1-\Delta)A - \Delta E\left[(1-\Delta)A \mid L\right]/\widehat{S}$, $\widehat{\Lambda}(u)$, $\varepsilon(\beta) = Y - g(X,\beta)$, and $\widehat{E}[\cdot \mid L]$ and $\widehat{S}$ are determined by the estimates based on (4.4). Under mild regularity conditions for each choice of $d(X)$, $\widehat{\beta}(d)$ will be a RAL estimator and the asymptotic variance of $n^{\frac{1}{2}}\left(\widehat{\beta}(d) - \beta_0\right)$ can be estimated using the bootstrap (Gill, 1989). However, the analytic sandwich estimator of the asymptotic variance

$$\widehat{I}^{-1}(d)\left[n^{-1}\sum_i \widehat{N}_{1i}^{O,\perp}(\beta, d)^{\otimes 2}\right]\widehat{I}(d)^{-1T} \tag{4.28}$$

evaluated at $\beta = \widehat{\beta}(d)$ with $\widehat{I}(d) = n^{-1}\sum_i \partial\widehat{N}_{1i}^{O,\perp}(\beta, d)/\partial\beta$ will be inconsistent for the asymptotic variance of $n^{\frac{1}{2}}\left(\widehat{\beta}(d) - \beta_0\right)$ unless A is equal to $A_m = a_m\left(C, \overline{L}(C)\right)$ solving (4.14) with $m(L) = d(X)\varepsilon$ (so that $N_1^{O,\perp}(\beta_0, d)$ is in $\mathcal{N}^{O,\perp}$ as well). However, the above analytic estimator can be used if we replace A by a consistent estimator $\widehat{A}_m$ of A_m obtained by solving the Volterra integral equation (4.14) with *(i)* $\widehat{\Lambda}(s)$ and $\widehat{S}(u)$ based on (4.4) replacing $\Lambda(s)$ and $S(s)$ and *(ii)* for any random H, $E\left[H \mid \overline{L}(u)\right]$ is consistently estimated, by $\left\{\sum_i I\left[\overline{L}_i(u) = \overline{L}(u)\right]\Delta_i H_i \widehat{S}_i(u)/\widehat{S}_i\right\} / \left\{\sum_i I\left[\overline{L}_i(u) = \overline{L}(u)\right]\Delta_i \widehat{S}_i(u)/\widehat{S}_i\right\}$. Replacement of A_m by $\widehat{A}_m$ does not change the asymptotic distribution of the estimator. Note that the Volterra integral equation (4.14) becomes a finite dimensional matrix equation in its estimated form. (Since we are continuing to assume that $\overline{L}(u)$ has only a few levels, the expectations from the Volterra integral equation can be estimated by sample averages.) Finally, a semiparametric efficient estimator can be obtained by estimating $d_{eff}(X)$ based on a consistent preliminary estimators of β_0.

4.4. Estimation in model $\mathbf{a}_r$. Model $\mathbf{a}_r$ differs from model $\mathbf{a}$ by imposing (4.1). As in Sec. 2, we allow F_L to follow a semiparametric model indexed by finite dimensional parameter β and infinite dimensional parameter θ. Thus in model $\mathbf{a}_r$, $\psi = (\beta', \gamma')'$ is the parametric component. The infinite dimensional component η associated with $F_{C|L}$ indexes functions $h(u)$ of u. If $h(u)$ were known, we would consider estimating equations based on $N_1^{O,\perp} \equiv N_1^{O,\perp}(\psi_0)$ of (4.5) indexed by $p+q$ dimensional functions $m(L) \in \mathcal{N}_1^{\perp}$ and $a(O) \in \mathcal{N}_{car}$. That is, we would solve $0 = \sum_i N_{1i}^{O,\perp}(\psi)$. Since $h(u)$ is unknown, we instead solve $0 = \sum_i \widehat{N}_{1i}^{O,\perp}(\psi)$ in which an estimator $\widehat{h}(u, \gamma)$ of $h(u)$ depending on γ has been substituted in $N_{1i}^{O,\perp}(\psi)$. For example, if F_L follows the model characterized by (4.10), $\widehat{N}_{1i}^{O,\perp}(\psi) = \Delta d(X)\varepsilon(\beta)/\widehat{S}(\gamma) - \widehat{N}_{car}(a, \gamma)$ where $\widehat{N}_{car}(a, \gamma)$ and $\widehat{S}(\gamma)$ are $N_{car}(a)$ and S with $\widehat{h}(u, \gamma)$ substituted for $h(u)$.

Specifically, let $Z(u, \gamma) = \exp\left[\nu\left(u, \overline{L}(u); \gamma\right) + q(u, L)\right]$ and again renumber subjects so that if $C_i < C_j$ that $i < j$. Then we recursively define estimators $\widehat{h}(u, \gamma)$ and thus $\widehat{\Lambda}(u; \gamma)$ as follows. Set $\exp\{\widehat{h}(u; \gamma)\} = 0$ unless $u = C_i < \tau_i$ for some i. For $C_i < \tau_i$, recursively define $\exp\{\widehat{h}(C_i; \gamma)\}$ starting from the largest C_i as $\left[\sum_{j=1}^{n} \Delta_j Z_j(C_i; \gamma) / \prod_{k=i+1}^{n} [1 - \widehat{\Lambda}_j(C_k; \gamma)] I(C_k \neq \tau_k)\right]^{-1}$.

Our goal is now to determine the orthogonal complement to the nuisance tangent space in model $\mathbf{a}_r$ which includes all influence functions IF for ψ_0. In model $\mathbf{a}_r$,

$$\mathcal{N}_2 = \left\{N_2 = N_2(a) = \int_0^{\tau} dM(u)\, a(u)\right\} . \tag{4.29}$$

Define $Z(u) = Z(u, \gamma_0)$. It follows by the results of Ritov and Wellner (1988) that

$$\begin{aligned} \mathcal{N}_2^{\perp} = \Big\{N_2^{\perp} = \int_0^{\tau} d\mathcal{M}(u)\, b(u, L) + m(L) \;;\; E[m(L)] = 0 \\ \textit{and } E[b(u, L)\, S(u)\, Z(u)] = 0\Big\} . \end{aligned} \tag{4.30}$$

Furthermore, $N_2^{O,\perp}$ is still defined in terms of $\mathcal{N}_2^{\perp}$ by (4.6), $\mathcal{N}_1^{O,\perp}$ is still given by (4.9) with $\mathcal{N}_1^{\perp}$ as in model $\mathbf{a}$ and $\mathcal{N}^{O,\perp}$ still $\mathcal{N}_1^{O,\perp} \bigcap \mathcal{N}_2^{O,\perp}$.

We now prove a lemma characterizing $\mathcal{N}^{O,\perp}$ in greater detail.

Given any function $m(L)$ and any function $a^*\left(u,\overline{L}(u)\right)$, let $a_{m,a^*}(u, \overline{L}(u))$ be the unique solution $a\left(u,\overline{L}(u)\right)$ to the "Volterra-like" recursive integral equation

$$\begin{aligned} a\left(u,\overline{L}(u)\right) &= a^*\left(u,\overline{L}(u)\right) \\ &- \{E[S(u)Z(u)]\}^{-1}\Big\{E\left[a^*\left(u,\overline{L}(u)\right)S(u)Z(u)\right] \\ &- E[m(L)Z(u)]+E\Big[\Big\{\int_0^u a\left(s,\overline{L}(s)\right)\Lambda(s)S(s)\,ds\Big\}Z(u)\Big]\Big\}. \end{aligned} \tag{4.31}$$

LEMMA 4.3. *In model* $\mathbf{a}_r$, $\mathcal{N}^{O,\perp} = \{N^{O,\perp} = N^{O,\perp}(m,a^*) = \Delta m(L)/S + N_{car}(a_{m,a^*})\,;\ a^*\left(u,\overline{L}(u)\right)$ *arbitrary,* $m(L)\in\mathcal{N}_1^{\perp}\}$.

Proof. We first follow the proof of Theorem (4.1) to obtain that the LHS of (4.18) is in $\mathcal{N}_2^{\perp}$ as given by (4.30) if and only if $b(u,L)$ given by (4.19) satisfies $E[b(u,L)S(u)Z(u)]=0$. But this is true if and only if

$$\begin{aligned} &E\left[a\left(u,\overline{L}(u)\right)S(u)Z(u)\right] = \\ &\qquad E[m(L)Z(u)] - E\left[\left\{\int_0^u a\left(s,\overline{L}(s)\right)\Lambda(s)S(s)\,ds\right\}Z(u)\right]. \end{aligned} \tag{4.32}$$

Now $a(u,\overline{L}(u))$ solving (4.31) clearly satisfies (4.32). Conversely, if $a(u,\overline{L}(u))$ satisfies (4.32), then if we define $a^{\dagger}\left(u,\overline{L}(u)\right) = a\left(u,\overline{L}(u)\right) - \{E[m(L)Z(u)] - E[\{\int_0^u a(s,\overline{L}(s))\Lambda(s)S(s)ds\}Z(u)]\}/E\big(S(u)Z(u)\big)$, then $E\left[a^{\dagger}\left(u,\overline{L}(u)\right)S(u)Z(u)\right]=0$. The Hilbert space projection of any function $a^*\left(u,\overline{L}(u)\right)$ on the space of functions $a^{\dagger}\left(u,\overline{L}(u)\right)$ satisfying the last equality is given by $a^*(u,\overline{L}(u)) - \{E[S(u)Z(u)]\}^{-1}E[a^*(u,\overline{L}(u))S(u)Z(u)]$ which proves the theorem. □

We now explain how to use Lemma 4.3 to construct asymptotic variance estimators. For concreteness, we continue to consider the model for F_L characterized by the sole restriction (4.10). Then the asymptotic variance of $n^{\frac{1}{2}}\left(\widehat{\psi}(d)-\psi_0\right)$ solving $0=\sum_i \widehat{N}_{1i}^{O,\perp}(\psi,d)$ based on $d(X)\varepsilon\in N_1^{\perp}$ can be consistently estimated by (4.28) [with ψ replacing β] only if the term $N_{car}(a)$ in $N_1^{O,\perp}(\psi,d)$ has $a=a_{m,a^*}$ for $m(L)=d(X)\varepsilon$ and some $a^*\left(u,\overline{L}(u)\right)$ [so that $N_1^{O,\perp}(\psi_0,d)$ is also $N^{O,\perp}$]. However, the analytic variance estimator (4.28) can be used if we use $N_{car}(\widehat{a}_{m,a})$ where $\widehat{a}_{m,a^*}$ is a consistent estimator of a_{m,a^*} which we obtain by *(i)* calculating an estimator $\widetilde{\psi}$ of ψ_0 based on any initial $\widehat{N}_1^{O,\perp}(\psi,d)$ and then *(ii)* solving (4.31) with $\widehat{\Lambda}(s;\widetilde{\gamma})$ and $S(s;\widetilde{\gamma})$ replacing $\Lambda(s)$ and $S(s)$ and with inverse-probability-of-remaining-uncensored-weighted sample averages replacing expectations.

REMARK 4.5. We have not as yet characterized the efficient score in model $\mathbf{a}_r$. However, if as recommended in Remark 2.7, γ_0 is a high-dimensional parameter and β_0 is the parameter of interest, then the semiparametric efficiency bound for β_0 in model $\mathbf{a}_r$ and model $\mathbf{a}$ should be similar. Thus we suggest using an estimator for β_0 that would be efficient in model $\mathbf{a}$. We can construct such an estimator, because we can know the form of the efficient estimator in model $\mathbf{a}$.

To clarify this proposal, suppose our model for F_L is still characterized by restriction (4.10). As with model $\mathbf{a}$, it is necessary to estimate $d_{eff}(X)$ of Eq. (4.26) and $a_{eff}\left(u, \overline{L}(u)\right)$ as defined in the paragraph preceding Eq. (4.26) from the data. This requires we solve an estimated version of the Volterra integral Equation (4.14). However, (4.14) requires that we compute conditional expectations given $\overline{L}(u)$ and X, both of which may now be high-dimensional and continuous. Thus, we suggest first one specify a fully parametric model for the joint distribution of (C, L), estimate the model by maximum likelihood from the observed data and construct estimators $\widehat{d}_{eff}(X)$ and $\widehat{a}_{eff}\left(u, \overline{L}(u)\right)$ based on the estimated law of (C, L). Then let $\widehat{a}_{m,a^*}$ be the estimated version of a_{m,a^*} calculated as described in the previous paragraph with $m(L) = \widehat{d}_{eff}(X)\,\varepsilon\left(\widetilde{\beta}\right)$, $a^*\left(u, \overline{L}(u)\right) = \widehat{d}_{eff}(X)\,\widehat{a}_{eff}\left(u, \overline{L}(u)\right)$ where $\widetilde{\beta}$ is a preliminary $n^{\frac{1}{2}}$ - consistent estimator of β_0. Finally, obtain $\widehat{\psi}(\widehat{d}_{eff}) = \left(\widehat{\beta}(\widehat{d}_{eff})^T, \widehat{\gamma}(\widehat{d}_{eff})^T\right)^T$ solving $0 = \sum_i \widehat{N}_{1i}^{O,\perp}\left(\psi, \widehat{d}\right)$ with the first p components of the $p+q$ - dimensional estimating function $N_{1i}^{O,\perp}\left(\psi, \widehat{d}\right)$ being $\Delta \widehat{d}_{eff}(X)\,\varepsilon(\beta)/\widehat{S}(\gamma) - \widehat{N}_{car}\left(\widehat{a}_{m,a^*}, \gamma\right)$ with $\widehat{a}_{m,a^*}$ as just defined. If the parametric model for (C, L) is correctly specified, then $\widehat{a}_{m,a^*}$ is consistent for $d_{eff}(X)\,a_{eff}(u, \overline{L}(u))$ and $\widehat{d}_{eff}(X)$ is consistent for $d_{eff}(X)$ [defined by Eq. (4.26)]. Furthermore, the solutions $\widehat{\beta}(\widehat{d}_{eff})$ and $\widehat{\gamma}(\widehat{d}_{eff})$ will be asymptotically independent and the asymptotic variance of $\widehat{\beta}(\widehat{d}_{eff})$ will attain the semiparametric variance bound for model $\mathbf{a}$ and thus, as argued above, be nearly efficient in model $\mathbf{a}_r$.

Even if the parametric model for (C, L) is misspecified, $\widehat{\psi}(\widehat{d}_{eff})$ is still a RAL estimator under model $\mathbf{a}_r$ with asymptotic variance that is consistently estimated by the analytic estimator (4.28) with β replaced by ψ. However, the asymptotic variance of $\widehat{\beta}\left(\widehat{d}_{eff}\right)$ will no longer equal that of the efficient estimator under model $\mathbf{a}$, although one would expect that the difference would not be large provided the parametric model for (C, L) is richly parameterized.

5. Selection odds models and the selection bias G-computation algorithm formula.

5.1. Selection bias g-computation algorithm formula.

5.1. Selection bias g-computation algorithm formula. In this subsection, we derive the non-ignorable selection bias g-computation algorithm formula. We return to the setting where drop-out occurs only at fixed times $k, k = 0, 1, \ldots, K$ and $L = \left(\overline{L}_{K+1}\right) = (L_0, \ldots, L_{K+1})$.

Define

$$
\begin{aligned}
& B_k\left(\underline{y}_{k+1}\right)=b_k\left(\underline{y}_{k+1}, \overline{L}_k\right)=f_{\underline{Y}_{k+1}}\left(\underline{y}_{k+1} \mid \overline{L}_k, C>k\right), \\
(5.1) \quad & B_k^*\left(\underline{y}_{k+1}\right)=b_k^*\left(\underline{y}_{k+1}, \overline{L}_k\right)=f_{\underline{Y}_{k+1}}\left(\underline{y}_{k+1} \mid \overline{L}_k, C \geq k\right) \text{ and} \\
& \Lambda_k^*=pr\left[C=k \mid C \geq k, \overline{L}_k\right].
\end{aligned}
$$

Consider now the selection bias g-computation algorithm formula identity

$$
\begin{aligned}
& f_{\underline{Y}_{k+1}}\left(\underline{y}_{k+1} \mid \bar{\ell}_k, C>k\right) \equiv b_k\left(\underline{y}_{k+1}, \bar{\ell}_k\right) \\
(5.2) \quad & =\int \cdots \iint \prod_{m=k+1}^{K+1} f\left[y_m \mid \bar{\ell}_{m-1}, C \geq m\right] dF\left[v_m \mid y_m,\right. \\
& \qquad \left.\bar{\ell}_{m-1}, C \geq m\right]\left\{\prod_{m=k+1}^{K} j\left(\bar{\ell}_m, \underline{y}_{m+1}\right)\right\}
\end{aligned}
$$

with

$$
\begin{aligned}
(5.3) \quad j\left(\overline{L}_m, \underline{Y}_{m+1}\right) & \equiv b_m^*\left(\underline{Y}_{m+1}, \overline{L}_m\right) / b_m\left(\underline{Y}_{m+1}, \overline{L}_m\right) \\
& =\left(1-\Lambda_k^*\right) / \left(1-\Lambda_k\right),
\end{aligned}
$$

where the last identity is by Bayes' theorem and Λ_k is as in Theorem 3.2. It follows from (5.2) that to make $b_k\left(\underline{y}_{k+1}, \bar{\ell}_k\right)$ identifiable from data on O, we need to make the $j\left(\bar{\ell}_k, \underline{y}_{k+1}\right)$ or, equivalently, the Λ_k identifiable which, by Theorem 3.2, can be accomplished by imposing the semiparametric model b for (C, L) characterized by the restrictions (3.5), (3.6). Indeed, Eq. (5.2) is essentially Eq. (3.7d) with the expectation in (3.7d) written out explicitly as an integral. Similarly Eqs. (3.7b) and (5.2) (evaluated at $k=-1$) are alternative representations for $F_Y(y)$ as a functional of F_O.

REMARK 5.1. We refer to the RHS of (5.2) as the selection bias G-computation algorithm formula. Under semiparametric model **b** of Theorem (3.2), if the $q_k\left(\bar{\ell}_k, \underline{y}_{k+1}\right) \equiv 0$ for all k so that there is no non-ignorable selection bias for Y, then $j\left(\bar{\ell}_k, \underline{y}_{k+1}\right)=1$ for all k and we obtain the standard g-computation algorithm formula of Robins (1986).

REMARK 5.2. Scharfstein, Rotnitzky, and Robins (1999) obtain a selection bias continuous time g-computation algorithm formula by explicitly writing out the expectation in Eq. (3.11) in terms of the joint distribution of the observables under semiparametric model **b** of Theorem 3.3 in the special case where the $\overline{L}(u)$ process jumps only at a finite number of nonrandom times. Richard Gill has generalized this result by allowing for $\overline{L}(u)$ processes that can jump in continuous time.

5.2. Selection odds model. Consider semiparametric model **b** for (Δ, L) of Theorem 3.2 with Y the outcome of interest. The odds ratio function of Y and Δ, $OR_{Y\Delta}(y)$ is defined to be $OR_{Y\Delta}(y) = \{pr[\Delta = 1 \mid Y = y]/pr[\Delta = 0 \mid Y = y]\}/\{pr[\Delta = 1 \mid Y = 0]/pr[\Delta = 0 \mid Y = 0]\} = \{f_Y[y \mid \Delta = 1]/f_Y[y \mid \Delta = 0]\}/\{f_Y[0 \mid \Delta = 1]/f_Y[0 \mid \Delta = 0]\}$. $OR_{Y\Delta}(y)$ is the unique functional of the distribution of $F_{Y,\Delta}$ that is a functional of both the conditional distribution of Y given Δ and of the distribution of Δ given Y. We refer to the semiparametric model **b** as a non-parametric selection odds model if we choose $\Phi(x)$ to be the logistic function $e^x/(1+e^x)$ since then $\ln OR_{Y\Delta}(y) = q(y)$. In the literature, a "selection" model is a model for selection bias that models the law of Δ given Y, and a pattern mixture model is a model for the law of Y given Δ. We see that our non-parametric selection odds model is the unique model that has both a pattern mixture and selection model interpretation and thus is of some independent interest. It is also of interest because, in general, physicians and other investigators have a fairly good intuitive sense of the meaning of the function $q(y)$ in a selection odds model because of the two equivalent useful ways to think about the meaning of $q(y)$ as encoded in the above equivalent definitions of $OR_{Y\Delta}(y)$.

We will now extend our study of selection odds models to the semiparametric model **b** of Theorem 3.2 for monotone missing data in discrete time with $\Phi(x)$ the logistic function. In this model, the chosen functions $q_k(\overline{L}_k, \underline{Y}_{k+1})$ represent the log odds ratio for drop-out at k. In the following, as discussed in Remark 2.10, we standardize our choice of q_k such that $q_k(\overline{L}_k, \underline{Y}_{k+1}) = 0$ if $\underline{Y}_{k+1} \equiv 0$. An alternative representation of our selection odds model is given in the following.

LEMMA 5.1. *Eq. (3.5) is true with $\Phi(x)$ logistic if and only if for $k = 0, \ldots, K$ $f_{\underline{Y}_{k+1}}(\underline{y}_{k+1} \mid \overline{L}_k, C = k) = f_{\underline{Y}_{k+1}}(\underline{y}_{k+1} \mid \overline{L}_k, C > k)\exp\{-q_k(\overline{L}_k, \underline{y}_{k+1})\}/c_k(\overline{L}_k)$ where*

$$c_k(\overline{L}_k) \equiv \int f_{\underline{Y}_{k+1}}\left(\underline{y}_{k+1} \mid \overline{L}_k, C > k\right)\exp\left\{-q_k\left(\overline{L}_k, \underline{y}_{k+1}\right)\right\} d\mu\left(\underline{y}_{k+1}\right). \tag{5.4}$$

We will now use the following lemma.

LEMMA 5.2. $B_K\left(\underline{y}_{K+1}\right) = f\left[\underline{y}_{K+1} \mid \overline{L}_K, C > K\right]$, $B_k^*\left(\underline{y}_{k+1}\right) = B_k\left(\underline{y}_{k+1}\right)\left[\{1 - \Lambda_k^*\} + \Lambda_k^* e^{-q_k\left(\overline{L}_k, \underline{y}_{k+1}\right)}/c_k\left(\overline{L}_k\right)\right]$, *and* $B_{m-1}\left(\underline{y}_m\right) = \int b_m^*\left(\underline{y}_{m+1}, \{\overline{L}_{m-1}, \ell_m = (v_m, y_m)\}\right) f(y_m \mid \overline{L}_{m-1}, C \geq m) dF\left[v_m \mid \overline{L}_{m-1}, Y_m = y_m, C \geq m\right]$.

REMARK 5.3. Note if $q_k(\overline{L}_k, \underline{y}_{k+1}) \equiv 0$ for all k so that there is no selection bias for Y, then $c_k(\overline{L}_k) \equiv 1$ and $B_k(\underline{y}_{k+1}) = B_k^*(\underline{y}_{k+1})$. For a selection odds model, $j(\overline{L}_k, \underline{y}_{k+1})$ has a particularly nice form. Specifically, if, in Eq. (3.5), $\Phi(x)$ is logistic, then

$$\begin{aligned} j\left(\overline{L}_m, \underline{y}_{m+1}\right) &\equiv b_m^*\left(\underline{y}_{m+1}, \overline{L}_m\right) / b_m\left(\underline{y}_{m+1}, \overline{L}_m\right) \\ &= \left(1-\Lambda_m^*\right)+\Lambda_m^* \exp\left\{-q_k\left(\overline{L}_m, \underline{y}_{m+1}\right)\right\} / c_m\left(\overline{L}_m\right) \end{aligned}$$

where the $c_m\left(\overline{\ell}_m\right)$ are obtained recursively starting with $m = K$ from Eq. (5.4).

6. Identification in causal inference problems.

6.1. The data and counterfactual data. Consider a study where we observe n i.i.d. copies of data $O = \left(\overline{A}(\tau), \overline{L}(\tau)\right)$, where τ is an administrative end of follow-up time, $\overline{A}(\tau)$ is a treatment process, $\overline{L}(\tau)$ is an outcome or response process and, for any $Z(u), \overline{Z}(t) \equiv \{Z(u); 0 \le u \le t\}$. We assume τ is an element of $L(0)$ since it is assumed known at time 0.

For purposes of causal inference, we assume the existence of an underlying treatment process $\overline{A} = \{A(u); 0 \le u < \infty\}$ with $A(u)$ taking values in a set $\mathcal{A}(u)$ and the existence of underlying counterfactual random variables

$$\{\overline{L}_{\overline{a}};\ \overline{a} \in \overline{\mathcal{A}}\} \tag{6.1}$$

where $\overline{L}_{\overline{a}} = \{L_{\overline{a}}(u); 0 \le u < \infty\}$, $\overline{a} = a(\cdot) = \{a(t); 0 \le t < \infty$ and $a(t) \in \mathcal{A}(t)\}$ is a treatment plan (equivalently, regime or function) lying in a set of functions $\overline{\mathcal{A}}$. Given a regime $\overline{a}$, let $\overline{L}_{\overline{a}(u),\mathbf{0}}$ be counterfactual history under a regime $\overline{a}^*$ that agrees with $\overline{a}$ through time u and is 0 thereafter, where 0 is the baseline value of $a(t)$. Then we assume that the $\overline{L}_{\overline{a}}$ satisfy the following consistency assumption with probability 1:

$$\overline{L}_{\overline{a}(u),\mathbf{0}}(u) = \overline{L}_{\overline{a}(t),\mathbf{0}}(u) = \overline{L}_{\overline{a}}(u) = \overline{L}_{\overline{a}^\dagger}(u) \tag{6.2}$$

for all $t > u$ and all $\overline{a}^\dagger$ with $\overline{a}^\dagger(u) = \overline{a}(u)$. This assumption essentially says that the future does not determine the past. The observed data are linked to the counterfactual data by

$$\overline{L}(\tau) = \overline{L}_{\overline{A}(\tau),0}(\tau) \ . \tag{6.3}$$

Eq. (6.3) states that a subject's observed outcome history through end of follow-up is equal to their counterfactual outcome history corresponding to the treatment they did indeed receive. We assume $\overline{L}_{\overline{a}} = \left(\overline{Y}_{\overline{a}}, \overline{V}_{\overline{a}}\right)$ where $\overline{Y}_{\overline{a}}$ is an outcome process of interest and $\overline{V}_{\overline{a}}$ is the process of other recorded variables. Robins (1987, 1997b) considers the sequential randomization (i.e., ignorable treatment assignment) assumption that for all t and $\overline{a} \in \overline{\mathcal{A}}$,

$$\underline{Y}_{\overline{a}}(t) \coprod A(t) \mid \overline{L}(t^-), \overline{A}(t^-) \tag{6.4}$$

where for any variable $\underline{Z}(t) = \{Z(u); u \ge t\}$ is the history of that variable from t onwards. We also refer to (6.4) as the assumption of no unmeasured confounders given prognostic factors $L(t)$. Because of measurability issues, (6.4) is not well-defined. If the $A(t)$ process can only jump at discrete non-random times $t_1, t_2, \ldots$ and the $\overline{L}(t)$ process has left-hand limits, i.e., $\overline{L}(t^-) \equiv \lim_{u \uparrow t} \overline{L}(u)$, (6.4) is formally, for each t_k,

$$(6.5) \quad f\left[A(t_k) \mid \overline{L}(t_k^-), \overline{A}(t_k^-), \underline{Y}_{\overline{a}}(t_k)\right] = f\left[A(t_k) \mid \overline{L}(t_k^-), \overline{A}(t_k^-)\right] .$$

where $f(\cdot \mid \cdot)$ is the conditional density of $A(t_k)$ with respect to a dominating measure $\mu(\cdot)$. If $A(t)$ is a marked point process that can jump in continuous time with CADLAG (continuous from the right with left-hand limits) step-function sample paths, then Eq. (6.4) is formally that

$$(6.6a) \qquad \lambda_A\left[t \mid \overline{L}(t^-), \overline{A}(t^-), \underline{Y}_{\overline{a}}(t)\right] = \lambda_A\left[t \mid \overline{L}(t^-), \overline{A}(t^-)\right]$$

and

$$(6.6b) \qquad \begin{aligned} &f\left[A(t) \mid \overline{L}(t^-), \overline{A}(t^-), A(t) \neq A(t^-), \underline{Y}_{\overline{a}}(t)\right] = \\ &\qquad\qquad f\left[A(t) \mid \overline{L}(t^-), \overline{A}(t^-), A(t) \neq A(t^-)\right] . \end{aligned}$$

Here, the intensity process $\lambda_A(t \mid \cdot)$ is $\lim_{\delta t \to 0} pr[A(t+\delta t) \neq A(t^-) \mid A(t^-), \cdot]/\delta t$. Eq. (6.6a) says that given past treatment and confounder history, the probability that the A process jumps at t does not depend on the future counterfactual history of the outcome of interest. Eq. (6.6b) says that given that the covariate process did jump at t, the probability it jumped to a particular value of $A(t)$ does not depend on the future counterfactual history of the outcome of interest. Given (6.4), Robins (1987) shows that the marginal distribution of $Y_{\overline{a}}$ is identified by the g-computation algorithm formula, as discussed further below.

Following Heitjan and Rubin (1991), we say the data are coarsened at random (CAR) if

$$(6.7) \quad f\left[\overline{A}(\tau) \mid \{\overline{L}_{\overline{a}}; \overline{a} \in \overline{\mathcal{A}}\}\right] \textit{ depends only on } O = \left(\overline{A}(\tau), \overline{L}(\tau)\right) .$$

Note that we can use ideas from the "missing data" literature because one's treatment history $\overline{A}(\tau)$ determines which components of one's counterfactual history $\{\overline{L}_{\overline{a}}; \overline{a} \in \overline{\mathcal{A}}\}$ one observes. Thus we can view causal inference as a missing data problem (Rubin, 1976). We shall make the following non-identifiable assumption concerning the statistical models for the full data $\left(A, \{\overline{L}_{\overline{a}}; \overline{a} \in \overline{\mathcal{A}}\}\right)$ considered in this section. Given $\overline{a}_1$ and $\overline{a}_2$, let u_{12} be the smallest time u with $a_1(u) \neq a_2(u)$. Thus consider the following non-identifiable assumption.

ASSUMPTION A. For all $\overline{a}_1$ and $\overline{a}_2$ the conditional distribution of $\left(\overline{L}_{\overline{a}_1}, \overline{L}_{\overline{a}_2}\right)$ given $\overline{L}_{\overline{a}_1}\left(u_{12}^-\right)$ is non-degenerate.

LEMMA 6.1. *If Assumption A and CAR hold, then so does sequential randomization (6.4).*

Proof. Ignoring measured theoretic subtleties, we can assume without loss of generality that the $A(t)$ process jumps only at $t = 0, A(t) \in \{0, 1\}$, the $L_{\overline{a}} = Y_{\overline{a}}$ process jumps only a $t = 1$, and that (6.4) is false because

$$f[A(0) = 1 \mid Y_1(1)] = q[Y_1(1)] \ .$$

Although the last display does not violate the CAR assumption (6.7), nonetheless, it also implies $f[A(0) = 0 \mid Y_1(1)] = 1 - q[Y_1(1)]$ which does violate (6.7) unless $Y_1(1) = Y_0(1)$ w.p.1, which is prohibited by Assumption A. □

Lemma 6.1 has the following obvious partial converse if we strengthen (6.4).

LEMMA 6.2. *Suppose that (6.4) holds with* $\{\overline{L}_{\overline{a}}; \overline{a} \in \overline{\mathcal{A}}\}$ *replacing* $\underline{Y}_{\overline{a}}(t)$. *Then CAR holds.*

However, if (6.4) is not so strengthened, then, even under Assumption A, the converse to Lemma 6.1 is not true. Specifically, Robins (1997b, p. 83) gives examples where one would expect (6.4) to be true even when (6.7) is false. However, if (6.7) is the sole restriction imposed, this essentially places no restrictions on the joint distribution of the observable random variables O (Gill, van der Laan, Robins, 1997) and, thus, is not subject to empirical test. Thus, once (6.4) is assumed, we can impose (6.7) without affecting our (non-parametric) inference. In the following remark, we show by counterexample that without Assumption A, CAR (i.e., 6.7) does not imply sequential randomization (i.e., 6.4), in which case the g-computation algorithm formula cannot be used to compute the marginal distribution of $\overline{Y}_{\overline{a}}$.

REMARK 6.1. Suppose that $A(t)$ process jumps only at time $1^-, 2^-$ and $A(t)$ is a dichotomous $(0,1)$ variable. Let $Y_{ij} = (Y_{ij}(1), Y_{ij}(2))$ be $Y_{\overline{a}=(i,j)}$ [i.e., $\overline{Y}_{\overline{a}=(a(1^-),a(2^-))}$ with $a(1^-) = i$ and $a(2^-) = j$]. Suppose, in violation of Assumption A, that $Y_{01}(2) = Y_{11}(2)$ with probability 1. That is, $a(1^-)$ has no direct effect on Y at time 2 when $a(2^-)$ is set to 1. Further suppose: $Y_{0j}(1) = Y_{i0}(2) = 0$ with probability 1 for all i and j. That is, Y is zero at time 1 or 2 if one receives treatment level 0 at times 1^- or 2^-, respectively. For notational convenience, write $A(1^-)$ and $A(2^-)$ as A_1 and A_2 respectively. Finally assume $Y_{10}(1)$ and $Y_{01}(2)$ are highly correlated and that

$$pr[A_1 = 1, A_2 = 0 \mid \{Y_{ij}; i, j = 1, 2\}] = \frac{1}{8} + \left(\frac{1}{8}\right) Y_{10}(1) \tag{6.8a}$$

$$pr[A_1 = 0, A_2 = 1 \mid \{Y_{ij}; i, j = 1, 2\}] = \frac{1}{8} + \left(\frac{1}{8}\right) Y_{01}(2) \tag{6.8b}$$

and

$$pr\big[A_1 = 1, A_2 = 1 \mid \{Y_{ij}; i, j = 1, 2\}\big] = \frac{3}{4} - \frac{1}{8} Y_{10}(1) - \frac{1}{8} Y_{01}(2) \ . \tag{6.8c}$$

Now, by (6.2), $Y_{10}(1) = Y_{11}(1)$ w.p.1 and, by assumption, $Y_{01}(2) = Y_{11}(2)$. Thus one can substitute Y_{11} for Y_{10} and Y_{01} in (6.8c) and check that the data are CAR. However, we now show that $pr[A_1 = 0 \mid Y_{10}(1)] \neq pr[A_1 = 0]$ in violation of (6.4). Specifically, $pr[A_1 = 0 \mid Y_{01}(2)]$ depends on $Y_{01}(2)$ by (6.8b). Furthermore, $pr[A_1 = 0 \mid Y_{10}(1)] = pr[A_1 = 0, A_2 = 1 \mid Y_{10}(1)] = 1/8 + (1/8) E[Y_{01}(2) \mid Y_{10}(1)]$ which depends, by the correlation assumption, on $Y_{10}(1)$.

This example was derived as follows. There are underlying dichotomous variables $Y^{(1)}, Y^{(2)}$. Furthermore, $Y_{10}(1) \equiv Y_{11}(1) \equiv Y^{(1)}$ and $Y_{01}(2) \equiv Y_{11}(2) \equiv Y^{(2)}$. Also $Y_{0i}(1) = Y_{i0}(2) = 0$ for $i \in \{1,2\}$. We observe $(A(1^-), A(1^-) Y^{(1)}, A(2^-), A(2^-) Y^{(2)})$ with the CAR probabilities given above. Under the CAR assumption, Gill, van der Laan, and Robins (1997) show that the joint distribution of $\{Y_{ij}; i,j = 1,2\}$ is identified but not by the g-computation algorithm formula.

REMARK 6.2. Assumptions concerning the joint distribution of $(\overline{L}_{\overline{a}_1}, \overline{L}_{\overline{a}_2})$ given $\overline{L}_{\overline{a}_1}(u_{\overline{1}2})$ plus the assumption that the data are CAR place no restriction on the joint distribution of the observed data O. However, as the above example shows, such assumptions may be sufficient to rule out sequential randomization. Indeed, in the example of Remark 6.1, the assumption that $Y_{01}(2) = Y_{11}(2)$ w.p.1 alone is sufficient to rule out the sequential randomization assumption, since the two assumptions together imply the restriction on the joint distribution of the observed data that $\Omega(j) \equiv \int E[Y(2) \mid A_1 = j, A_2 = 1, Y(1)]\, dF[Y(1) \mid A_1 = j]$ is not a function of j. However, assuming both CAR and that Assumption A is violated is not sufficient to conclude that sequential randomization is false. To see this, consider the example of Remark 6.1 but assume that the probability of the event $A_1 = A_2 = 1$ was zero. Then it is easy to check that CAR is equivalent to sequential randomization even though Assumption A is assumed false.

REMARK 6.3. The example of Remark 6.1 can be viewed as a discrete-time version of interval censored data in which we assume there is an underlying failure time variable T and we define $Y^{(1)} = I(T \leq 1), Y^{(2)} = I(T \leq 2)$ and $A_j = 1$ if a subject was monitored at time j. On the other hand, when the probability of the event $A_1 = A_2 = 1$ is zero, we can view the example as a discrete-time version of current status data in which each subject is monitored only once. We can then conclude from our previous discussion that if we wish to estimate the distribution of our failure time random variable T under the sole assumption that the data are CAR, the distribution of T can be obtained using the g-computation algorithm formula in the case of current status data but cannot be so obtained in the case of interval censored data. This fact underlies the observation that the efficient score for estimating functionals of the distribution of T has an elegant closed form martingale representation in the case of current status data but not in the case of interval censored data (van der Laan and Robins, 1998).

We now consider identification of the law of $Y_{\overline{a}}$ when (6.4) is false due to confounding by unmeasured factors.

6.2. Identification with unmeasured confounders. Suppose the A-process jumps only at fixed times $0, 1, 2, \ldots, K$ and the L-process jumps only at times $0^-, 1^-, \ldots, K+1^-$. Write, for notational convenience, $A_k = A(k)$ and $L_k = L(k^-)$. $\overline{A}_k \equiv (A_0, \ldots, A_k) \underline{Y}_{\overline{a},k} = (Y_{\overline{a},k}, Y_{\overline{a},k+1}, \ldots, Y_{\overline{a},K+1})$. We then have the following theorem.

THEOREM 6.1. *Suppose that A_k is discrete and*

$$f_{A_k}\left[a_k \mid \overline{A}_{k-1} = \overline{a}_{k-1}, \overline{L}_k\right] > 0 \text{ w.p.1} \tag{6.9}$$

for all $\overline{a}_k \in \overline{\mathcal{A}}_k, k = 0, \ldots, K$. Then, the semiparametric model **b** *for $\left(\overline{A}, \left\{\overline{L}_a; \overline{a} \in \overline{\mathcal{A}}\right\}\right)$ characterized by the sole restriction*

$$\begin{aligned} &f_{A_k}\left[a_k \mid \overline{A}_{k-1} = \overline{a}_{k-1}, \overline{L}_k, \underline{Y}_{\overline{a},k+1}\right] \\ &\quad = 1 - \Phi\left[h_k\left(\overline{L}_k, \overline{a}\right) + q_k\left(\overline{L}_k, \underline{Y}_{\overline{a},k+1}, \overline{a}\right)\right] \end{aligned} \tag{6.10}$$

with (i) $\Phi(x)$ a known continuous, monotone increasing, distribution function, (ii) $q_k\left(\overline{\ell}_k, \underline{y}_{k+1}, \overline{a}\right)$ a known function, and (iii) $h_k\left(\overline{\ell}_k, \overline{a}\right)$ unknown is a non-parametric model for the law F_O of $O = \left(\overline{A}(\tau), \overline{L}(\tau)\right)$ and the distributions $B_m\left(\underline{y}_{m+1}, \overline{a}\right) \equiv b_m\left(\underline{y}_{m+1}, \overline{L}_m, \overline{a}\right) \equiv f_{\underline{Y}_{\overline{a},m+1}}\left(\underline{y}_{m+1} \mid \overline{L}_m, \overline{A}_m = \overline{a}_m\right)$, $B^*_m\left(\underline{y}_{m+1}, \overline{a}\right) \equiv b^*_m\left(\underline{y}_{m+1}, \overline{L}_m, \overline{a}\right) \equiv f_{\underline{Y}_{\overline{a},m+1}}\left(\underline{y}_{m+1} \mid \overline{L}_m, \overline{A}_m = \overline{a}_{m-1}\right)$, and $f_{\overline{Y}_{\overline{a}}}(y)$ and the functions $h_k\left(\overline{L}_k, \overline{a}\right)$ are identified from data on O. Specifically, suppress the dependence on $\overline{a}$ in the notation and write, for a given $\overline{a}$, $h_k\left(\overline{\ell}_k\right) \equiv h_k\left(\overline{\ell}_k, \overline{a}\right), q_k\left(\overline{\ell}_k, \underline{y}_{k+1}\right) \equiv q_k\left(\overline{\ell}_k, \underline{y}_{k+1}, \overline{a}\right)$, etc., and define C to be the minimum of $K+1$ and the first time for which $A_k \neq a_k$. Write $\Delta = I\left(C = K+1\right)$. Then, with Λ_k defined as in (3.5), $h_m\left(\overline{L}_m\right)$ is the unique solution to (3.7a) and $F_{\overline{Y}_{\overline{a}}}(y)$ and $F_{\underline{Y}_{\overline{a},m+1}}\left(\underline{y}_{m+1} \mid \overline{L}_m, \overline{A}_{m-1} = \overline{a}_{m-1}\right)$, $F_{\underline{Y}_{\overline{a},m+1}}\left(\underline{y}_{m+1} \mid \overline{L}_m, \overline{A}_m = \overline{a}_m\right)$ are given by the RHS of (3.7b), (3.7c), and (3.7d) respectively. Further, $f_{\underline{Y}_{\overline{a},k+1}}\left(\underline{y}_{k+1} \mid \overline{\ell}_k, \overline{A}_k = \overline{a}_k\right)$ is given by the selection bias g-computation algorithm formula [i.e., the RHS of (5.2)] with $j(\cdot,\cdot)$ given by (5.3). In particular, if $\Phi(x)$ is logistic, $j(\cdot,\cdot)$ is given by (5.5). Note this implies that

$$c_k(\overline{L}_k) \equiv \int f_{\underline{Y}_{\overline{a},k+1}}(\underline{y}_{k+1} \mid \overline{L}_k, \overline{A}_k = \overline{a}_k) \exp[-q_k(\overline{L}_k, \underline{y}_{k+1})] d\mu(\underline{y}_{k+1}) . \tag{6.11}$$

REMARK 6.4. Although we do not give the proof of Theorem 6.1, we do here address an important issue. Although true, it is not obvious that given any F_O, there exists a law for $\left(\overline{A}, \left\{\overline{L}_{\overline{a}}; \overline{a} \in \overline{\mathcal{A}}\right\}\right)$ satisfying (6.10). We take the simplest possible setting to make clear why indeed there is such a law. The general setting follows by arguing recursively. Consider the case where $K=0$, $L_1=Y_1$, and $L_0=\emptyset$ and define $A=A_0$ and $Y=Y_1$. Then (6.10) says

$$f_A\left[a\mid Y_a\right]=1-\Phi\left[h\left(a\right)+q\left(Y_a,a\right)\right]$$

which, by Bayes' Theorem, is equivalent to

$$\text{(6.12a)}\quad \begin{aligned} f_{Y_a}\left(y\mid A\neq a\right)=f_{Y_a}\left(y\mid A=a\right)\left\{pr\left(A\neq a\right)/pr\left(A=a\right)\right\}\\ \left\{\left[1-\Phi\left(h\left(a\right)+q\left(y,a\right)\right)\right]/\Phi\left(h\left(a\right)+q\left(y,a\right)\right)\right\}\end{aligned}$$

where $h\left(a\right)$ is the unique solution to

$$\text{(6.12b)}\quad \begin{aligned} &pr\left(A=a\right)/pr\left(A\neq a\right)=\\ &\int f_{Y_a}\left(y\mid A=a\right)\left\{\left[1-\Phi\left(h\left(a\right)+q\left(y,a\right)\right)\right]/\Phi\left(h\left(a\right)+q\left(y,a\right)\right)\right\}d\mu\left(y\right).\end{aligned}$$

Note, by Φ being a strictly increasing distribution function and assuming as we do throughout that the integral is finite, (6.12b) is guaranteed to have a unique solution $h\left(a\right)$. Since the RHS of (6.12a) thus only depends on the law F_O of the observed data and the known function $q\left(y,a\right)$, it is obvious that we can generate a joint distribution for $\left(A,\left\{Y_a;a\in\mathcal{A}\right\}\right)$ satisfying (6.12a).

7. Arbitrary continuous or discrete treatments.

7.1. Selection odds models for discrete or continuous treatments. We will generalize the selection odds model of Section 6 by allowing A_k to be discrete or continuous. Write $\Pi_k^*(\overline{a}_k)=\pi_k^*(\overline{L}_k,\overline{a}_k)=f_{A_k}(a_k\mid\overline{L}_k,\overline{A}_{k-1}=\overline{a}_{k-1})$ and $\Pi_k(\underline{y}_{k+1},\overline{a})\equiv\pi_k(\overline{L}_k,\underline{y}_{k+1},\overline{a})=f_{A_k}(a_k\mid\overline{L}_k,\overline{A}_{k-1}=\overline{a}_{k-1},\underline{Y}_{\overline{a},k+1}=\underline{y}_{k+1})$. Again define $B_k(\underline{y}_{k+1},\overline{a})\equiv b_k(\underline{y}_{k+1},\overline{L}_k,\overline{a})=f_{\underline{Y}_{\overline{a},k+1}}(\underline{y}_{k+1}\mid\overline{L}_k,\overline{A}_k=\overline{a}_k)$, $B_k^*(\underline{y}_{k+1},\overline{a})=b_k^*(\underline{y}_{k+1},\overline{L}_k,\overline{a})=f_{\underline{y}_{\overline{a},k+1}}(\underline{y}_{k+1}\mid\overline{L}_k,\overline{A}_{k-1}=\overline{a}_{k-1})$. Let $J_k(\underline{y}_{k+1},\overline{a})\equiv j_k(\overline{L}_k,\underline{y}_{k+1},\overline{a})\equiv\Pi_k^*(\overline{a}_k)/\Pi_k(\underline{y}_{k+1},\overline{a})=B_k^*(\underline{y}_{k+1},\overline{a})/B_k(\underline{y}_{k+1},\overline{a})$ where the last equality is by Bayes' theorem. Consider now the selection-bias g-computation algorithm formula identity

$$\text{(7.1a)}\quad \begin{aligned} b_k\left(\underline{y}_{k+1},\overline{\ell}_k,\overline{a}\right)&=\int\cdots\iint\prod_{m=k+1}^{K+1}f_{Y_m}\left[y_m\mid\overline{\ell}_{m-1},\overline{a}_{m-1}\right]dF\Big[v_m\mid\\ &\qquad y_m,\overline{\ell}_{m-1},\overline{a}_{m-1}\Big]\prod_{m=k+1}^{K}j_m\left(\overline{\ell}_m,\underline{y}_{m+1},\overline{a}\right)\\ &=\int\cdots\iint f\Big[\underline{y}_{k+1},\underline{v}_{k+1},\underline{a}_{k+1}\mid\\ &\qquad\overline{\ell}_k,\overline{a}_k\Big]\left\{\prod_{m=k+1}^{K}\pi_m\left(\overline{\ell}_m,\underline{y}_{m+1},\overline{a}\right)\right\}^{-1}\prod_{m=k+1}^{K+1}d\mu\left(v_m\right)\end{aligned}$$

and

$$b_k^*\left(\underline{y}_{k+1},\overline{\ell}_k,\overline{a}\right)=\int\cdots\iint\prod_{m=k+1}^{K+1}f_{Y_m}\left[y_m\mid\overline{\ell}_{m-1},\overline{a}_{m-1}\right]dF\left[v_m\mid y_m,\overline{\ell}_{m-1},\overline{a}_{m-1}\right]\prod_{m=k}^{K}j_m\left(\overline{\ell}_m,\underline{y}_{m+1},\overline{a}\right)$$

$$(7.1b)\qquad =\int\cdots\iint f\left[\underline{y}_{k+1},\underline{v}_{k+1},\underline{a}_{k+1}\mid\overline{\ell}_k,\overline{a}_k\right]\left\{\prod_{m=k}^{K}\pi_m\left(\overline{\ell}_m,\underline{y}_{m+1},\overline{a}\right)\right\}^{-1}\pi_k^*\left(\overline{\ell}_k,\overline{a}_k\right)\prod_{m=k+1}^{K+1}d\mu\left(v_m\right).$$

It follows from (7.1a) that to make $b_k\left(\underline{y}_{k+1},\overline{\ell}_k,\overline{a}\right)$ identifiable from data on O, we need to make the $j_k\left(\overline{\ell}_k,\underline{y}_{k+1},\overline{a}\right)$ or equivalently the $\pi_k\left(\overline{\ell}_k,\underline{y}_{k+1},\overline{a}\right)$ identifiable. One approach to doing so is given in the following lemma.

LEMMA 7.1. *Consider the semiparametric selection odds model for the distribution of* $\left(\overline{A},\left\{\overline{L}_{\overline{a}};\overline{a}\in\overline{\mathcal{A}}\right\}\right)$ *that imposes the sole restriction that*

$$(7.2)\qquad f_{\underline{Y}_{\overline{a},k+1}}\left(\underline{y}_{k+1}\mid\overline{L}_k,A_k\neq a_k,\overline{A}_{k-1}=\overline{a}_{k-1}\right)=\mathcal{C}_k\left(\overline{a}\right)B_k\left(\underline{y}_{k+1},\overline{a}\right)Q_k^*\left(\underline{y}_{k+1},\overline{a}\right)$$

where (i) $Q_k^*\left(\underline{y}_{k+1},\overline{a}\right)\equiv q_k^*\left(\overline{L}_k,\underline{y}_{k+1},\overline{a}\right)$ *is a known non-negative function, and (ii)* $\mathcal{C}_k\left(\overline{a}\right)=c_k\left(\overline{L}_k,\overline{a}\right)$ *is a normalizing constant chosen to make the LHS of (7.2) a density. Then, if (6.9) holds, the* $\mathcal{C}_k\left(\overline{a}\right)$ *and the* $J_k\left(\underline{y}_{k+1},\overline{a}\right)$ *are identified.*

In particular, it follows immediately from its definition that

$$(7.3a)\qquad J_k\left(\underline{y}_{k+1},\overline{a}\right)=\Pi_k^*\left(\overline{a}_k\right)+\left\{1-\Pi_k^*\left(\overline{a}_k\right)\right\}Q_k^*\left(\underline{y}_{k+1},\overline{a}\right)\left\{\mathcal{C}_k\left(\overline{a}\right)\right\}^{-1}$$

if

$$(7.3b)\qquad pr\left[A_k=a_k\mid\overline{L}_k,\overline{A}_{k-1}=\overline{a}_{k-1}\right]\neq0,$$

and

$$(7.3c)\qquad J_k\left(\underline{y}_{k+1},\overline{a}\right)=Q_k^*\left(\underline{y}_{k+1},\overline{a}\right)\left\{\mathcal{C}_k\left(\overline{a}\right)\right\}^{-1},\quad\textit{otherwise}.$$

[For example, if A_k is continuous and was measured at each occasion k, we would expect (7.3b) to be false and $f_{a_k}\left(a_k\mid\overline{L}_k,\overline{A}_{k-1}=\overline{a}_{k-1}\right)$ to be a density with respect to Lesbesgue measure.] Then all necessary quantities can be calculated from the distribution of the observed data O by the following backward recursion. First, $B_K\left(\underline{y}_{K+1},\overline{a}\right)=f_{\underline{Y}_{K+1}}\left(\underline{y}_{K+1}\mid\overline{L}_K,\overline{A}_K=\right.$

$\overline{a}_K)$. Then, given $B_k\left(\underline{y}_{k+1}, \overline{a}\right)$, we can calculate $C_k\left(\overline{a}\right)$, $J_k\left(\underline{y}_{k+1}, \overline{a}\right)$, and $B_{k-1}\left(\underline{y}_k, \overline{a}\right)$ as follows. By its definition as a normalizing constant, we calculate $C_k\left(\overline{a}\right) = \int B_k\left(\underline{y}_{k+1}, \overline{a}\right) Q_k^*\left(\underline{y}_{k+1}, \overline{a}\right) d\mu\left(\underline{y}_{k+1}\right)$. We then calculate $J_k\left(\underline{y}_{k+1}, \overline{a}\right)$ by (7.3a)–(7.3c). Finally, we calculate $B_{k-1}\left(\underline{y}_k, \overline{a}\right)$ from (7.1).

REMARK 7.1. If $Q_k^*\left(\underline{y}_{k+1}, \overline{a}\right)$ does not depend on $\underline{y}_{k+1}$ so that (5.4) holds, then the $j_k\left(\overline{\ell}_k, \underline{y}_{k+1}, \overline{a}\right)$ are all identically 1 and (7.1) reduces to the usual g-computation algorithm formula.

REMARK 7.2. A selection odds model is a non-parametric model for F_O in the sense that even though $Q_k^*\left(\underline{y}_{k+1}, \overline{a}\right)$ is a known function, the model is compatible with any law F_O of O since the restriction (7.2) is not identifiable from data O. It is interesting to note that if there is selection bias due to unmeasured confounding (i.e., $Q_k^*\left(\underline{y}_{k+1}, \overline{a}\right)$ depends on $\underline{y}_{k+1}$), then the conditional densities $b_k\left(\underline{y}_{k+1}, \overline{\ell}_k, \overline{a}\right)$ of the counterfactuals do not depend on the densities of the treatment process $f\left(a_k \mid \overline{\ell}_k, \overline{a}_{k-1}\right)$ if and only if (7.3b) is false with probability 1 for each $\overline{a}_k$.

REMARK 7.3. We can restate restriction (7.2) in a manner closely related to (6.10). Indeed, its correspondence is exact when (7.3b) is true w.p.1. Specifically, the NPI model defined by restriction (7.2) is equivalent to the following NPI model:

(i) If (7.3b) is true,

$$\pi_k\left(\overline{L}_k, \underline{y}_{k+1}, \overline{a}\right) = 1 - expit\left[h_k\left(\overline{L}_k, \overline{a}\right) + q_k\left(\overline{L}_k, \underline{y}_{k+1}, \overline{a}\right)\right] \tag{7.4}$$

with $h_k(\cdot,\cdot)$ unrestricted and $q_k(\cdot,\cdot,\cdot)$ known. Specifically, the models are related by

$$h_k\left(\overline{L}_k, \overline{a}\right) = \ln\left[\left\{\Pi_k^*\left(\overline{a}_k\right)\right\}^{-1}\left\{1 - \Pi_k^*\left(\overline{a}_k\right)\right\} C_k\left(\overline{a}\right)^{-1}\right] \tag{7.5}$$

and

$$q_k\left(\overline{L}_k, \underline{y}_{k+1}, \overline{a}\right) = \ln Q_k^*\left(\underline{y}_{k+1}, \overline{a}\right) . \tag{7.6}$$

(ii) If (7.3b) is false,

$$\Pi_k\left(\underline{y}_{k+1}, \overline{a}\right) = \exp\left[-\left\{h_k\left(\overline{L}_k, \overline{a}\right) + q_k\left(\overline{L}_k, \underline{y}_{k+1}, \overline{a}\right)\right\}\right] \tag{7.7}$$

with $h_k(\cdot,\cdot)$ unrestricted and $q_k(\cdot,\cdot,\cdot)$ known. Specifically, the models are related by $q_k\left(\overline{L}_k, \underline{y}_{k+1}, \overline{a}\right)$ being given by (7.6) and

$$h_k\left(\overline{L}_k, \overline{a}\right) = -\ln\left[\Pi_k^*\left(\overline{a}_k\right) C_k\left(\overline{a}\right)\right] . \tag{7.8}$$

Furthermore, whether or not (7.3b) is true, the $h_k\left(\overline{\ell}_k, \overline{a}\right)$ and thus the $\pi_k\left(\overline{\ell}_k, \underline{y}_{k+1}, \overline{a}\right)$ are identified from the law F_O of O and the known function $q_k^*\left(\overline{\ell}_k, \underline{y}_{k+1}, \overline{a}\right)$ as the unique solution to the identity

$$E_O\left[w_k\left(\underline{A}_k\right) / \prod_{m=k}^{K} \pi_m\left(\overline{L}_m, \underline{Y}_{m+1}, \overline{A}\right) \mid \overline{L}_k=\overline{\ell}_k, \overline{A}_{k-1}=\overline{a}_{k-1}\right] = \int w_k\left(\underline{a}_k\right) d\mu\left(\underline{a}_k\right) \tag{7.9}$$

for all functions $w_k\left(\underline{a}_k\right), k=K, K-1, \ldots, 0$. Specifically, we proceed recursively and first identify $h_K\left(\overline{L}_K, \overline{a}\right)$ by (7.9) with $k=K$. We then identify $h_{K-1}\left(\overline{L}_{K-1}, \overline{a}\right)$ by (7.9) with $k=K-1$, etc.

Proof. That (7.9) is true follows from the fact that by (7.1b), (7.9) equals $\int\left\{\int b_k^*\left(\underline{y}_{k+1}, \overline{\ell}_k, \underline{a}\right) d\mu\left(\underline{y}_{k+1}\right)\right\} w_k\left(\underline{a}_k\right) d\mu\left(\underline{a}_k\right)=\int w_k\left(\underline{a}_k\right) d\mu\left(\underline{a}_k\right)$. Finally it is straightforward to show that the solution $h_k\left(\overline{\ell}_k, \overline{a}\right)$ must be unique. □

By a similar argument, given the $\pi_k\left(\overline{\ell}_k, \underline{y}_{k+1}, \overline{a}\right)$, the $b_k\left(\underline{y}_{k+1}, \overline{\ell}_k, \overline{a}\right)$ are the unique solutions to the identity

$$E_O\left[w\left(\underline{Y}_{k+1}, \underline{A}_{k+1}\right) / \prod_{m=k+1}^{K} \Pi_m\left(\underline{Y}_{m+1}, \overline{A}\right) \mid \overline{L}_k=\overline{\ell}_k, \overline{A}_k=\overline{a}_k\right] = \int w_k\left(\underline{y}_{k+1}, \underline{a}_{k+1}\right) b_k\left(\underline{y}_{k+1}, \overline{\ell}_k, \overline{a}\right) d\mu\left(\underline{a}_{k+1}\right) d\mu\left(\underline{y}_{k+1}\right) \tag{7.10}$$

for all functions $w\left(\underline{y}_{k+1}, \underline{a}_{k+1}\right)$. We thus have the following theorem, which is almost a perfect analog of Theorem 3.2.

THEOREM 7.1. *The semiparametric model* **b** *for* $\left(\overline{a},\left\{\overline{L}_a ; \overline{a} \in \overline{\mathcal{A}}\right\}\right)$ *characterized by the sole restrictions (7.4) and (7.7) with the* $q_k(\cdot, \cdot, \cdot)$ *known functions and the* $h_k(\cdot, \cdot)$ *completely unknown, is a non-parametric model for the law* F_O *for the observed data* $O=(\overline{A}(C), \overline{L}(C))$. *Furthermore, if (6.9) holds, the* $h_k\left(\overline{\ell}_k, \overline{a}\right)$ *and* $b_k\left(\underline{y}_{k+1}, \overline{\ell}_k, \overline{a}\right)$ *are identified from the law of* O *as the unique solutions to (7.9) and (7.10). Further, the unique solution to (7.10) is Eq. (7.1a) with* $j_k\left(\overline{\ell}_k, \underline{y}_{k+1}, \overline{a}\right)$ *given by (7.3).*

7.2. Difficulty with semiparametric inference selection odds models in high-dimensional problems.

7.2.1. Difficulty with modeling $h_k(\cdot, \cdot)$.

When the covariates L_k are high-dimensional with continuous components, we might hope, as in Sec. 4, to respond to the curse of dimensionality by modeling the functions $h_k\left(\overline{\ell}_k, \overline{a}\right)$ in the representation (7.4) or (7.7) of our NPI selection odds model. Unfortunately, this approach fails.

To see why, consider the simplest setting where $K=0$, $Y_1=L_1$ and A_0 are dichotomous $(0,1)$ variables. Write $Y \equiv Y_1, L=L_0, A=A_0$. Then our NPI selection odds model defined by restriction (7.4) can be written for $a \in\{0,1\}$

$$pr\left[A=a \mid L, Y_a=y\right]=\pi(L, y, a)=1-expit[h(L, a)+q(L, y, a)] \tag{7.11}$$

$$q(L, y, a) \text{ known} \tag{7.12}$$

and $h(L,a)$ completely unrestricted. Now suppose L is high-dimensional with continuous components. Suppose that the contrast $E(Y_1) - E(Y_0)$ is the parameter of interest. We might hope, in analogy with our approach in Sec. 4, to estimate our contrast of interest using semiparametric augmented inverse probability of treatment weighted estimators as follows. First, in analogy to Eq. (4.1), we impose the additional restriction that the function $h(\ell,a)$ lies in a parametric family, i.e., for $a \in \{0,1\}$

$$h(\ell,a) = h(\ell,a;\gamma_a^*) \tag{7.13}$$

where $h(\cdot,\cdot,\cdot)$ is a known function and γ_0^* and γ_1^* are unknown parameter vectors to be estimated. Then, by Eq. (7.9), for $a \in \{0,1\}$, we estimate γ_a^* by $\widehat{\gamma}_a^*$ satisfying

$$0 = n^{-1} \sum_i \{I(A_i = a)/\pi(L_i, Y_i, a; \widehat{\gamma}_a) - 1\} w(a, L_i) \tag{7.14}$$

where $w(a,L_i)$ is a user-supplied vector function of the dimension of γ_a and $\pi(\ell,y,a;\widehat{\gamma}_a)$ is defined as in Eq. (7.11) with $h(\ell,a;\widehat{\gamma}_a)$ replacing $h(\ell,a)$. We then estimate $E(Y_a)$ by

$$\widehat{E}(Y_a) = n^{-1} \sum_i I(A_i = a) Y_i / \pi(L_i, Y_i, a; \widehat{\gamma}_a) \ . \tag{7.15}$$

The difficulty with this approach is that in general there will exist no joint distribution for (Y_1, Y_0, A, L) compatible with our estimates

$$\left(\widehat{E}(Y_1), \widehat{E}(Y_0), \widehat{\gamma}_0, \widehat{\gamma}_1\right) \ . \tag{7.16}$$

This is because $pr[A = 0 \mid L]$ is separately identifiable from data on L_i, A_i, $A_i Y_i$, $i = 1, \ldots, n$ and also identifiable from the data L_i, A_i, $(1 - A_i) Y_i$, $i = 1, \ldots, n$.

Specifically, in order that there exists a joint distribution, say $\widehat{F}$ for (Y_1, Y_0, A, L) compatible with our estimate Eq. (7.16), requires that there exist densities $\widehat{F}_{Y_a}(1 \mid \ell) \equiv \widehat{F}_{Y|A,L}(y \mid \ell, a)$ and $\widehat{f}(\ell)$ such that

$$\widehat{E}(Y_a) = \int \widehat{f}_{Y_a}(1 \mid \ell)\, d\widehat{F}(\ell), a \in \{0,1\} \tag{7.17}$$

for which the following two equations are equal with probability one.

$$\widehat{pr}[A = 0 \mid L] = \sum_{y=0}^{1} \pi(L, y, 0; \widehat{\gamma}_0) \widehat{f}_{Y_0}(y \mid L) \tag{7.18}$$

and

$$\widehat{pr}[A=0 \mid L] = 1 - \widehat{pr}[A=1 \mid L] = 1 - \sum_{y=0}^{1} \pi(L, y, 1; \widehat{\gamma}_1) \widehat{f}_{Y_1}(y \mid L) \ . \tag{7.19}$$

In general, there will not exist any joint law satisfying (7.17) and having (7.18) and (7.19) equal for all L.

There are several possible philosophical and/or practical views we might take of this inconvenient fact.

1. View the models $\{h(\ell, a; \gamma_a)\}$ as a "sieve" in which we allow the dimension of γ_a to increase with sample size n such that, as $n \to \infty$, the model becomes dense in all functions $h(\ell, a)$. We then content ourselves with the notion that as $n \to \infty$, our incompatibility problem disappears, since we know that if $h(\ell, a)$ unrestricted, our selection odds model is a non-parametric model for the law of the observed data $O = (Y, L, A)$. We simply accept that, with any finite sample size, we have an incompatible model. One could argue that this approach is related to similar approaches taken in other parts of statistics. For example, the Dabrowska estimator (Dabrowska, 1988) of a bivariate survival function for independently right-censored data is not a true survival function at sample size n, although, as $n \to \infty$, it converges to a survival function. Similarly, Edgeworth or higher order kernel approximations to densities are not densities for any fixed sample size n, since for certain values of x they may be negative. Nonetheless, for each fixed x, they become positive as $n \to \infty$.
2. A second approach is that we could try to modify our estimates (7.16) by replacing them with new estimates based on those obtained from the closest (in some metric) joint distribution for (Y_1, Y_0, L, A).

This second option we do not know how to implement. The first option seems quite unsatisfactory, especially as we do not even know how to pick a model for $h(\ell, a)$ so that we are even close to a joint distribution at finite sample sizes.

7.2.2. Difficulty with modeling $C_k(\overline{a})$. An alternative approach would be to still use the augmented inverse probability of treatment weighted estimators (7.14)–(7.15) to obtain the estimates (7.16), except that we now model directly the $C_k(\overline{a}) = c_k(\overline{L}_k, \overline{a})$ and the $\Pi^*(\overline{a}_k)$ rather than the $h_k(\overline{L}_k, \overline{a})$. We then estimate the $h_k(\overline{L}_k, \overline{a})$ using the identity (7.5). To fix ideas, again consider our simple model with $O = (A, L, Y)$ used in the previous subsection. Then it is unproblematic to specify and fit a parametric model $\pi(L, a; \eta)$ for $\Pi^*(a) \equiv \pi^*(L, a) \equiv pr[A = a \mid L]$ by maximizing $\prod_{i=1}^{n} \pi^*(L_i, A_i; \eta)$ with respect to η. We also specify a parametric model

$$c(L, a) = c(L, a; \gamma_a^*) \tag{7.20}$$

for $c(L, a)$. We then precede as in the last subsection, where now $\pi(\ell, y, a; \widehat{\gamma}_a)$ is again as defined in Eq. (7.11) but with $h(\ell, a; \widehat{\gamma}_a, \widehat{\eta})$ [via (7.5)] replacing $h(\ell, a)$ and $\widehat{\eta}$ suppressed in the notation. As argued in the last subsection, in general, then there will exist no joint law for (Y_1, Y_0, A, L) consistent with the estimators (7.16) and $\widehat{\eta}$.

Thus, in general, our attempt to use augmented inverse probability of treatment weighted estimators to estimate our selection odds model has failed. There are two options. Either we keep the selection odds model but change our estimation procedure or we replace the selection odds model with another NPI model which allows a simple semiparametric inverse probability of treatment weighted estimator while avoiding incompatible models.

We shall consider both approaches in Sec. 8.

8. Sensitivity analysis for multivariate structural models. In this section, we discuss sensitivity analysis for both multivariate structural nested models and multivariate marginal structural models. In Sections 8.1–8.4, we consider structural nested models.

8.1. Structural nested models.

8.1.1. Structural nested distribution models (SNDMs). In this section, we suppose the outcome $\underline{Y}_m = (Y_m, \ldots, Y_{K+1})$ has a continuous multivariate distribution given $\overline{L}_{m-1}, \overline{A}_{m-1}$ with probability 1. Then we can do a sensitivity analysis based on g-estimation of multivariate structural nested distribution models. The foundations of this analysis are again formed by a class of non-parametric (just) identified (NPI) models which we shall call SNDMs.

Given a history $\overline{a}$, the history $(\overline{a}_m, 0)$ is the history $\overline{a}^*$ that agrees with $\overline{a}$ through time m and is zero thereafter, where zero is the baseline level of treatment. Following Robins et al. (1992, Appendix 2), we define the multivariate blip-down functions $\gamma_m(\underline{y}_{m+1}, \overline{\ell}_m, \overline{a}_m) = [\gamma_{m,m+1}(\underline{y}_{m+1}, \overline{\ell}_m, \overline{a}_m), \ldots, \gamma_{m,K+1}(\underline{y}_{m+1}, \overline{\ell}_m, \overline{a}_m)]$ as the unique solution to

$$\text{(8.1a)} \quad F_{\underline{Y}_{(\overline{a}_{m-1},0),m+1}|\overline{\ell}_m,\overline{a}_m}[\gamma_m(\underline{y}_{m+1}, \overline{\ell}_m, \overline{a}_m)] = F_{\underline{Y}_{(\overline{a}_m,0),m+1}||\overline{\ell}_m,\overline{a}_m}(\underline{y}_{m+1})$$

satisfying

$$\text{(8.1b)} \qquad \gamma_{m,k}\left(\underline{y}_{m+1}, \overline{\ell}_m, \overline{a}_m\right) \textit{ is a function of } \overline{y}_{K+1} \textit{ only through } \overline{y}_k$$

for $m = 0, \ldots, K$. To be specific, define $z^{m:k} = (z_m, \ldots, z_k)$. Then

$$\gamma_{m,m+1}\left(\underline{y}_{m+1}, \overline{\ell}_m, \overline{a}_m\right) = F^{-1}_{Y_{(\overline{a}_{m-1},0),m+1}|\overline{\ell}_m,\overline{a}_m} \circ F_{Y_{(\overline{a}_m,0),m+1}|\overline{\ell}_m,\overline{a}_m}(y_{m+1}),$$

and

$$\gamma_{m,k}\left(\underline{y}_{m+1}, \overline{\ell}_m, \overline{a}_m\right) = F^{-1}_{Y_{(\overline{a}_{m-1},0),k}|\overline{\ell}_m,\overline{a}_m, Y^{m+1:k-1}_{(\overline{a}_{m-1},0)} = \gamma^{m+1:k-1}_m\left(\underline{y}_{m+1},\overline{\ell}_m,\overline{a}_m\right)} \circ$$
$$\times F_{Y_{(\overline{a}_m,0),k}|\overline{\ell}_m,\overline{a}_m, Y^{m+1:k-1}_{(\overline{a}_m,0)} = (y_{m+1},\ldots,y_{k-1})}(y_k).$$

Many functions satisfy (8.1a). The restriction (8.1b) picks out a particular multivariate quantile-quantile function. Any alternative to (8.1b) that picked out a unique solution to (8.1a) would also serve for our purposes. Next recursively define, for $m = K-1, ..., 0$,

$$u_m\left(\overline{y}_{K+1}, \overline{\ell}_K, \overline{a}_K\right) = \gamma_m\left[\left\{y_{m+1}, u_{m+1}\left(\overline{y}_{K+1}, \overline{\ell}_K, \overline{a}_K\right)\right\}, \overline{\ell}_m, \overline{a}_m\right] \tag{8.2}$$

with $u_K\left(\overline{y}_{K+1}, \overline{\ell}_K, \overline{a}_K\right) \equiv \gamma_K\left(\underline{y}_{K+1}, \overline{\ell}_K, \overline{a}_K\right)$. Define

$$U_m = u_m\left(\overline{Y}_{K+1}, \overline{L}_K, \overline{A}_K\right).$$

Note U_m is a random vector of the same dimension as $\underline{Y}_{m+1}$.

The following theorem can be proved analogously to the proof of Theorem A1.1 in Robins (1993, Appendix 1).

THEOREM 8.1. $pr\left[U_m > \underline{y}_{m+1} \mid \overline{\ell}_m, \overline{a}_m\right] = pr\left[\underline{Y}_{(\overline{a}_{m-1},0),m+1} > \underline{y}_{m+1} \mid \overline{\ell}_m, \overline{a}_m\right]$.

We shall consider the model defined by the sole restriction that

$$\begin{aligned} f&\left[a_m \mid \overline{\ell}_m, \overline{a}_{m-1}, \underline{Y}_{(\overline{a}_{m-1},0),m+1} = \underline{y}_{m+1}\right] \\ &= \frac{t\left(a_m \mid \overline{\ell}_m, \overline{a}_{m-1}\right)\exp\left[q_m\left(\underline{y}_{m+1}, \overline{\ell}_m, \overline{a}_m\right)\right]}{\int t\left(a_m \mid \overline{\ell}_m, \overline{a}_{m-1}\right)\exp\left[q_m\left(\underline{y}_{m+1}, \overline{\ell}_m, \overline{a}_m\right)\right] d\mu\left(a_m\right)} \end{aligned} \tag{8.3a}$$

with

(8.3b) $q_m(\underline{y}_{m+1}, \overline{\ell}_m, \overline{a}_m)$ *known, satisfying* $q_m(\underline{y}_{m+1}, \overline{\ell}_m, \overline{a}_{m-1}, a_m{=}0){=}0$

and

(8.3c) $\quad t\left(a_m \mid \overline{\ell}_m, \overline{a}_{m-1}\right)$ *an unknown conditional density.*

The following theorem, proved in Appendix A, states that the SNDM model (8.3) is a NPI model.

THEOREM 8.2. *The model characterized by the sole restriction (8.3) on the law of* $\left(\overline{A}, \left\{\overline{L}_{\overline{a}}(K+1); \overline{a} \in \overline{\mathcal{A}}\right\}\right)$ *is a non-parametric model for the law of* $O = \left(\overline{L}_{K+1}, \overline{A}_K\right)$. *Furthermore, the functions* γ_m, *the density* $t(\cdot \mid \cdot, \cdot)$, *the law of* $\overline{Y}_{(0)}$, *and the conditional law* $\underline{Y}_{(\overline{A}_{m-1},0),m+1} \mid \overline{L}_m, \overline{A}_m$ *are all identified. Specifically, the identifying formulas are as follows. Let* γ_m^{-1} *be the inverse of the function* γ_m *with respect to the argument* $\underline{y}_{m+1}$. *Define* $U_m^* = (Y_m, U_m')'$; *note* U_m^* *is a vector of the dimension of* $\underline{Y}_m$. *Then by definition*

$$F_{U_{K+1}^* \mid \overline{L}_K, \overline{A}_K}\left(y_{K+1}\right) = F_{Y_{K+1} \mid \overline{L}_K, \overline{A}_K}\left(y_{K+1}\right).$$

We then have for $m = K, K-1, \ldots, 0$ *that* $\gamma_m^{-1}\left(\underline{y}_{m+1}, \overline{\ell}_m, \overline{a}_m\right)$ *is the unique solution to*

$$\text{(8.4a)} \quad F_{U_{m+1}^{*}|\overline{\ell}_m,\overline{a}_m}\left[\gamma_m^{-1}(\underline{y}_{m+1}, \overline{\ell}_m, \overline{a}_m)\right] = \tau(\underline{y}_{m+1}, \overline{\ell}_m, \overline{a}_m)/\tau(\infty, \overline{\ell}_m, \overline{a}_m)$$

satisfying

$$\text{(8.4b)} \qquad \gamma_{m,k}^{-1}\left(\underline{y}_{m+1}, \overline{\ell}_m, \overline{a}_m\right) \text{ depends on } \overline{y}_{K+1} \text{ only through } \overline{y}_k$$

where

$$\tau\left(\underline{y}_{m+1}, \overline{\ell}_m, \overline{a}_m\right) \equiv$$

$$\int_{-\infty}^{\underline{y}_{m+1}} f_{U_{m+1}^{*}|\overline{\ell}_m,\overline{a}_{m-1},a_m=0}\left(\underline{x}_{m+1}\right) \exp\left\{q_m\left(\underline{x}_{m+1}, \overline{\ell}_m, \overline{a}_m\right)\right\} d\underline{x}_{m+1} \ .$$

Furthermore,

$$\text{(8.5)} \quad \begin{aligned} & f_{U_m|\overline{\ell}_m,\overline{a}_{m-1}}\left(\underline{y}_{m+1}\right) \\ & = f_{U_{m+1}^{*}|\overline{\ell}_m,\overline{a}_{m-1},a_m=0}\left(\underline{y}_{m+1}\right) \int_{-\infty}^{\infty} f\left[a_m \mid \overline{\ell}_m, \overline{a}_{m-1}\right] \\ & \times \exp\left[q_m(\underline{y}_{m+1}, \overline{\ell}_m, \overline{a}_m)\right]\left\{\tau\left(\infty, \overline{\ell}_m, \overline{a}_m\right)\right\}^{-1} d\mu(a_m) \end{aligned}$$

$$\text{(8.6)} \quad t\left(a_m \mid \overline{\ell}_m, \overline{a}_{m-1}\right) = \frac{f\left(a_m \mid \overline{\ell}_m, \overline{a}_{m-1}\right) \tau\left(\infty, \overline{\ell}_m, \overline{a}_m\right)}{\int f\left(a_m \mid \overline{\ell}_m, \overline{a}_{m-1}\right) \tau\left(\infty, \overline{\ell}_m, \overline{a}_m\right) d\mu\left(a_m\right)}$$

$$f_{U_m^{*}|\overline{\ell}_{m-1},\overline{a}_{m-1}}\left(\underline{y}_{m+1}\right) =$$

$$\int f_{U_m|\overline{\ell}_m=(y_m,v_m,\overline{\ell}_{m-1}),\overline{a}_{m-1}}\left(\underline{y}_{m+1}\right) f\left(y_m, v_m \mid \overline{\ell}_{m-1}, \overline{a}_{m-1}\right) d\mu\left(v_m\right) \ .$$

REMARK 8.1. If we do not impose the equality restriction in (8.3b), Theorem (8.2) still holds provided we replace $q_m\left(\underline{y}_{m+1}, \overline{\ell}_m, \overline{a}_m\right)$ by $q_m\left(\underline{y}_{m+1}, \overline{\ell}_m, \overline{a}_m\right) - q_m\left(\underline{y}_{m+1}, \overline{\ell}_m, \overline{a}_{m-1}, a_m = 0\right)$.

Theorem 8.2 has the following dual which is proved in Appendix A.

THEOREM 8.3. *The model for the joint law of* $\left(\overline{A}, \left\{\overline{L}_{\overline{a}}(K+1); \overline{a} \in \overline{\mathcal{A}}\right\}\right)$ *characterized by the sole restriction that*

$$\text{(8.7)} \qquad \gamma_m\left(\underline{y}_{m+1}, \overline{\ell}_m, \overline{a}_m\right) \text{ is known for each } m$$

with $\gamma_m\left(\underline{y}_{m+1}, \overline{\ell}_m, \overline{a}_m\right)$ *defined as in (8.1) is a non-parametric model for the distribution of the observed data* $O = \left(\overline{L}_{K+1}, \overline{A}_K\right)$. *Furthermore,*

$f\left[a_m \mid \overline{\ell}_m, \overline{a}_{m-1}, \underline{Y}_{(\overline{a}_{m-1,0}),m+1} = \underline{y}_{m+1}\right]$ *is identified and given by Eq. (8.3a) with*

$$\exp\left[q_m\left(\underline{y}_{m+1}, \overline{\ell}_m, \overline{a}_m\right)\right] = \frac{f_{U_m \mid \overline{\ell}_m, \overline{a}_m}\left[\underline{y}_{m+1}\right] f_{U_m \mid \overline{\ell}_m, \overline{a}_{m-1}, a_m=0}\left(\underline{0}_{m+1}\right)}{f_{U_m \mid \overline{\ell}_m, \overline{a}_m}\left[\underline{0}_{m+1}\right] f_{U_m \mid \overline{\ell}_m, \overline{a}_{m-1}, a_m=0}\left(\underline{y}_{m+1}\right)} . \tag{8.8}$$

In addition, $t\left(a_m \mid \overline{\ell}_m, \overline{a}_{m-1}\right)$ *and the densities of* $U_m \mid \overline{\ell}_m, \overline{a}_{m-1}$ *and* $U_m^* \mid \overline{\ell}_{m-1}, \overline{a}_{m-1}$ *are identified recursively by Eqs. (8.5) and (8.6).*

8.1.2. Structural nested mean models (SNMMs). For SNMMs, we shall redefine $\gamma_m\left(\underline{y}_{m+1}, \overline{\ell}_m, \overline{a}_m\right)$ and U_m. Robins (1994, 1997b) has previously considered two types of SNMMs: multiplicative SNMMs and additive SNMMs. For an additive SNMM, define

$$\gamma_m^*\left(\overline{\ell}_m, \overline{a}_m\right) = E\left[\underline{Y}_{(\overline{a}_m,0),m+1} - \underline{Y}_{(\overline{a}_{m-1},0),m+1} \mid \overline{\ell}_m, \overline{a}_m\right] \tag{8.9a}$$

and

$$\gamma_m\left(\underline{y}_{m+1}, \overline{\ell}_m, \overline{a}_m\right) = \underline{y}_{m+1} - \gamma_m^*\left(\overline{\ell}_m, \overline{a}_m\right) . \tag{8.9b}$$

For a multiplicative SNMM, define

$$\gamma_m\left(\underline{y}_{m+1}, \overline{\ell}_m, \overline{a}_m\right)' = \left(\gamma_{m,m+1}\left(y_{m+1}, \overline{\ell}_m, \overline{a}_m\right), \ldots, \gamma_{m,K+1}\left(y_{K+1}, \overline{\ell}_m, \overline{a}_m\right)\right) \tag{8.10a}$$

where

$$\gamma_{m,k}\left(y_k, \overline{\ell}_m, \overline{a}_m\right) = y_k \exp\left[-\left\{\gamma_{m,k}^*\left(\overline{\ell}_m, \overline{a}_m\right)\right\}\right] \tag{8.10b}$$

and

$$\gamma_{m,k}^*(\overline{\ell}_m, \overline{a}_m) = \log\left\{E[Y_{(\overline{a}_m,0),k} \mid \overline{\ell}_m, \overline{a}_m] / E[Y_{(\overline{a}_{m-1},0),k} \mid \overline{\ell}_m, \overline{a}_m]\right\} . \tag{8.10c}$$

Now define $u_m, U_m = \left(U_{m,m+1}, \ldots, U_{m,K+1}\right)', U_m^*$ in terms of γ_m as above. Then we have for both additive and multiplicative SNMMs the following easily proved theorem.

THEOREM 8.4. *With* $\gamma_m\left(\underline{y}_{m+1}, \overline{\ell}_m, \overline{a}_m\right)$ *as defined in either (8.9) or (8.10),*

$$E\left[U_m \mid \overline{\ell}_m, \overline{a}_m\right] = E\left[\underline{Y}_{(\overline{a}_{m-1},0),m+1} \mid \overline{\ell}_m, \overline{a}_m\right] .$$

Next, consider the model defined by the sole restrictions that for $k = m+1, \ldots, K+1$ and $m = 0, \ldots, K$,

$$\text{(8.11a)} \quad E\left[Y_{(\overline{a}_{m-1},0),k} \mid \overline{\ell}_m, \overline{a}_m\right] = \Phi\left\{t\left(k, \overline{\ell}_m, \overline{a}_{m-1}\right) + q_m\left(k, \overline{\ell}_m, \overline{a}_m\right)\right\}$$

(8.11b) *with* $q_m(k, \overline{\ell}_m, \overline{a}_m)$ *known, satisfying* $q_m(k, \overline{\ell}_m, \overline{a}_{m-1}, a_m{=}0){=}0$,

(8.11c) $t\left(k, \overline{\ell}_m, \overline{a}_{m-1}\right)$ *an unknown function*

and

(8.11d) $\Phi(x)$ *a known one-to-one function.*

Note $\Phi(x)$ no longer needs to be a distribution function. The following theorem, whose proof is omitted, gives conditions under which our model in a NPI model.

THEOREM 8.5. *Under Consistency Assumption 1, the model characterized by the sole restriction (8.11) is a non-parametric model for the law of* $O = \left(\overline{L}_{K+1}, \overline{A}_K\right)$
(a) with $\Phi(x)$ *the identity, provided* $E\left[Y_{k+1} \mid \overline{\ell}_k, \overline{a}_k\right]$ *may take values anywhere in* $(-\infty, \infty)$*;*
(b) with $\Phi(x) = \exp(x)$*, provided* $E\left[Y_{k+1} \mid \overline{L}_k, \overline{A}_k\right]$ *can take values anywhere in* $(0, \infty)$*;*
(c) with $\Phi(x) = e^x / \{1 + e^x\}$ *if the* Y_k *are dichotomous* $(0,1)$ *variables.*

Further, the functions γ^*_m (defined by either (8.9) or (8.10)) and t as well as $E\left[\overline{Y}_{(0)}\right]$ and the conditional expectations $E[\underline{Y}_{(\overline{a}_{m-1},0),m+1} \mid \overline{\ell}_m, \overline{a}_m]$ are identified. We give identifying formulae for two important cases. For $m = K, K-1, \ldots, 0$ and $k = m+1, \ldots, K+1$
(i) for an additive SNMM (i.e., γ^*_m given by (8.9)) with $\Phi(x) = x$

$$\text{(8.12a)} \quad \begin{aligned} \gamma^*_{m,k}\left(\overline{\ell}_m, \overline{a}_m\right) &= E\left[U^*_{m+1,k} \mid \overline{\ell}_m, \overline{a}_m\right] \\ &\quad - E\left[U^*_{m+1,k} \mid \overline{\ell}_m, \overline{a}_{m-1}, a_m = 0\right] - q_m\left(k, \overline{\ell}_m, \overline{a}_m\right) \end{aligned}$$

and $t\left(k, \overline{\ell}_m, \overline{a}_{m-1}\right) = E\left[U_{m,k} \mid \overline{\ell}_m, \overline{a}_{m-1}, a_m = 0\right]$,
(ii) for a multiplicative SNMM (i.e., γ^*_m given by (8.10)) with $\Phi(x) = e^x$

$$\text{(8.12b)} \quad \begin{aligned} \gamma^*_{m,k}\left(\overline{\ell}_m, \overline{a}_m\right) &= \log\left\{E\left[U^*_{m+1,k} \mid \overline{\ell}_m, \overline{a}_m\right]\right\} \\ &\quad - \log\left\{E\left[U^*_{m+1,k} \mid \overline{\ell}_m, \overline{a}_{m-1}, a_m = 0\right]\right\} - q_m\left(k, \overline{\ell}_m, \overline{a}_m\right) \end{aligned}$$

and

$$\text{(8.12c)} \quad t\left(k, \overline{\ell}_m, \overline{a}_{m-1}\right) = \log\left\{E\left[U_{m,k} \mid \overline{\ell}_m, \overline{a}_{m-1}, a_m = 0\right]\right\} .$$

REMARK 8.2. Conditions (a)–(c) of Theorem 8.5 characterize a priori restrictions on the possible laws of O. For example, in the restriction (b), we are considering all laws of the observed data O in which the Y_{k+1} have positive conditional means. We largely restrict attention to the additive SNMM with $\Phi(x) = x$ and the multiplicative SNMM with $\Phi(x) = e^x$ because these are the SNMMs for which we can later estimate the $\gamma_m^*(\overline{\ell}_m, \overline{a}_m)$ by the method of g-estimation based on modelling the law of A_m given $(\overline{A}_{m-1}, \overline{L}_m)$.

Theorem 8.5 has the following dual.

THEOREM 8.6. *If $E\left[Y_k \mid \overline{L}_k, \overline{A}_k\right]$ can take any value in $(-\infty, \infty)$, then the model characterized by the sole restriction that*

$$\gamma_m^*\left(\overline{\ell}_m, \overline{a}_m\right) \text{ is known for each } m \tag{8.13}$$

with $\gamma_m^*\left(\overline{\ell}_m, \overline{a}_m\right)$ as defined in (8.9) is a non-parametric model for the distribution F_O of the observed data. Furthermore, if $\Phi(x) = x$, then $q_m\left(k, \overline{\ell}_m, \overline{a}_m\right)$ defined by Eq. (8.11) is identified from Eq. (8.12a) applied recursively.

In addition, if $E\left[Y_k \mid \overline{L}_k, \overline{A}_k\right]$ can take any value in the interval $[0, \infty)$, then the model characterized by the sole restriction (8.13) with $\gamma_m^*\left(\overline{\ell}_m, \overline{a}_m\right)$ defined by (8.10) is a non-parametric model for the distribution of the observed data. Furthermore, if $\Phi(x) = e^x$, then $q_m\left(k, \overline{\ell}_m, \overline{a}_m\right)$ defined by (8.11a) is identified from Eq. (8.12b) applied recursively.

8.2. Inference and the curse of dimensionality.

8.2.1. Structural nested distribution models. In practice, due to the curse of dimensionality, in order to estimate, in a sensitivity analysis, $\gamma_m(\underline{y}_{m+1}, \overline{\ell}_m, \overline{a}_m)$ under model (8.3) when we vary the selection bias function $q_m(\underline{y}_{m+1}, \overline{\ell}_m, \overline{a}_m)$, we must consider a submodel of our NPI model (8.3) in which we impose parametric models

$$\gamma_m\left(\underline{y}_{m+1}, \overline{\ell}_m, \overline{a}_m\right) \in \left\{\gamma_m\left(\underline{y}_{m+1}, \overline{\ell}_m, \overline{a}_m; \psi\right); \psi \in \boldsymbol{\psi}\right\}, \tag{8.14}$$

$$t\left(a_m \mid \overline{\ell}_m, \overline{a}_{m-1}\right) \in \left\{t\left(a_m \mid \overline{\ell}_m, \overline{a}_{m-1}; \eta\right); \eta \in \boldsymbol{\eta}\right\} \tag{8.15}$$

where ψ and η are unknown finite dimensional parameters taking values in sets $\boldsymbol{\psi}$ and $\boldsymbol{\eta}$ and $\gamma_m\left(\underline{y}_{m+1}, \overline{\ell}_m, \overline{a}_m; \psi\right)$ and $t\left(a_m \mid \overline{\ell}_m, \overline{a}_{m-1}; \eta\right)$ are respectively a known function and a known density.

We then estimate (ψ, η) by g-estimation. That is, given a vector of functions $g_m\left(\underline{y}_{m+1}, \overline{\ell}_m, \overline{a}_m\right)$ of the dimension of ψ chose by the data analyst, we maximize an artificial likelihood (defined below) that depends on the selection bias function q_m of model (8.3), η, ψ and the artificial parameter θ. Specifically, we maximize

$$\prod_i \prod_m \mathcal{L}ik_{m,i}(\theta, \eta, \psi) \tag{8.16a}$$

with respect to η and θ with ψ held fixed to obtain estimates $\widehat{\eta}(\psi)$ and $\widehat{\theta}(\psi)$. We then define our g-estimate $\widehat{\psi}$ to be the value of ψ for which $\widehat{\theta}(\psi) = 0$ and define $\widehat{\eta} = \widehat{\eta}\left(\widehat{\psi}\right)$. Here

$$\text{(8.16b)} \qquad \mathcal{L}ik_{m,i}(\theta, \eta, \psi) = \nu_i(A_{m,i}) \Big/ \int \nu_i(a_m)\, d\mu(a_m)$$

where $\nu(a_m) = t\left[a_m \mid \overline{L}_m, \overline{A}_{m-1}; \eta\right] \exp\left\{q_m\left[U_m(\psi), \overline{L}_m, \overline{A}_{m-1}, a_m\right] + \theta' g_m\left[U_m(\psi), \overline{L}_m, \overline{A}_{m-1}, a_m\right]\right\}$ and g_n is a user-supplied function, $U_m(\psi)$ is defined like U_m except with $\gamma_m\left(\underline{y}_{m+1}, \overline{\ell}_m, \overline{a}_m; \psi\right)$ in place of $\gamma_m\left(\underline{y}_{m+1}, \overline{\ell}_m, \overline{a}_m\right)$. In conducting a sensitivity analysis, we will often choose a class of selection bias functions indexed by a parameter α of the form $q_m\left[\underline{y}_{m+1}, \overline{\ell}_m, \overline{a}_m, \alpha\right]$ satisfying $q_m\left[\underline{y}_{m+1}, \overline{\ell}_m, \overline{a}_m, 0\right] = 0$ so that $\alpha = 0$ corresponds to the absence of selection bias. We would then plot $\widehat{\psi}$ (or some functional of $\widehat{\psi}$) as a function of the selection bias parameter α. That is, we plot the function $\widehat{\psi}(\alpha)$ as the function of the selection bias parameter α. If our model characterized by (8.3), (8.14), and (8.15) is correctly specified for some particular α, then, for that α, $\widehat{\psi}(\alpha)$ will be a consistent asymptotically normal estimator of the true value of ψ. The optimal choice of g_m, say $g_{m,opt}$, is given in Sec. 9 of Robins (1997b) and results in a semiparametric efficient estimator of ψ under our model.

Consider the model in which we replace the assumption (8.3b) that the selection bias function is known with the weaker assumption that the true selection bias function is a member of the parametric family $\left\{q_m\left[\underline{y}_{m+1}, \overline{\ell}_m, \overline{a}_m, \alpha\right]; \alpha \in \boldsymbol{\alpha}\right\}$ where α is a finite dimensional parameter space. Since we have imposed restrictions (8.14), and (8.15), it is possible that (η, ψ, α) will be jointly identifiable. However, as discussed earlier, when the dimension of the parameters ψ and η are reasonably large, there will be little independent information about the three parameters, and their joint estimation will require truly huge sample sizes. Furthermore, the identification of α is strictly a consequence of our imposition of parametric models (8.14), and (8.15). Therefore, even with large sample sizes, if we carry out joint estimation of (α, ψ, η), any estimator of ψ will be highly sensitive to misspecification of both models (8.9) and (8.10), and there will be little power to detect such misspecification. As a consequence, we continue to recommend that one regard α as fixed and known and estimate (η, ψ) in a sensitivity analysis in which α is varied.

8.2.2. Structural nested mean models. For our SNMM, we consider a submodel of our NPI model (8.11) in which we impose parametric models for γ_m^* and for the conditional density of A_m given $\left(\overline{L}_m, \overline{A}_{m-1}\right)$. That is, we assume

$$\text{(8.17)} \qquad \gamma_m^*\left(\overline{\ell}_m, \overline{a}_m\right) \in \left\{\gamma_m^*\left(\overline{\ell}_m, \overline{a}_m; \psi\right); \psi \in \boldsymbol{\psi}\right\}$$

and

$$(8.18)\qquad f\left(a_m \mid \overline{\ell}_m, \overline{a}_{m-1}\right) \in \left\{f\left(a_m \mid \overline{\ell}_m, \overline{a}_{m-1}; \eta\right); \eta \in \boldsymbol{\eta}\right\}$$

with ψ and η unknown finite dimensional parameters. To estimate ψ by g-estimation under the model characterized by (8.11), (8.17), and (8.18), we first estimate η by the maximizer $\widehat{\eta}$ of the partial likelihood $\prod_{i=1}^{n} PL_i(\eta)$ where $PL(\eta) = \prod_{m=0}^{K} f\left[A_m \mid \overline{L}_m, \overline{A}_{m-1}; \eta\right]$. We then estimate ψ as follows. For $m = 0, \ldots, K$, let $g_m(a_m, \overline{\ell}_m, \overline{a}_{m-1})$ be a $(K+1-m) \times \dim \psi$ matrix-valued function chosen by the analyst and let $D'_m(\eta) = g'_m\left(A_m, \overline{L}_m, \overline{A}_{m-1}\right) - \int g'\left(a_m, \overline{L}_m, \overline{A}_{m-1}\right) dF\left(a_m \mid \overline{\ell}_m, \overline{A}_{m-1}; \eta\right)$. Then for $m = 0, \ldots, K$ and $k = m+1, \ldots, K+1$, let $c\left(k, \overline{\ell}_m, \overline{a}_{m-1}\right)$ be functions chosen by the analyst. For an additive SNMM with $\Phi(x) = x$, define $H_{m,k}(\psi) = U_{m,k}(\psi) - q_m\left(k, \overline{L}_m, \overline{A}_m\right) - c\left(k, \overline{L}_m, \overline{A}_{m-1}\right)$. Define $H_{m,k}(\psi) = U_{m,k}(\psi) \exp\left[-q_m\left(k, \overline{L}_m, \overline{A}_m\right) - c\left(k, \overline{L}_m, \overline{A}_{m-1}\right)\right]$ for a multiplicative SNMM with $\Phi(x) = e^x$. Here $q_m\left(k, \overline{\ell}_m, \overline{a}_m\right)$ is the known selection bias function in (8.11).

Then $\widehat{\psi}$ solves $0 = \sum_i W_i(\psi, \widehat{\eta})$ where $W(\psi, \eta) = \sum_{m=0}^{K} D'_m(\eta) \times \left(H_{m,m+1}(\psi), \ldots, H_{m,K+1}(\psi)\right)'$. It is easy to check that $E[W(\psi, \eta)] = 0$ at the true values of ψ and η under the model characterized by (8.11), (8.17), and (8.18). For readers conversant with the theory of semiparametric models, it will be of interest to note that in this model, the orthogonal complement to the nuisance tangent space is random vectors of the form $W(\psi, \eta) + S(\psi, \eta)$ where $S(\eta) = \sum_{m=0}^{K} r\left(\overline{A}_m, \overline{L}_m\right) - \int r\left(\overline{A}_m, \overline{L}_m\right) dF\left[A_m \mid \overline{L}_m, \overline{A}_{m-1}; \eta\right]$ for some user-supplied function $r(\cdot, \cdot)$.

It is interesting to note in the model characterized by (8.11), (8.17), and (8.18), in contrast to the model specified by (8.3), (8.14), and (8.15) studied in the last section, is that the density of A_m given $\overline{L}_m, \overline{A}_{m-1}$ is no longer ancillary when the selection bias function q_m is not identically zero. That is, the estimate of η obtained by maximizing the above partial likelihood is not an efficient estimator of η. The reason for this is that when the selection bias function q_m is not identically zero, $H_{m,k}(\psi)$ is not a deterministic function of $H_{m+1,k}(\psi), \overline{L}_{m+1}, \overline{A}_m$. In contrast, when the q_m are identically zero (i.e., there is no confounding), $H_{m,k}(\psi) = U_{m,k}(\psi)$ and $H_{m,k}(\psi)$ is therefore a deterministic function of the quantities mentioned above.

8.2.3. An alternative sensitivity analysis for continuous Y. The approach of Sec. 8.1.2 suggests the following alternative nonparametric identified model in the case of continuous Y. Define γ_m, $U_m = \left(U_{m,m+1}, \ldots, U_{m,K+1}\right)$ and U^*_m as in Sec. 8.1.1. Redefine $q_m\left(\underline{y}_{m+1}, \overline{\ell}_m, \overline{a}_m\right)$ as the unique solution to

(8.19a)
$$F_{\underline{Y}_{(\overline{a}_{m-1},0),m+1}|\overline{\ell}_m,\overline{a}_{m-1},a_m=0}\left[q\left(\underline{y}_{m+1},\overline{\ell}_m,\overline{a}_m\right)\right] = F_{\underline{Y}_{(\overline{a}_{m-1},0),m+1}|\overline{\ell}_m,\overline{a}_m}\left(\underline{y}_{m+1}\right)$$

satisfying

(8.19b) $q_{m,k}\left(\underline{y}_{m+1},\overline{\ell}_m,\overline{a}_m\right)$ *is a function of* $\overline{y}_{K+1}$ *only through* $\overline{y}_k$.

Let $H_m \equiv q_m\left(U_m,\overline{L}_m,\overline{A}_m\right)$. We then have the following obvious lemma.

LEMMA 8.1.

(8.20)
$$H_m \coprod A_m \mid \overline{L}_m,\overline{A}_{m-1}$$

and the following theorem.

THEOREM 8.7. *The model characterized by the sole restriction that, for each* m,

(8.21) $q_m\left(\underline{y}_{m+1},\overline{\ell}_m,\overline{a}_m\right)$ *defined by (8.19) is a known function*

is a non-parametric model for the law of F_O *of* O. *Furthermore, the functions* γ_m *are identified from the law of* F_O. *Specifically,* $\gamma_m = q_m^{-1} \circ \rho_m$, *where* $\rho_m\left(\underline{y}_{m+1},\overline{\ell}_m,\overline{a}_m\right)$ *is defined to be the function* $\gamma_m\left(\underline{y}_{m+1},\overline{\ell}_m,\overline{a}_m\right)$ *that would be obtained from the given law* F_O *under model (8.3) in the absence of confounding, i.e., when* $q_m\left(\underline{y}_{m+1},\overline{\ell}_m,\overline{a}_m\right)$ *as defined in (8.3b) is identically zero.*

REMARK 8.3. Since under the conditions of Theorem 8.7, γ_m is identified, it follows from Theorems 8.3 and 8.1 that under Assumption (8.21), the law of $\overline{Y}_{(0)}$ and the conditional laws of $\underline{Y}_{(\overline{A}_{m-1},0),m+1}$ given $\left(\overline{L}_m,\overline{A}_m\right)$ are identified.

Implications for g-estimation: It follows that given a parametric model $\gamma_m\left(\underline{y}_{m+1},\overline{\ell}_m,\overline{a}_m,\psi\right)$ for $\gamma_m\left(\underline{y}_{m+1},\overline{\ell}_m,\overline{a}_m\right)$ and a parametric model $f\left(a_m \mid \overline{\ell}_m,\overline{a}_{m-1};\eta\right)$ for $f\left(a_m \mid \overline{\ell}_m,\overline{a}_{m-1}\right)$, we can estimate ψ by standard g-estimation as in Robins (1997b). That is, $\widehat{\psi}$ is the vector ψ for which $\widehat{\theta}(\psi) = 0$ when maximizing (8.16a) with respect to θ and η with $\nu(a_m)$ in (8.16b) redefined to be

(8.22)
$$\nu(a_m) = f\left(a_m \mid \overline{L}_m,\overline{A}_{m-1};\eta\right)\exp\left\{\theta' g_m(H_m(\psi),\overline{L}_m,\overline{A}_{m-1},a_m)\right\}$$

with $H_m(\psi) = q_m\left(U_m(\psi),\overline{L}_m,\overline{A}_m\right)$. Again, if the function q_m is not identically zero (i.e., there is confounding), the partial likelihood estimator of η described following (8.18) is not efficient. This reflects the fact that $H_0(\psi)$ is not a deterministic function of $H_m(\psi),\overline{L}_m,\overline{A}_{m-1}$ except when the functions q_m are identically zero, in which case $H_m(\psi) = U_m(\psi)$. This also implies that the score equations for g-estimation described in Robins (1992) no longer have the uncorrelated increments property of a "martingale."

8.3. Identification of $\overline{Y}_{\overline{a}}$. Under the conditions of Theorem 8.2, 8.3, and 8.7, given a law F_O of the observed data, the distribution of $\overline{Y}_{\overline{a},K+1}$ is not identified except for $\overline{a} \equiv 0$. Similarly, in Theorems 8.5 and 8.6, the mean of $\overline{Y}_{\overline{a},K+1}$ is not identified except for $\overline{a} \equiv 0$. We shall now give sufficient and non-identifiable conditions to identify the above means and laws for any $\overline{a}$.

In fact, we give sufficient conditions to identify the mean and law of $\overline{Y}_{g,K+1}$, where $\overline{Y}_{g,K+1}$, as defined below, is the outcome under a possibly dynamic regime g.

Definition of Regimes: A treatment regime g is a collection of $K+1$ functions $g = (g_0, \dots, g_K)$ where $g_m \equiv g_m(\overline{\ell}_m)$ maps an outcome history $\overline{\ell}_m$ into a treatment $g_m(\overline{\ell}_m) \in \mathcal{A}_m$. If, for each m, $g_m(\overline{\ell}_m)$ is a constant, say, a_m^* not depending on $\overline{\ell}_m$, we say the regime g is non-dynamic and write $g = \overline{a}^* = (a_0^*, \dots, a_K^*)$. Otherwise we say the regime g is dynamic. The treatment at time m under a dynamic regime depends on the evolution of one's covariate history under that regime. We let $\mathcal{G}$ denote the set of all treatment regimes.

We let $\overline{L}_{g,K+1}$ be the subject's outcome history when, possibly contrary to fact, the subject follows regime g. Now define $g(\overline{\ell}_m) \equiv \{g_0(\ell_0), \dots, g_m(\overline{\ell}_m)\}$ so $g(\overline{\ell}_m) \in \overline{\mathcal{A}}_m$. The counterfactual data $\overline{L}_{g,K+1}$ is linked to the observed data by the following consistency assumption.

Consistency Assumption 1:

$$\text{(8.23)} \qquad \textit{If } g(\overline{L}_m) = \overline{A}_m, \textit{ then } \overline{L}_{g,m+1} = \overline{L}_{m+1}\ .$$

This consistency assumption states that if the subject has actually followed regime g until time t_{m+1}, then his counterfactual outcome under that regime and his observed outcome will agree through time t_{m+1}.

Consistency Assumption 2: If $g(\overline{\ell}_m) = g^*(\overline{\ell}_m)$ for regimes g and g^*, then $\overline{L}_{g,m+1} = \overline{L}_{g^*,m+1}$.

We shall now need to define various current treatment interaction functions. We adopt the convention

$$\text{(8.24)} \qquad E\left[Z \mid \overline{\ell}_m, g(\overline{\ell}_m)\right] \equiv E\left[Z \mid \overline{L}_m = \overline{\ell}_m, \overline{A}_m = g(\overline{\ell}_m)\right].$$

DEFINITION 8.1. *The additive current treatment interaction function* $r_m(\overline{\ell}_m, g)$ *is*

$$\text{(8.25)} \qquad \begin{aligned} r_m(\overline{\ell}_m, g) &= E\left[\underline{Y}_{g,m+1} - \underline{Y}_{(g(\overline{\ell}_{m-1}),0),m+1} \mid \overline{\ell}_m, g(\overline{\ell}_m)\right] \\ &\quad - E\left[\underline{Y}_{g,m+1} - \underline{Y}_{(g(\overline{\ell}_{m-1}),0),m+1} \mid \overline{\ell}_m, g(\overline{\ell}_{m-1}), A_m \neq g_m(\overline{\ell}_m)\right]. \end{aligned}$$

If $r_m(\overline{\ell}_m, g) = 0$ for all $\overline{\ell}_m$, we say we have no additive current treatment interaction for regime g.

DEFINITION 8.2. *The multiplicative current treatment interaction function is* $r_m\left(\overline{\ell}_m, g\right) = \left(r_{m,m+1}\left(\overline{\ell}_m, g\right), \ldots, r_{m,K+1}\left(\overline{\ell}_m, g\right)\right)$ *where*

$$\begin{aligned} r_{m,k}\left(\overline{\ell}_m, g\right) = & \log\left\{E\left(Y_{g,k} \mid \overline{\ell}_m, g\left(\overline{\ell}_m\right)\right)\right\} \\ & - \log\left\{E\left(Y_{\left(g\left(\overline{\ell}_{m-1}\right),0\right),k} \mid \overline{\ell}_m, g\left(\overline{\ell}_m\right)\right)\right\} \\ & - \left[\log\left\{E\left(Y_{g,k} \mid \overline{\ell}_m, g\left(\overline{\ell}_{m-1}\right), A_m \neq g_m\left(\overline{\ell}_m\right)\right)\right\}\right. \\ & \left. - \log\left\{E\left(Y_{\left(g\left(\overline{\ell}_{m-1}\right),0\right),k} \mid \overline{\ell}_m, g\left(\overline{\ell}_{m-1}\right), A_m \neq g_m\left(\overline{\ell}_m\right)\right)\right\}\right] . \end{aligned}$$

DEFINITION 8.3. *Define* $\nu_m^{\dagger}(\underline{y}_{m+1}, \overline{\ell}_m, g)$ *to be the unique solution to*

$$\begin{aligned} & F_{\underline{Y}_{\left(g\left(\overline{\ell}_{m-1}\right),0\right),m+1} \mid \overline{\ell}_m, g\left(\overline{\ell}_{m-1}\right), A_m \neq g_m\left(\overline{\ell}_m\right)}\left[\nu_m^{\dagger}\left(\underline{y}_{m+1}, \overline{\ell}_m, \overline{a}_m\right)\right] \\ \text{(8.26a)} \qquad & = F_{\underline{Y}_{g,m+1} \mid \overline{\ell}_m, g\left(\overline{\ell}_{m-1}\right), A_m \neq g_m\left(\overline{\ell}_m\right)}\left(\underline{y}_{m+1}\right) \end{aligned}$$

satisfying

(8.26b) $\quad \nu_{m,k}^{\dagger}\left(\underline{y}_{m+1}, \overline{\ell}_m, g\right)$ *is a function of* $\overline{y}_{K+1}$ *only through* $\overline{y}_k$.

Define $\nu_m\left(\underline{y}_{m+1}, \overline{\ell}_m, g\right)$ similarly, except with conditioning events being $\overline{\ell}_m, g\left(\overline{\ell}_m\right)$.

DEFINITION 8.4. *The distribution current treatment interaction function is* $r_m\left(\underline{y}_{m+1}, \overline{\ell}_m, g\right) \equiv r_m \equiv \nu_m^{\dagger} \circ \nu_m^{-1}$ *where* ν_m^{-1} *is the inverse of the function* ν_m *with respect to the argument* $\underline{y}_{m+1}$. *We now state our main theorems.*

THEOREM 8.8. *Under the consistency assumption 1, given (i) a law* F_O *of the observed data* $O = \left(\overline{A}_K, \overline{L}_{K+1}\right)$, *(ii) the conditional means* $E\left[\underline{Y}_{\left(g\left(\overline{\ell}_{m-1}\right),0\right),m+1} \mid \overline{\ell}_m, \overline{a}_m\right]$ *and (iii) either the additive or multiplicative current treatment interaction functions* $r_m\left(\overline{\ell}_m, g\right)$, *then* $E\left[\overline{Y}_{g,K+1}\right]$ *and* $E\left[\underline{Y}_{g,m+1} \mid \overline{\ell}_m, g\left(\overline{\ell}_m\right)\right]$ *are determined (i.e., identified).*

THEOREM 8.9. *Under the consistency assumption 1, given (i) a law* F_O *of the observed data* O, *(ii) the conditional laws* $\underline{Y}_{\left(g\left(\overline{\ell}_{m-1}\right),0\right),m+1}$ *given* $\left(\overline{\ell}_m, \overline{a}_m\right)$, *and the distribution current treatment interaction functions* $r_m\left(\underline{y}_{m+1}, \overline{\ell}_m, g\right)$, *the law of* $\overline{Y}_{g,K+1}$, *and the conditional laws of* $\underline{Y}_{g,m+1}$ *given* $\left(\overline{\ell}_m, g\left(\overline{\ell}_m\right)\right)$ *are determined (i.e., identified).*

Proof of Theorem 8.8. We first note that

$$E\left[Y_{g,m+1} \mid \overline{\ell}_m, g\left(\overline{\ell}_m\right)\right] = E\left[Y_{m+1} \mid \overline{\ell}_m, g\left(\overline{\ell}_m\right)\right]$$

by Consistency Assumption 1. Further, $E\left[Y_m \mid \bar{\ell}_m, g\left(\bar{\ell}_m\right)\right]$ is identified, since F_O is given. Thus, arguing recursively in reverse, beginning at $m = K$, if we can show that

$$E\left[\underline{Y}_{g,m+1} \mid \bar{\ell}_m, g\left(\bar{\ell}_m\right)\right] \textit{ identified} \tag{8.27}$$

implies, under our assumptions, that $E\left[\underline{Y}_{g,m+1} \mid \bar{\ell}_m, g\left(\bar{\ell}_{m-1}\right)\right]$ is identified, then the theorem is proved since *(i)*, by F_O given, we can then conclude that $E\left[\underline{Y}_{g,m+1} \mid \bar{\ell}_{m-1}, g\left(\bar{\ell}_{m-1}\right)\right]$ is identified, and thus, by the first display in the proof, $E\left[\underline{Y}_{g,m} \mid \bar{\ell}_{m-1}, g\left(\bar{\ell}_{m-1}\right)\right]$ is identified. Now,

$$\begin{aligned} E\big[&\underline{Y}_{g,m+1} \mid \bar{\ell}_m, g(\bar{\ell}_{m-1})\big] \\ &= E\big[\underline{Y}_{g,m+1} \mid \bar{\ell}_m, g(\bar{\ell}_m)\big] pr\big[A_m = g(\bar{\ell}_m) \mid \bar{\ell}_m, g(\bar{\ell}_{m-1})\big] \\ &+ E\big[\underline{Y}_{g,m+1} \mid \bar{\ell}_m, g(\bar{\ell}_{m-1}), A_m \neq g_m(\bar{\ell}_m)\big] pr\big[A_m \neq g_m(\bar{\ell}_m) \mid \bar{\ell}_m, g(\bar{\ell}_{m-1})\big] \end{aligned} \tag{8.28}$$

Given (8.27) and F_O, $E\left[\underline{Y}_{g,m+1} \mid \bar{\ell}_m, g\left(\bar{\ell}_{m-1}\right), A_m \neq g_m\left(\bar{\ell}_m\right)\right]$ is the only unknown on the RHS of Eq. (8.27). However, $E\big[\underline{Y}_{g,m+1} \mid \bar{\ell}_m, g\left(\bar{\ell}_{m-1}\right),$ $A_m \neq g_m\left(\bar{\ell}_m\right)\big]$ is a function of $E\left[\underline{Y}_{g,m+1} \mid \bar{\ell}_m, g\left(\bar{\ell}_m\right)\right]$, the given F_O, $r_m\left(\bar{\ell}_m, g\right)$ and $E\left[Y_{\left(g\left(\bar{\ell}_{m-1}\right),0\right)} \mid \bar{\ell}_m, \bar{a}_m\right]$ and thus is determined (i.e., identified), which completes the proof. □

The proof of Theorem 8.9 is similar and is omitted.

We next take up the question whether specifying particular current treatment interaction functions places any restrictions on the joint law of the observed data.

DEFINITION 8.5. *We say that any given function $r_m\left(\bar{\ell}_m, g\right)$ is a potential additive or multiplicative current treatment interaction function if $r_m\left(\bar{\ell}_m, g\right)$ satisfies*

$$\textit{if } g_k\left(\bar{\ell}_k\right) = 0 \textit{ for } k \geq m \text{ , } \textit{then } r_m\left(\bar{\ell}_m, g\right) = 0. \tag{8.29a}$$

$$g_m^*\left(\bar{\ell}_m\right) = g_m\left(\bar{\ell}_m\right) \quad \textit{then} \quad r_{m,m+1}\left(\bar{\ell}_m, g\right) = r_{m,m+1}\left(\bar{\ell}_m, g^*\right). \tag{8.29b}$$

Note that the Equations (8.29a) and (8.29b) hold for any additive or multiplicative current treatment interaction function by the Consistency Assumptions 1 and 2.

REMARK 8.4. Any function satisfying (8.29) can be represented as follows. Given a collection of functions $g = (g_0, \ldots, g_K)$ as defined previously, let $r_m^*\left(\bar{\ell}_m, \bar{a}_m, g\right) = \big(r_{m,m+1}^*\left(\bar{\ell}_m, \bar{a}_m\right), r_{m,m+2}^*\left(\bar{\ell}_m, \bar{a}_m, g_{m+1}\right), \ldots,$ $r_{m,K+1}^*\left(\bar{\ell}_m, \bar{a}_m, g_{m+1}, \ldots, g_K\right)\big)$. Then the set of functions $r_m\left(\bar{\ell}_m, g\right)$ satisfying (8.29) is precisely the set $\{r_m^*\left(\bar{\ell}_m, g\left(\bar{\ell}_m\right), g\right); r_{m,k}^*\big(\bar{\ell}_m, \bar{a}_m, g_{m+1},$ $\ldots, g_k\big) = 0$ *if* $a_m = 0$ and $g_{m+1}, \ldots, g_k$ *are all the zero function*$\}$.

Similarly,

DEFINITION 8.6. *We say a function $r_m\big(\underline{y}_{m+1}, \bar{\ell}_m, g\big)$ is a potential current treatment interaction function if (i) $r_{m,k}\big(\underline{y}_{m+1}, \bar{\ell}_m, g\big)$ depends on*

$\overline{y}_{K+1}$ *only through* $\overline{y}_k$ *and is increasing in* y_k, *(ii)* $r_m\left(\underline{y}_{m+1}, \overline{\ell}_m, g\right) = \underline{y}_{m+1}$ *if* $g_k\left(\overline{\ell}_k\right) = 0$ *for* $k \geq m$, *and (iii) if* $g^*\left(\overline{\ell}_m\right) = g\left(\overline{\ell}_m\right)$ *then* $r_{m,m+1}\left(\underline{y}_{m+1}, \overline{\ell}_m, g\right) = r_{m,m+1}\left(\underline{y}_{m+1}, \overline{\ell}_m, g^*\right)$.

Consider the following theorem.

THEOREM 8.10. *Under Consistency Assumptions 1 and 2, given any law* F_O *for the observed data, any function* $r_m\left(\overline{\ell}_m, g\right)$ *satisfying (8.29), and any function* $q_m\left(k, \overline{\ell}_m, \overline{a}_m\right)$, *there exists a joint law for* $\left(\overline{A}, \left\{\overline{L}_{g,K+1};\, g \in \mathcal{G}\right\}\right)$ *satisfying model (8.11) with* $\Phi(x) = x$ *and with* $r_m\left(\overline{\ell}_m, g\right)$ *the additive current treatment interaction function, provided* $E\left[Y_{k+1} \mid \overline{\ell}_k, \overline{a}_k\right]$ *may take values anywhere in* $\left(-\infty, \infty\right)$.

REMARK 8.5. Note by Consistency Assumption 2, $\left\{\overline{L}_{\overline{a},K+1}; \overline{a} \in \overline{\mathcal{A}}\right\}$ completely determines $\overline{L}_{g,K+1}$ for each $g \in \mathcal{G}$. Thus, in the statement of Theorem 8.10, we could have replaced $\left\{\overline{L}_{g,K+1}; g \in \mathcal{G}\right\}$ by $\left\{\overline{L}_{\overline{a},K+1}; \overline{a} \in \overline{\mathcal{A}}\right\}$.

REMARK 8.6. Note, it follows from Theorem 8.5 that under the conditions of Theorem 8.10, $\gamma_m^*\left(\overline{\ell}_m, \overline{a}_m\right)$ defined by (8.9a) as identified as a function of $q_m\left(k, \overline{\ell}_m, \overline{a}_m\right)$. Suppose for a particular choice of q_m, $\gamma_m^*\left(\overline{\ell}_m, \overline{a}_m\right)$ is identically zero. This implies according to (8.9a) that there is no effect of a final brief blip of treatment a_m at time t_m on subjects with history $\overline{\ell}_m, \overline{a}_m$. Often it would seem reasonable to have strong prior beliefs $\gamma_m^*\left(\overline{\ell}_m, \overline{a}_m\right) = 0$, then the g-null hypothesis that $E\left[\overline{Y}_{g,K+1}\right]$ is the same for all $g \in \mathcal{G}$ was true. This prior will be satisfied if we choose the potential additive current treatment interaction function $r_m\left(\overline{\ell}_m, g\right)$ in Theorem 8.10 to be identically zero whenever $\gamma_m^*\left(\overline{\ell}_m, \overline{a}_m\right)$ is identically zero.

For multiplicative current treatment interaction functions, we have the following similar weaker result.

THEOREM 8.11. *Under Consistency Assumptions 1 and 2, given a law* F_O, *a function* $q_m\left(k, \overline{\ell}_m, \overline{a}_m\right)$, *and a function* $r_m\left(\overline{\ell}_m, g\right)$ *satisfying Eq. (8.29), there exists a joint law for* $\left(\overline{A}, \left\{\overline{L}_{\overline{a}}; \overline{a} \in \overline{\mathcal{A}}\right\}\right)$ *satisfying (8.11) with* $\Phi(x) = e^x$ *and with* $r_m\left(\overline{\ell}_m, g\right)$ *the multiplicative current treatment interaction function for non-dynamic regimes* $g = \overline{a}$, *provided* $E\left[\, Y_{k+1} \mid \overline{\ell}_k, \overline{a}_k\right]$ *may take values anywhere in* $[0, \infty)$.

REMARK 8.7. Unlike Theorem 8.10, Theorem 8.11 cannot be extended to include dynamic regimes. Specifically, if $E\left[Y_{g,k} \mid \overline{\ell}_m, g\left(\overline{\ell}_m\right)\right]$ only takes values in $[0, \infty)$, then $E\left[\underline{Y}_{g,m+2} \mid \overline{\ell}_m, g\left(\overline{\ell}_{m-1}\right), A_m \neq g_m\left(\overline{\ell}_m\right)\right]$ must be zero if

$$E\left[\underline{Y}_{\left(g\left(\overline{\ell}_m\right), a_{m+1}, 0\right), m+2} \mid \overline{\ell}_m, g\left(\overline{\ell}_{m-1}\right), A_m \neq g\left(\overline{\ell}_m\right)\right] = 0$$
$$\text{for all } a_{m+1} \in \mathcal{A}_{m+1}\,.$$

This follows by the fact that, under Consistency Assumption 2, the last display implies $\underline{Y}_{g,m+2} = 0$ on $L_m, \overline{A}_{m-1} = g\left(\overline{\ell}_{m-1}\right), A_m \neq g\left(\overline{\ell}_m\right)$.

It follows that knowledge of $r_m\left(\overline{\ell}_m, g\right)$ for non-dynamic regimes can place various kinds of restrictions on $r_m\left(\overline{\ell}_m, g\right)$ for dynamic regimes.

For similar reasons, for continuous Y, the best we can obtain is the following for continuous $\overline{Y}$.

THEOREM 8.12. *Under Consistency Assumptions 1 and 2, given a law F_O and a potential current treatment interaction function $r_m\left(\underline{y}_{m+1}, \overline{\ell}_m, g\right)$, there exists a joint law for $\left(\overline{A}, \left\{\overline{L}_{(\overline{a})}; \overline{a} \in \overline{\mathcal{A}}\right\}\right)$ satisfying the constraints imposed by either model (8.3) or model (8.21) with $r_m\left(\underline{y}_{m+1}, \overline{\ell}_m, g\right)$ the current treatment interaction function for non-dynamic regimes $g = \overline{a}$.*

REMARK 8.8. If $K = 0$ so we only have a single time-independent treatment A_0, Theorems 8.11 and 8.12 are true with $r_m(\overline{\ell}_m, g)$ and $r_m(\underline{y}_{m+1}, \overline{\ell}_m, g)$ the multiplicative and distribution current treatment interaction functions for all regimes g, both dynamic and non-dynamic. Here of course m takes only the value 0.

8.4. Logistic structural nested mean models. In this subsection, we introduce Logistic Structural Nested Mean Models (SNMMs) for dichotomous Y_k. Redefine

$$\gamma^*_{m,k}\left(\overline{\ell}_m, \overline{a}_m\right) = \text{logit}\left\{E\left[Y_{(\overline{a}_m,0),k} \mid \overline{\ell}_m, \overline{a}_m\right]\right\} - \text{logit}\left\{E\left[Y_{(\overline{a}_{m-1},0)} \mid \overline{\ell}_m, \overline{a}_m\right]\right\} . \tag{8.30}$$

Then Theorem 8.5 is obviously still true with γ^*_m redefined by (8.30). Indeed, the identifying formulas (8.12b) and (8.12c) remain true with "*log*" replaced by "*logit*" and $U^*_{m+1,k}$ and $U_{m,k}$ replaced by $Y_{(\overline{a}_m,0),k}$ and $Y_{(\overline{a}_{m-1},0),k}$ respectively. Note that we obtain identification because $Y_{\overline{a}_K,K+1} = Y_{K+1}$ by Consistency Assumption 1.

However, there is no longer a function U_m of $\underline{Y}_{m+1}$ and the redefined γ^*_m such that Theorem 8.4 holds. Thus, we cannot estimate a parametric logistic SNMM $\gamma^*_m\left(\overline{\ell}_m, \overline{a}_m, \psi\right)$ by g-estimation. See Remark 8.13 in Sec. 8.5 for further discussion of this point. Fully parametric likelihood based and Bayesian approaches to estimation of this model are considered in Secs. 8.5 and 11.

Now define the logistic current treatment interaction function like a multiplicative current treatment interaction function except with "*logit*" replacing "*log*" in the definition. Then Theorem 8.8 remains true with $r_m\left(\overline{\ell}_m, g\right)$ the logistic current treatment interaction function. Further, the following analog of Theorem 8.11 holds.

THEOREM 8.13. *Suppose Y_k is dichotomous. Under Consistency Assumptions 1 and 2, given a law F_O, a function $q_m\left(k, \overline{\ell}_m, \overline{a}_m\right)$, and a function $r_m\left(\overline{\ell}_m, g\right)$ satisfying Eq. (8.29), there exists a joint law for $\left(\overline{A}, \left\{\overline{L}_{\overline{a}}; \overline{a} \in \overline{\mathcal{A}}\right\}\right)$ satisfying (8.11) with $\Phi(x) = e^x / (1 + e^x)$ and with $r_m\left(\overline{\ell}_m, g\right)$ the logistic current treatment interaction function for non-dynamic regimes $g = \overline{a}$.*

8.5. Likelihood inference for structural nested models. The likelihood function for the structural nested distribution model of Sec. 8.1.1 has been given in Robins (1997b) and is quite straightforward. We shall next, therefore, consider the likelihood function for structural nested mean models. In the following, $\Phi^{-1}(x)$ is x, $\log x$, and *logit* $x = \log\{x/(1-x)\}$ for additive multiplicative and logistic models respectively. Thus, $\Phi(x)$ is respectively x, e^x, and $e^x/(1+e^x)$. Recall the definitions:

$$\begin{aligned}\gamma^*_{m,k+1}\left(\overline{\ell}_m,\overline{a}_m\right) = {} & \Phi^{-1}\left\{E\left[Y_{(\overline{a}_m,0),k+1} \mid \overline{\ell}_m,\overline{a}_m\right]\right\} \\ & - \Phi^{-1}\left\{E\left[Y_{(\overline{a}_{m-1},0),k+1} \mid \overline{\ell}_m,\overline{a}_m\right]\right\}\end{aligned} \tag{8.31}$$

$$\begin{aligned}q_m\left(k+1,\overline{\ell}_m,\overline{a}_m\right) = {} & \Phi^{-1}\left\{E\left[Y_{(\overline{a}_{m-1},0),k+1} \mid \overline{\ell}_m,\overline{a}_m\right]\right\} \\ & - \Phi^{-1}\left\{E\left[Y_{(\overline{a}_{m-1},0),k+1} \mid \overline{\ell}_m,\overline{a}_{m-1},a_m=0\right]\right\}.\end{aligned} \tag{8.32}$$

Define

$$\begin{aligned}\nu^*_m\left(k+1,\overline{\ell}_m,\overline{a}_{m-1}\right) = {} & \Phi^{-1}\left\{E\left[Y_{(\overline{a}_{m-1},0),k+1} \mid \overline{\ell}_m,\overline{a}_{m-1}\right]\right\} \\ & - \Phi^{-1}\left\{E\left[Y_{(\overline{a}_{m-1},0),k+1} \mid \overline{\ell}_{m-1},\overline{a}_{m-1},\ell_m=0\right]\right\}.\end{aligned} \tag{8.33}$$

To construct the likelihood function, we need an expression for the following.

$$\begin{aligned}& \Phi^{-1}\left\{E\left[Y_{(\overline{a}_{m-1},0),k+1} \mid \overline{\ell}_m,\overline{a}_m\right]\right\} - \Phi^{-1}\left\{E\left[Y_{(\overline{a}_{m-1},0),k+1} \mid \overline{\ell}_m,\overline{a}_{m-1}\right]\right\} \\ & \qquad \equiv q_m\left(k+1,\overline{\ell}_m,\overline{a}_m\right) - \Gamma\left(k+1,\overline{\ell}_m,\overline{a}_{m-1}\right)\end{aligned} \tag{8.34}$$

where

$$\begin{aligned}\Gamma\left(k+1,\overline{\ell}_m,\overline{a}_{m-1}\right) \equiv {} & -\Phi^{-1}\left\{E\left(Y_{(\overline{a}_{m-1},0),k+1} \mid \overline{\ell}_m,\overline{a}_{m-1},a_m=0\right)\right\} \\ & + \Phi^{-1}\left\{E\left[Y_{(\overline{a}_{m-1},0),k+1} \mid \overline{\ell}_m,\overline{a}_{m-1}\right]\right\},\end{aligned} \tag{8.35}$$

and

$$\begin{aligned}& \Phi^{-1}\left\{E\left[Y_{(\overline{a}_{m-1},0),k+1} \mid \overline{\ell}_m,\overline{a}_{m-1}\right]\right\} - \Phi^{-1}\left\{E\left[Y_{(\overline{a}_{m-1},0),k+1} \mid \overline{\ell}_{m-1},\overline{a}_{m-1}\right]\right\} \\ & \qquad \equiv \nu^*_m\left(k+1,\overline{\ell}_m,\overline{a}_{m-1}\right) - \Gamma^*\left(k+1,\overline{\ell}_{m-1},\overline{a}_{m-1}\right)\end{aligned} \tag{8.36}$$

where

$$\begin{aligned}\Gamma^*\left(k+1,\overline{\ell}_{m-1},\overline{a}_{m-1}\right) = {} & -\Phi^{-1}\left\{E\left[Y_{(\overline{a}_{m-1},0),k+1} \mid \overline{\ell}_{m-1},\ell_m=0,\overline{a}_{m-1}\right]\right\} \\ & + \Phi^{-1}\left\{E\left[Y_{(\overline{a}_{m-1},0),k+1} \mid \overline{\ell}_{m-1},\overline{a}_{m-1}\right]\right\}.\end{aligned} \tag{8.37}$$

Note for $\Phi(x) = e^x$ *or* $\Phi(x) = x$, one can calculate that

$$\Gamma\left(k+1, \bar{\ell}_m, \bar{a}_{m-1}\right) = \Phi^{-1} \int \Phi\left\{q_m\left(k+1, \bar{\ell}_m, \bar{a}_m\right)\right\} dF\left(a_m \mid \bar{\ell}_m, \bar{a}_{m-1}\right) \tag{8.38}$$

and

$$\Gamma^*\left(k+1, \bar{\ell}_{m-1}, \bar{a}_{m-1}\right) = \Phi^{-1} \int \Phi\left[\nu_m^*\left(k+1, \bar{\ell}_m, \bar{a}_{m-1}\right)\right] dF\left[\ell_m \mid \bar{\ell}_{m-1}, \bar{a}_{m-1}\right] . \tag{8.39}$$

For $\Phi(x) = e^x / (1+e^x)$, $\exp\left\{-\Gamma^*\left(k+1, \bar{\ell}_{m-1}, \bar{a}_{m-1}\right)\right\}$ is the unique solution x to the equation

$$(1-p)^2 = \int \left\{(1-p)\nu_m^*(k+1, \bar{\ell}_m, \bar{a}_{m-1})^{-1} x^{-1} + p\right\}^{-1} dF\left[\ell_m \mid \bar{\ell}_{m-1}, \bar{a}_{m-1}\right] \tag{8.40}$$

with

$$p \equiv E\left[Y_{(\bar{a}_{m-1},0),k+1} \mid \bar{\ell}_{m-1}, \bar{a}_{m-1}\right] . \tag{8.41}$$

Further, $\exp\left[-\Gamma\left(k+1, \bar{\ell}_m, \bar{a}_{m-1}\right)\right]$ is the unique solution x to

$$(1-p)^2 = \int \left\{(1-p)\, q_m\left(k+1, \bar{\ell}_m, \bar{a}_m\right)^{-1} x^{-1} + p\right\}^{-1} dF\left[a_m \mid \bar{\ell}_m, \bar{a}_{m-1}\right] \tag{8.42}$$

with

$$p \equiv E\left[Y_{(\bar{a}_{m-1},0),k+1} \mid \bar{\ell}_m, \bar{a}_{m-1}\right] . \tag{8.43}$$

To construct the likelihood function for non-parametric, semiparametric, and/or parametric versions of our model, we shall consider sets of densities indexed by (possibly infinite dimensional parameters) η and $\gamma' = (\gamma_1', \gamma_2')$

$$\left\{f\left[a_m \mid \bar{\ell}_m, \bar{a}_{m-1}; \eta\right];\ \eta \in \boldsymbol{\eta},\ 0 \le m \le K\right\} \tag{8.44a}$$

$$\left\{f\left(\varepsilon_{k+1} \mid \bar{\ell}_k, \bar{a}_k; \gamma_1\right);\ \int \varepsilon_{k+1} dF\left(\varepsilon_{k+1} \mid \bar{\ell}_k, \bar{a}_k; \gamma_1\right) = 0 \text{ and } \gamma_1 \in \boldsymbol{\gamma}_1,\ -1 \le k \le K\right\} \tag{8.44b}$$

$$\left\{f\left(v_{k+1} \mid \bar{\ell}_k, \bar{a}_k, Y_{k+1}; \gamma_2\right);\ \gamma_2 \in \boldsymbol{\gamma}_2,\ -1 \le k \le K\right\} . \tag{8.44c}$$

We use the convention that for any $\overline{Z}$, $\overline{Z}_{-1} \equiv 0$ with probability 1. We shall also need to consider sets of functions indexed by parameters ψ, μ_1, and μ_2.

$$\text{(8.44d)} \quad \left\{\gamma^*_{m,k+1}\left(\overline{\ell}_m, \overline{a}_m; \psi\right); \ \gamma^*_{m,k+1}\left(\overline{\ell}_m, \overline{a}_{m-1}, a_m = 0; \psi\right) = 0, \right. \\ \left. \psi \in \boldsymbol{\psi}, \ K \geq k \geq m, \ 0 \leq m \leq K\right\}$$

$$\text{(8.44e)} \quad \left\{q_m(k+1, \overline{\ell}_m, \overline{a}_m; \mu_1); \ q_m(k+1, \overline{\ell}_m, \overline{a}_{m-1}, a_m = 0; \mu_1) = 0, \right. \\ \left. \mu_1 \in \boldsymbol{\mu}_1, \ K \geq k \geq m, \ 0 \leq m \leq K\right\}$$

$$\text{(8.44f)} \quad \left\{\nu^*_m(k+1, \overline{\ell}_1, \overline{a}_{m-1}; \mu_2); \ \nu^*_m(k+1, \overline{\ell}_{m-1}, \ell_m = 0, \overline{a}_{m-1}; \mu_2) = 0, \right. \\ \left. \mu_2 \in \boldsymbol{\mu}_2, \ K \geq k \geq m, \ 0 \leq m \leq K\right\}.$$

Finally, we need to consider a set of vectors

$$\text{(8.44g)} \quad \left\{\omega = (\omega_0, \ldots, \omega_{K+1}); \omega \in \boldsymbol{\omega} \subset R^{K+2}\right\}.$$

We shall consider a model in which the unknown parameters, functions, and densities lie in the sets specified in (8.44). We derive the likelihood function for our model by considering the following algebraic identity, $K \geq k \geq 0$.

$$\text{(8.45)} \quad \begin{aligned} \Phi^{-1}\left\{E\left(Y_{k+1} \mid \overline{\ell}_k, \overline{a}_k\right)\right\} = \sum_{m=0}^{k} & \gamma^*_{m,k+1}\left(\overline{\ell}_m, \overline{a}_m\right) \\ + & \left\{q_m\left(k+1, \overline{\ell}_m, \overline{a}_m\right) - \Gamma\left(k+1, \overline{\ell}_m, \overline{a}_{m-1}\right)\right\} \\ + & \left\{\nu^*_m\left(k+1, \overline{\ell}_m, \overline{a}_{m-1}\right) - \Gamma^*\left(k+1, \overline{\ell}_{m-1}, \overline{a}_{m-1}\right)\right\} \\ + & E\left(Y_{(0),k+1}\right). \end{aligned}$$

Write, for $k = -1, \ldots, K$,

$$\text{(8.46)} \quad \varepsilon_{k+1} = Y_{k+1} - E\left(Y_{k+1} \mid \overline{L}_k, \overline{A}_k\right).$$

Then the likelihood for $O = \left(\overline{A}_K, \overline{L}_{K+1}\right)$ with $L_k \equiv (V_k, Y_k)$ can be written as follows, in terms of the parameter $\rho = (\psi, \eta, \gamma, \mu, \omega)$.

$$\text{(8.47)} \quad \begin{aligned} f[O; \rho] = & \prod_{m=0}^{K+1} f\left[\varepsilon_k(\rho) \mid \overline{L}_{k-1}, \overline{A}_{k-1}; \gamma_1\right] f\left(V_k \mid \overline{L}_{k-1}, \overline{A}_{k-1}, Y_k; \gamma_2\right) \\ & \times \prod_{m=0}^{K} f\left[A_k \mid \overline{L}_k, \overline{A}_{k-1}; \eta\right] \end{aligned}$$

where, for $k = -1, \dots, K$,

$$\varepsilon_{k+1}(\rho) = Y_{k+1} - E\left(Y_{k+1} \mid \overline{L}_k, \overline{A}_k; \rho\right), \tag{8.48}$$

$\Phi^{-1}\left\{E\left[Y_0 \mid \overline{L}_{-1}, \overline{A}_{-1}; \rho\right]\right\} = \omega_0$ and $\Phi^{-1}\left\{E\left[Y_{k+1} \mid \overline{L}_k, \overline{A}_k; \rho\right]\right\}$ for $k \geq 0$ is given by the RHS of (8.45) except with the parameterized versions of γ^*, q, and ν^*, as defined in (8.44), replacing the unparameterized versions and ω_{k+1} replacing $\Phi^{-1}\left\{E\left[Y_{(0),k+1}\right]\right\}$.

Note by (8.38), (8.39), (8.40), and (8.42), Γ and Γ^* on the RHS of (8.45) can be parameterized in terms of the parameter ρ, although, in the logistic case, the dependence on ρ will be quite complex. Note that if Y_k is dichotomous and $\Phi(x) = e^x/(1+e^x)$, there is no parameter γ_1, since the conditional law of $\varepsilon_{k+1} \mid \overline{\ell}_k, \overline{a}_k$ is determined by the remaining components of ρ.

REMARK 8.9. The parameter ρ will have variation-independent components (i.e., ρ will take values in the product space $\boldsymbol{\rho} = \boldsymbol{\psi} \times \boldsymbol{\eta} \times \boldsymbol{\gamma} \times \boldsymbol{\mu} \times \boldsymbol{\omega}$) if *(i)* $\Phi(x) = e^x/(1+e^x)$ and Y_k is dichotomous or *(ii)* $\Phi(x) = x$ and Y_k is absolutely continuous with respect to Lesbesgue measure with support on the entire real line. If $\Phi(x) = e^x$ and Y_k is absolutely continuous with respect to Lesbesgue measure with support on the positive half line, then $\boldsymbol{\rho}$ will be variation independent if we (a) redefine $\varepsilon_{k+1} = Y_{k+1}/E\left(Y_{k+1} \mid \overline{L}_k, \overline{A}_k\right)$, (b) restrict the integral in (8.44b) to be 1 rather than 0 and require ε_{k+1} to be supported on the positive half line, and (c) add the Jacobian terms $\partial\, \varepsilon_k/\partial Y_k$ to the likelihood (8.47).

Now consider the model in which the parameter space for $\rho = (\psi, \eta, \gamma, \mu, \omega)$ is unrestricted in the sense that the spaces $\boldsymbol{\psi}, \boldsymbol{\eta}, \boldsymbol{\gamma}_1, \boldsymbol{\gamma}_2, \boldsymbol{\mu}_1, \boldsymbol{\mu}_2, \boldsymbol{\omega}$ are as large as possible, subject to the restrictions specified in (8.44). In this model, ψ, μ_1, μ_2, and ω are not identified.

REMARK 8.10. Consider the model in which q_m is known [i.e., the set $\boldsymbol{\mu}_1$ in (8.44) has a single element] but the other components of ρ remain unrestricted as above. It then follows from Theorem 8.5 and Sec. 8.4 that the remainder of ρ is identified, since this is a NPI model for the law F_O of the observed data if *(a)* $\Phi(x) = x$ and $E\left(Y_{k+1} \mid \overline{L}_k, \overline{A}_k\right)$ can potentially take any value in $(-\infty, \infty)$, *(b)* $\Phi(x) = e^x$ and $E\left(Y_{k+1} \mid \overline{L}_k, \overline{A}_k\right)$ can potentially take any value in $(0, \infty)$, or *(c)* $\Phi(x) = e^x/(1+e^x)$ and Y_k is dichotomous.

REMARK 8.11. Furthermore, by Theorem 8.5 and Sec. 8.4, if *(a)*, *(b)*, or *(c)* is true, then the model in which γ^* is known (i.e., $\boldsymbol{\psi}$ in (8.44d) has but a single element) with all the other parameters left unrestricted is also a NPI model. Fully parametric likelihood inference based on the likelihood (8.47) for the unknown components of ρ in either of the above two models is available if we further restrict the unknown parameters to lie in finite dimensional parameter spaces.

REMARK 8.12. The likelihood function (8.47) can be written as $\mathcal{L}_1(\rho_1)\,\mathcal{L}_2(\rho_2)$ with $\psi \in \rho_1, \eta \in \rho_2$, ρ_1 and ρ_2 variation independent, and

$\rho = (\rho_{1,}\rho_2)$ if and only if the functions q_m are identically zero (i.e., there is no confounding). It follows that, in the presence of confounding, the treatment process $f\left[a_m \mid \overline{\ell}_m, \overline{a}_{m-1}; \eta\right]$ is no longer ancillary for ψ in the model with q_m known.

In Sec. 8.2.2 we considered semiparametric inference for ψ in the model with q_m (i.e., μ_1) known and ψ and η unknown finite dimensional parameters with $\Phi(x)$ either x or e^x. The following remark considers this model further.

REMARK 8.13. No reasonable semiparametric inference (e.g., based on g-estimation) is available for ψ in the semiparametric models with q_m known and ψ and η finite dimensional when Y_k is dichotomous and $\Phi(x) = e^x/(1+e^x)$ (because all influence functions for ψ depend on a high-dimensional smooth, i.e., a conditional expectation or density which is left unrestricted by the model). Specifically, it can be shown that although the semiparametric information bound for ψ is finite when $\Phi(x) = e^x/(1+e^x)$, the curse of dimensionality appropriate (CODA) semiparametric variance bound in the sense of Robins and Ritov (1997b) is zero. In contrast, with $\Phi(x) = x$ or e^x, the CODA bound is finite [as evidenced by the existence of our semiparametric g-estimators for ψ that we were able to calculate without smoothing].

REMARK 8.14. In the special case in which $K = 0$, things simplify considerably. To be concrete, suppose Y is dichotomous and $\Phi(x) = e^x/(1+e^x)$. From our previous definitions, we have the identity

$$\begin{aligned} \Phi^{-1}\{E[Y_1 \mid A_0, L_0]\} = \; & \gamma^*_{0,1}(\ell_0, a_0) + q_0(1, \ell_0, a_0) \\ & + \Phi^{-1}\left\{E\left[Y_{(0),1} \mid \ell_0, a_0 = 0\right]\right\} . \end{aligned} \tag{8.49}$$

This is natural to consider a model in which we assume q_0 is known (which is then varied in a sensitivity analysis), $\gamma^*_{0,1}(\ell_0, a_0)$ is known up to a finite dimensional parameter ψ, and the function $\Phi^{-1}\left\{E\left[Y_{(0),1} \mid \ell_0, a_0 = 0\right]\right\}$ of ℓ_0 is assumed known up to a finite dimensional parameter ω. Then we can jointly estimate ψ and ω by maximum likelihood by maximizing the conditional likelihood given A_0 and L_0. Note here, because of the non-nested structure (on account of K being zero), the conditional law of A_0 given L_0 and the marginal law of L_0 are ancillary for (ψ, ω).

For example, we could consider fitting, using an off-the-shelf logistic regression program, the model

$$logit\,\{pr\,[Y_1 = 1 \mid A_0, L_0]\} = \omega_0 + \omega_1' L_0 + \psi_0 A_0 + \psi_1' A_0 L_0 + \alpha A_0 + \alpha_1' L_0 A_0$$

where α_0 and α_1 are known fixed offsets (which are then varied in a sensitivity analysis) and $\omega_0, \omega_1, \psi_0, \psi_1$ are unknown finite dimensional parameters to be estimated. In this set-up and $q_0(1, L_0, A_0) \equiv \alpha_0 A_0 + \alpha_1' L_0 A_0, \gamma'_{0,1}(L_0, A_0) = \psi_0 A_0 + \psi_1' A_0 L_0$ and $\Phi^{-1}\{E[Y_{(0),1} \mid L_0, A_0 = 0]\} = \omega_0 + \omega_1' L_0$.

8.6. Marginal structural mean models. A marginal structural model is a model for the law of $\overline{Y}_{\overline{a},K+1}$ given a subset V_0^* of L_0 for all $\overline{a} \in \overline{\mathcal{A}}$. A marginal structural mean model specifies that

$$\Phi^{-1}\left\{E\left[Y_{\overline{a},k+1} \mid V_0^*\right]\right\} \equiv \gamma_{k+1}^*\left(\overline{a}_k, V_0^*\right) \tag{8.50}$$

where Φ is a known $1-1$ function and

$$\gamma_{k+1}^*\left(\overline{a}_k, V_0^*\right) \in \left\{\gamma_{k+1}^*\left(\overline{a}_k, V_0^*; \psi\right); \psi \in \boldsymbol{\psi}\right\} \tag{8.51}$$

and ψ is a (possibly infinite dimensional) unknown parameter taking values in $\boldsymbol{\psi}$. Our ultimate goal is to construct a sensitivity analysis for ψ.

8.6.1. Likelihood inference for marginal structural mean models. We shall construct the likelihood for our model based on the following decomposition.

$$\begin{aligned}
\Phi^{-1}\left\{E\left[Y_{\overline{a},k+1} \mid \overline{a}_k, \overline{\ell}_k\right]\right\} &= \sum_{m=0}^{k} \Phi^{-1}\left\{E\left[Y_{\overline{a},k+1} \mid \overline{a}_m, \overline{\ell}_m\right]\right\} \\
&\quad - \Phi^{-1}\left\{E\left[Y_{\overline{a},k+1} \mid \overline{a}_{m-1}, \overline{\ell}_m\right]\right\} + \sum_{m=0}^{k} \Phi^{-1}\left\{E\left[Y_{\overline{a},k+1} \mid \overline{a}_{m-1}, \overline{\ell}_m\right]\right\} \qquad (8.52)\\
&\quad - \Phi^{-1}\left\{E\left[Y_{\overline{a},k+1} \mid \overline{a}_{m-1}, \overline{\ell}_{m-1}, v_0^*\right]\right\} + \Phi^{-1}\left\{E\left[Y_{\overline{a},k+1} \mid v_0^*\right]\right\} \\
&\equiv \sum_{m=0}^{k} m_{k+1}\left(\overline{\ell}_m, \overline{a}_k\right) + m_{k+1}^*\left(\overline{\ell}_m, \overline{a}_k\right) + \gamma_{k+1}^*\left(\overline{a}_k, v_0^*\right) \qquad (8.53)
\end{aligned}$$

where

$$\begin{aligned}
m_{k+1}\left(\overline{\ell}_m, \overline{a}_k\right) &= \Phi^{-1}\left\{E\left[Y_{\overline{a},k+1} \mid \overline{a}_m, \overline{\ell}_m\right]\right\} \\
&\quad - \Phi^{-1}\left\{E\left[Y_{\overline{a},k+1} \mid \overline{a}_{m-1}, \overline{\ell}_m\right]\right\}
\end{aligned} \tag{8.54}$$

and

$$\begin{aligned}
m_{k+1}^*\left(\overline{\ell}_m, \overline{a}_k\right) &= \Phi^{-1}\left\{E\left[Y_{\overline{a},k+1} \mid \overline{a}_{m-1}, \overline{\ell}_m\right]\right\} \\
&\quad - \Phi^{-1}\left\{E\left[Y_{\overline{a},k+1} \mid \overline{a}_{m-1}, \overline{\ell}_{m-1}, v_0^*\right]\right\} .
\end{aligned} \tag{8.55}$$

However, to obtain an unrestricted variation-independent parameterization, we cannot directly parameterize $m_{k+1}\left(\overline{\ell}_m, \overline{a}_k\right)$ and $m_{k+1}^*\left(\overline{\ell}_m, \overline{a}_k\right)$. However, we can take the following approach. Define

$$\begin{aligned}
q_m\left(k+1, \overline{\ell}_m, \overline{a}_k, a_m^*\right) &\equiv \Phi^{-1}\left\{E\left(Y_{\overline{a},k+1} \mid \overline{\ell}_m, \overline{a}_m\right)\right\} \\
&\quad - \Phi^{-1}\left\{E\left(Y_{\overline{a},k+1} \mid \overline{\ell}_m, \overline{a}_{m-1}, a_m^*\right)\right\}
\end{aligned} \tag{8.56}$$

and

(8.57a)
$$\nu_m^*\left(k+1,\overline{\ell}_m,\overline{a}_k\right)=\Phi^{-1}\left\{E\left(Y_{\overline{a},k+1}\mid\overline{\ell}_m,\overline{a}_{m-1}\right)\right\} - \Phi^{-1}\left\{E\left(Y_{\overline{a},k+1}\mid\overline{\ell}_{m-1},\overline{a}_{m-1},\ell_m=0\right)\right\},\ m>0$$

where $\ell_m=0$ is a baseline level of ℓ_m and

(8.57b)
$$\nu_m^*\left(k+1,\overline{\ell}_m,\overline{a}_k\right)=\Phi^{-1}\left\{E\left(Y_{\overline{a},k+1}\mid\overline{\ell}_m,\overline{a}_{m-1}\right)\right\} - \Phi^{-1}\left\{E\left(Y_{\overline{a},k+1}\mid v_0^*,\ell_0\backslash v_0^*=0\right)\right\},\ m=0$$

where $L_0\backslash V_0^*$ are those components of L_0 other than V_0^*.

We thus obtain that for $\Phi(x)=x$ or e^x

(8.58)
$$m_{k+1}\left(\overline{\ell}_m,\overline{a}_k\right)= -\Phi^{-1}\int\Phi\left[-q_m\left(k+1,\overline{\ell}_m,\overline{a}_k,a_m^*\right)\right]dF\left[a_m^*\mid\overline{\ell}_m,\overline{a}_{m-1}\right].$$

When $\Phi(x)=e^x/(1+e^x)$,

(8.59)
$$m_{k+1}\left(\overline{\ell}_m,\overline{a}_k\right)=\Phi^{-1}(p)-\Phi^{-1}\left\{E\left(Y_{\overline{a},k+1}\mid\overline{\ell}_m,\overline{a}_{m-1}\right)\right\}$$

where $p=p\left(k+1,\overline{\ell}_m,\overline{a}_k\right)$ is the unique solution to

(8.60)
$$E\left(Y_{\overline{a},k+1}\mid\overline{\ell}_m,\overline{a}_{m-1}\right)= \int\left\{1+(1-p)p^{-1}\exp\left[q_m(k+1,\overline{\ell}_m,\overline{a}_k,a_m^*)\right]\right\}^{-1}dF\left(a_m^*\mid\overline{\ell}_m,\overline{a}_{m-1}\right).$$

Furthermore, we have

(8.61)
$$m_{k+1}^*\left(\overline{\ell}_m,\overline{a}_k\right)=\nu_m^*\left(k+1,\overline{\ell}_m,\overline{a}_k\right)-\Gamma^*\left(k+1,\overline{\ell}_{m-1},\overline{a}_k,v_0^*\right)$$

where

(8.62a)
$$\Gamma^*\left(k+1,\overline{\ell}_{m-1},\overline{a}_k,v_0^*\right)=-\Phi^{-1}\left[E\left(Y_{\overline{a},k+1}\mid\overline{\ell}_{m-1},\ell_m=0,\overline{a}_{m-1}\right)\right] +\Phi^{-1}\left[E\left(Y_{\overline{a},k+1}\mid\overline{\ell}_{m-1},\overline{a}_{m-1}\right)\right],\ m>0$$

and

(8.62b)
$$\Gamma^*\left(k+1,\overline{\ell}_{m-1},\overline{a}_k,v_0^*\right)=-\Phi^{-1}\left[E\left(Y_{\overline{a},k+1}\mid v_0^*,\ell_0\backslash v_0^*=0\right)\right] +\Phi^{-1}\left[E\left(Y_{\overline{a},k+1}\mid v_0^*\right)\right],\ m=0\ .$$

For $\Phi(x)=x$ or e^x

(8.63)
$$\Gamma^*\left(k+1,\overline{\ell}_{m-1},\overline{a}_k,v_0^*\right)= \Phi^{-1}\left[\int\Phi\left[\nu_m^*\left(k+1,\overline{\ell}_m,\overline{a}_k\right)\right]dF\left[\ell_m\mid\overline{\ell}_{m-1},\overline{a}_{m-1},v_0^*\right]\right],$$

while, for $\Phi(x) = e^x/(1+e^x)$, $\exp\left\{-\Gamma^*\left(k+1,\bar{\ell}_{m-1},\bar{a}_k,v_0^*\right)\right\}$ is the unique solution x to

$$(8.64)\qquad \begin{aligned}&(1-p)^2 = \\ &\int\left[(1-p)\,\nu_m^*\left(k+1,\bar{\ell}_m,\bar{a}_k\right)x^{-1}+p\right]^{-1}dF\left[\ell_m \mid \bar{\ell}_{m-1},\bar{a}_{m-1},v_0^*\right]\end{aligned}$$

with

$$(8.65)\qquad p \equiv E\left[Y_{\bar{a},k+1} \mid \bar{\ell}_{m-1},\bar{a}_{m-1},v_0^*\right]\ .$$

To construct the likelihood function for non-parametric, semiparametric, and/or parametric versions of our marginal structural mean model, we consider again the sets of densities (8.44a)–(8.44c). We will also consider the following sets of functions.

$$(8.66a)\qquad \left\{\gamma_{k+1}^*\left(\bar{a}_k,v_0^*;\psi\right);\psi\in\boldsymbol{\psi}\right\}$$

$$(8.66b)\quad \left\{q_m(k+1,\bar{\ell}_m,\bar{a}_k,a_m^*;\mu_1);\ q_m(k+1,\bar{\ell}_m,\bar{a}_k,a_m)=0\ \textit{and}\ \mu_1\in\boldsymbol{\mu}_1\right\}$$

and

$$(8.66c)\qquad \begin{aligned}&\Big\{\nu_m^*\left(k+1,\bar{\ell}_m,\bar{a}_k;\mu_2\right);\\ &\qquad \nu_m^*\left(k+1,\bar{\ell}_{m-1},v_0^*,\ell_m\backslash v_0^*=0,\bar{a}_k;\mu_2\right)=0\ \textit{and}\ \mu_2\in\boldsymbol{\mu}_2\Big\}\ .\end{aligned}$$

$$(8.66d)\qquad \left\{s\left(v_0^*;\omega\right);\omega\in\boldsymbol{\omega}\right\}\ .$$

In (8.66c), we set $\ell_m\backslash v_0^*$ to be ℓ_m if $m\neq 0$. Then the likelihood function can be written again as (8.47) with $\varepsilon_{k+1}(\rho)$ as in (8.48), $\rho = (\psi,\eta,\gamma,\mu,\omega)$ with variation-independent components and ψ, μ, and ω as redefined in (8.66), with $E\left[Y_0 \mid \overline{L}_{-1},\overline{A}_{-1},V_0^*;\rho\right] = s\left(V_0^*;\omega\right)$, and $E\big[Y_{k+1} \mid \overline{L}_k,\overline{A}_k;\rho\big]$ for $k\geq 0$ given by the RHS of (8.53), except with the parameterized versions of $m_{k+1}\left(\bar{\ell}_m,\bar{a}_k\right)$, $m_{k+1}^*\left(\bar{\ell}_m,\bar{a}_k\right)$, and $\gamma_{k+1}^*\left(\bar{a}_k,v_0^*\right)$ replacing the unparameterized versions. Note by (8.58), (8.59), (8.61), (8.62), (8.63), and (8.64) $m_{k+1}\left(\bar{\ell}_m,\bar{a}_k\right)$ and $m_{k+1}^*\left(\bar{\ell}_m,\bar{a}_k\right)$ can be parameterized in terms of the parameter ρ. Again, there is no parameter γ_1 when Y_k is dichotomous and $\Phi(x) = e^x/(1+e^x)$. The components of ρ will be variation independent under the same conditions described in Remark 8.9.

REMARK 8.15. With the MSM-specific redefinitions of the various quantities, Remarks 8.9–8.13 of Sec. 8.5 continue to hold for MSMs. In the next section, we provide a semiparametric estimator for the parameter ψ of a marginal structural mean model with $\Phi(x) = x$ or e^x when the parameter η is finite-dimensional.

REMARK 8.16. The sharp null hypothesis that

$$\overline{Y}_{\overline{a},K+1} = \overline{Y}_{\overline{a}^*,K+1} \text{ w.p.1 for all } \overline{a} \text{ and } \overline{a}^* \tag{8.67}$$

implies

$$\gamma^*_{k+1}\left(\overline{a}_k, v^*_0\right) \text{ does not depend on } \overline{a}_k \tag{8.68a}$$

$$\nu^*_m\left(k+1, \overline{\ell}_m, \overline{a}_k\right) \text{ depends on } \overline{a}_k \text{ only through } \overline{a}_{m-1}\,. \tag{8.68b}$$

$$q_m\left(k+1, \overline{\ell}_m, \overline{a}_k, a^*_m\right) \equiv q_m\left(k+1, \overline{\ell}_m, \left\{\overline{a}_{m-1}, a_m\right\}, a^*_m\right) \text{ depends on } \overline{a}_k \text{ only through } \overline{a}_m \tag{8.68c}$$

$$q_m\left(k+1, \overline{\ell}_m, \{\overline{a}_{m-1}, a_m\}, a^*_m\right) = -q_m\left(k+1, \overline{\ell}_m, \{\overline{a}_{m-1}, a^*_m\}, a_m\right) \text{ is anti-symmetric in } a_m \text{ and } a^*_m\,. \tag{8.68d}$$

The above implies that, in contrast with SNMs, if we are performing a sensitivity analysis in which we fix the non-identifiable function q_m, then, in order to test the null hypothesis (8.67) it is necessary for us to restrict our choice of q_m. In particular, our choice of q_m must satisfy (8.68c) and (8.68d), which can be shown to be the only restrictions on q_m implied by (8.67).

Restrictions (8.68c) and (8.68d) together are equivalent to the condition that $r_m\left(k+1, \overline{\ell}_m, \overline{a}_k, a^*_m\right) = 0$ where $r_m\left(k+1, \overline{\ell}_m, \overline{a}_k, a^*_m\right) \equiv q_m\left(k+1, \overline{\ell}_m, \overline{a}_k, a^*_m\right) - q_m\left(k+1, \overline{\ell}_m\left(\overline{a}_{m-1}, 0\right), a^*_m\right) + q_m\left(k+1, \overline{\ell}_m, \left(\overline{a}_{m-1}, 0\right), a_m\right)$. Note, with $\Phi(x) = x$,

$$\begin{aligned}
&r_m\left(k+1, \overline{\ell}_m, \overline{a}_k, a^*_m\right)\\
&\quad= \left\{E\left[Y_{\overline{a},k+1} \mid \overline{\ell}_m, \overline{a}_m\right] - E\left[Y_{(\overline{a}_{m-1},0),k+1} \mid \overline{\ell}_m, \overline{a}_m\right]\right\}\\
&\qquad - \left\{E\left[Y_{\overline{a},k+1} \mid \overline{\ell}_m, \overline{a}_{m-1}, a^*_m\right] - E\left[Y_{(\overline{a}_{m-1},0),k+1} \mid \overline{\ell}_m, \overline{a}_{m-1}, a^*_m\right]\right\}
\end{aligned}$$

which has an interpretation as a type of current-treatment interaction function.

It would be unlikely to hold prior beliefs that (8.68a) is true but (8.67) is false. This implies it would be unlikely to hold prior beliefs that (8.68a) is true, but (8.68c) and/or (8.68d) were false. Thus, in conducting a sensitivity analysis which treats the selection bias function $q_m\left(k+1, \overline{\ell}_m, \overline{a}_k, a^*_m\right)$ as known and then tests (8.68a) from the data, it would be important to choose $q_m\left(k+1, \overline{\ell}_m, \overline{a}_k, a^*_m\right)$ to satisfy (8.68c) and (8.68d), which can be accomplish by setting $r_m\left(k+1, \overline{\ell}_m, \overline{a}_k, a^*_m\right) = 0$ and then choosing the single function $q_m\left(k+1, \overline{\ell}_m, \left(\overline{a}_{m-1}, 0\right), a_m\right)$. It follows that this same approach to choosing $q_m\left(k+1,\bar{\ell}_m,\bar{a}_k,a_m^*\right)$ should be used whenever one wishes to test the hypothesis (8.67).

REMARK 8.17. **Direct effect null hypothesis:** Suppose that $\overline{A}_K = \left(\overline{A}_{PK},\overline{A}_{ZK}\right)$ where P and Z refer to two different treatments. The sharp null hypothesis that $\overline{A}_{PK}$ has no direct effect on $\overline{Y}_{K+1}$ when treatment $\overline{A}_{ZK}$ is set to a particular value $\overline{a}_{ZK}$ is the hypothesis

$$\overline{Y}_{(\bar{a}_P,\bar{a}_Z)} = \overline{Y}_{\left(\bar{a}_P^*,\bar{a}_Z\right)} \ \textit{w.p.1 for all } \bar{a}_P,\bar{a}_P^*,\bar{a}_Z^* \ . \tag{8.69}$$

This implies that

$$\gamma_{k+1}^*\left(\bar{a}_k,v_0^*\right) = \gamma_{k+1}^*\left(\bar{a}_{Zk},v_0^*\right) \tag{8.70}$$

$$\nu_m^*\left(k+1,\bar{\ell}_m,\bar{a}_k\right) = \nu_m^*\left(k+1,\bar{\ell}_m,\left(\bar{a}_{m-1},\bar{a}_{Zk}\right)\right) \tag{8.71}$$

$$q_m^*\left(k+1,\bar{\ell}_m,\bar{a}_k,a_m^*\right) = q_m^*\left(k+1,\bar{\ell}_m,\left\{\bar{a}_{Zk},\bar{a}_{Pm}\right\},a_m^*\right) \tag{8.72}$$

and

$$\begin{aligned} &q_m^*\left(k+1,\bar{\ell}_m,\left(\bar{a}_{Zk},\bar{a}_{Pm}\right),\left(a_{Zm},a_{Pm}^*\right)\right) \\ &\quad = -q_m^*\left(k+1,\bar{\ell}_m,\left(\bar{a}_{Zk},\bar{a}_{P(m-1)},a_{Pm}^*\right),\left(a_{Zm},a_{Pm}\right)\right) \ . \end{aligned} \tag{8.73}$$

It is important to note in (8.73) that there is no a_{Zm}^* in addition to a_{Zm}.

REMARK 8.18. **Inadequacies of MSMs and SNMs for sensitivity analysis in randomized trials with non-compliance:** Consider a randomized trial with all or none compliance in which the observed data are $(A_0,A_1,Y=Y_2)$, all of which are dichotomous. $A_0 \equiv A_{P0}$ is a randomization indicator, $A_1 \equiv A_{Z1}$ is the actual treatment, and $Y=Y_2$ is the observed outcome. We make the exclusion restriction that A_0 has no direct effect on Y when A_1 is fixed, i.e.,

$$Y_{(0,a_1)} = Y_{(1,a_1)} \equiv Y_{a_1} \ \textit{w.p.1 for } a_1 \in \{0,1\} \ . \tag{8.74}$$

Further, since A_0 is randomized, we assume

$$A_0 \coprod \left(Y_1,Y_0\right) \ . \tag{8.75}$$

Now, given data $(A_0,A_1,Y\equiv Y_{A_1})$ all dichotomous, a marginal structural mean model with $\Phi(x) = e^x/(1+e^x)$ has 15 parameters: $f(a_0,a_1)$ has 3 parameters, and $\gamma_1^*(a_0,a_1)$, $q_0\left[(a_0,a_1),a_0^*=(1-a_0)\right]$, and $q_1\left[\left(a_0,a_1\right),a_1^*=(1-a_1)\right]$ have 4 each. Now our restrictions (8.74) and (8.75) imply that

$$\gamma_1^*\left(a_0,a_1\right) = \gamma_1^*\left(1-a_0,a_1\right) \equiv \gamma_1^*\left(a_1\right) \tag{8.76}$$

and

$$q_0 \left[(a_0, a_1), a_0^* = (1 - a_0) \right] = 0 \; . \tag{8.77}$$

However, in the absence of knowledge of the distribution of the observed data F_O, these restrictions (8.74)–(8.75) place no other functional equality constraints on the remaining 9 parameters $\gamma_1^*(a_1)$, $q_1\big((a_0, a_1), \; a_1^* = 1 - a_1\big)$, and $f(a_0, a_1)$. However, (8.74) plus the "marginal" randomization assumption

$$A_0 \coprod Y_{a_1}; a_1 \in \{0, 1\} \tag{8.78}$$

also imply (8.76) and (8.77). Now suppose we are given the distribution F_O of $O = (A_0, A_1, Y)$. This distribution has 7 parameters, so if we impose (8.76) and (8.77), we would not generally expect the parameter of interest $\gamma_1^*(a_1)$ to be identified. Now since (8.74) and (8.78) imply (8.76) and (8.77), the so-called natural bounds of Robins (1989) and Manski (1990) on $E(Y_1) - E(Y_0) = \gamma_1^*(1) - \gamma_1^*(0)$ determined by F_O, (8.74) and (8.78) will have width less than or equal to the bounds determined by F_O, (8.76), and (8.77). However, Balke and Pearl (1997) shows the natural bounds can, for certain F_O, be strictly wider than the bounds determined by F_O, (8.74) and (8.75). Thus, it follows that for such an F_O, (8.74) and (8.75) imply additional constraints on the parameters of our MSM beyond (8.76) and (8.77). However, it is not easy to write down these additional constraints implying that, in general, the use of our MSM parameterization is not particularly convenient for analyzing a randomized trial with all or none compliance. [Indeed, Balke and Pearl (1997) show that, given (8.74) and (8.75), for certain special F_O, the joint distribution of (Y_0, Y_1, A_0, A_1) is identified and thus $\gamma_1^*(a_1)$ and $q_1\left[(a_0, a_1), a_1^* = 1 - a_1\right]$ are precisely known.] It can be shown similarly that our logistic SNM parameterization is also inconvenient in the same sense. However, both our MSM and our logistic SNM parameterizations should be suitable for analyzing most observational studies or randomized equivalence trials with non-compliance since *(i)* as argued in Robins (1997b), in observational studies, practicing epidemiologists give zero prior probability to the event that (8.78) or the event (8.74) are true, and *(ii)* Robins (1998c) shows that randomized equivalence trials with noncompliance, that compare a known active therapy to a new therapy, can be viewed statistically as to observational studies. An exception would be observational studies in which one thinks there may be a "near instrument" such as studies of the effect of education on schooling where the month in which a student dropped out of high school is considered an instrument.

REMARK 8.19. In our parameterization of MSMs, we could have replaced the parameter $q_m\left(k+1, \overline{\ell}_m, \overline{a}_k, a_m^*\right)$ of (8.56) by

$$\begin{aligned} &q_m\left(k+1, \overline{\ell}_m, \overline{a}_k\right) \equiv \\ &\Phi^{-1}\big\{E(Y_{\overline{a},k+1} \mid \overline{\ell}_m, \overline{a}_m)\big\} - \Phi^{-1}\big\{E(Y_{\overline{a},k+1} \mid \overline{\ell}_m, \overline{a}_{m-1}, A_m \neq a_m)\big\}. \end{aligned} \tag{8.79}$$

With this parameterization, the marginal structural mean model with $\Phi(x) = e^x / (1 + e^x)$ is a special case of the selection odds model of Sec. 7 and thus remains, based on the results of that section, a NPI model. In addition, as noted in that section, if A_m is a continuous random variable and $pr\left[A_m = a_m \mid \bar{\ell}_m, \bar{a}_{m-1}\right] = 0$ for all a_m, then the density $f\left(a_m \mid \bar{\ell}_m, \bar{a}_{m-1}\right)$ remains ancillary for the parameter ψ. That is, Remark 8.12 of Sec. 8.5 holds for all functions $q_m\left(k+1, \bar{\ell}_m, \bar{a}_k\right)$, rather than just holding when the function is identically zero (i.e., when there is no confounding). It also follows that the MSM parameterization described in this section can be used as a parameterization of our selection odds model of Sec. 7, for purposes of fully parametric likelihood-based inference.

Unfortunately, as we now describe, there is a major difficulty with using the parameterization discussed in this remark if we wish to test the null hypothesis (8.67). Therefore, the approach described in the last paragraph of Remark 8.16 of this subsection should be used. The null hypothesis (8.67) implies not only that $q_m\left(k+1, \bar{\ell}_m, \bar{a}_k\right)$ is a function of $\bar{a}_k$ only through $\bar{a}_m$, but it also implies additional joint restrictions on $q_m\left(k+1, \bar{\ell}_m, \bar{a}_k\right)$ and the identifiable density $f\left(a_m \mid \bar{\ell}_m, \bar{a}_{m-1}\right)$. Suppose, therefore, that one takes the point of view that it is *a priori* unlikely that (8.68a) is true but (8.67) is false (although this is logically possible). Then it is not appropriate to simply use the parameterization $q_m\left(k+1, \bar{\ell}_m, \bar{a}_k\right)$ of (8.79) for the selection bias function in an estimation procedure which treats this function as known and then tests (8.68a) from the data, as there is no guarantee that the joint restriction on the chosen $q_m\left(k+1, \bar{\ell}_m, \bar{a}_k\right)$ and $f\left(a_m \mid \bar{\ell}_m, \bar{a}_{m-1}\right)$ implied by (8.67) will be fulfilled.

8.6.2. Semiparametric inference in marginal structural mean models. We consider a marginal structural mean model in which

(8.80a) $q_m\left(k+1, \bar{L}_m, \bar{A}_k, a_m^*\right)$ *is known*

(8.80b) ψ *in (8.66a) is a finite dimensional vector with true value* ψ^*

(8.80c) η *in (8.44a) is a finite dimensional vector with true value* η^* .

Let $g_k\left(\bar{A}_k, V_0^*\right)$ and $s_k\left(\bar{A}_k, \bar{L}_k\right)$ be, respectively, user-specified $\dim\psi + \dim\eta$ and $\dim\eta$ vector-valued functions. Let

$$W^\dagger(\eta) = W^\dagger(\eta, s) =$$

$$\left(0', \left[\sum_{k=0}^{K} s_k(\bar{A}_k, \bar{L}_k) - \int s(\bar{A}_k, \bar{L}_k) dF(A_k \mid \bar{A}_{k-1}, \bar{L}_k; \eta)\right]'\right)' \tag{8.81}$$

where 0 is a $\dim\psi$ vector of 0's. Let $g\left(\bar{A}, V_0^*\right)$ be the $(\dim\psi + \dim\eta) \times (K+1)$ matrix-valued function with columns $g_k\left(\bar{A}_k, V_0^*\right), k = 0, \ldots, K$.

Let

$$H_k(\psi,\eta) =$$

$$\left\{Y_{k+1} - \sum_{m=0}^{k} \int q_m\left(k+1, \overline{L}_m, \overline{A}_k, a_m^*\right) dF\left(a_m^* \mid \overline{L}_m, \overline{A}_{m-1}; \eta\right) - \gamma_{k+1}^*\left(\overline{A}_k, V_0^*; \psi\right)\right\} \Big/ \left\{\prod_{m=0}^{k} f\left[A_m \mid \overline{A}_{m-1}, \overline{L}_m\right]\right\}, \tag{8.82a}$$

for $\Phi(x) = x$

$$H_k(\psi,\eta) =$$

$$\left\{Y_{k+1} \prod_{m=0}^{k} \int \exp\left\{-q_m(k+1, \overline{L}_m, \overline{A}_k, a_m^*)\right\} dF(a_m^* \mid \overline{L}_m, \overline{A}_{m-1}; \eta) - \exp\left\{\gamma_{k+1}^*\left(\overline{A}_k, V_0^*; \psi\right)\right\}\right\} \Big/ \left\{\prod_{m=0}^{k} f\left[A_m \mid \overline{A}_{m-1}, \overline{L}_m\right]\right\}, \tag{8.82b}$$

for $\Phi(x) = e^x$.

Let

$$W(\psi,\eta) \equiv W(\psi,\eta,g) = g\left(\overline{A}, V_0^*\right)\left[H_0(\psi,\eta), \ldots, H_K(\psi,\eta)\right]' .$$

THEOREM 8.14. *In the semiparametric marginal structural mean model characterized by (8.80) if* $\Phi(x) = x$ *or* e^x*, then, subject to regularity conditions,*
(a). $E\left[W(\psi^*,\eta^*)\right] = 0$*, and* $E\left[W^\dagger(\eta^*)\right] = 0$*;*
(b). $\left(\widehat{\psi},\widehat{\eta}\right) = \left(\widehat{\psi}(g,s), \widehat{\eta}(g,s)\right)$ *solving*

$$0 = \sum_i W_i(\psi,\eta) + W_i^\dagger(\eta) \tag{8.83}$$

is a consistent asymptotically normal estimator of (ψ^*,η^*)*;*
(c). $\left\{W(\psi,\eta;g) + W^\dagger(\eta,s)\right\}$*, as g and s vary, is the orthogonal complement to the nuisance tangent space for the model; (d). There exists* g_{eff}, s_{eff} *such that the asymptotic variance of* $\left[\widehat{\psi}(g_{eff}, s_{eff}), \widehat{\eta}(g_{eff}, s_{eff})\right]$ *attains the semiparametric variance bound for the model. The crucial result 1 is proved in Appendix B.*

REMARK 8.20. An alternative estimation procedure is to first estimate η by the partial likelihood estimator $\widehat{\eta}$ maximizing $\prod_{i=1}^{n} PL_i(\eta)$ where

$$PL(\eta) = \prod_{m=0}^{K} f\left[A_m \mid \overline{L}_m, \overline{A}_{m-1}; \eta\right] . \tag{8.84}$$

We then estimate ψ by the solution to $0 = \sum_i W_i(\psi, \widehat{\eta}) = 0$ with each $g_k(\cdot, \cdot)$ now a $\dim \psi$ vector-valued function. This class will not contain a semiparametric efficient estimator. However, this class avoids the need to compute the integral in (8.81).

REMARK 8.21. The integral in (8.82a) and (8.82b) can be difficult to compute. The need to compute the integral can be avoided in two different ways. The first way is to change the model by replacing the known $q\left(k+1, \overline{L}_m, \overline{A}_k, a_m^*\right)$ by $q_m\left(k+1, \overline{L}_m, \overline{A}_k\right)$ of Eq. (8.79). Then, for example, in defining $H_k(\psi, \eta)$, we would replace the integral in (8.81a) by $\left\{f\left(A_m \mid \overline{L}_m, \overline{A}_{m-1}\right) + \left[1 - f\left(A_m \mid \overline{L}_m, \overline{A}_{m-1}\right)\right] q_m\left(k+1, \overline{L}_m, \overline{A}_k\right)\right\}$ if $pr\left[A_m = a_m \mid \overline{L}_m, \overline{A}_{m-1}\right] \neq 0$ for $a_m = A_m$ and by $q_m\left(k+1, \overline{L}_m, \overline{A}_k\right)$ if $pr\left[A_m = a_m \mid \overline{L}_m, \overline{A}_{m-1}\right] = 0$ for $a_m = A_m$. In this latter case, the partial likelihood estimator of η is efficient, $f\left(A_m \mid \overline{L}_m, \overline{A}_{m-1}\right)$ is ancillary for ψ, and the class of estimators in Remark 8.20 will include an efficient estimator.

A second approach to avoiding the integrals in (8.82a) and (8.92b) is to sample. Specifically, suppose $\Phi(x) = x$. Then we redefine $H_k(\psi, \eta)$ in (8.82a) as

$$H_k(\psi, \eta) = Y_{k+1} - J^{-1} \sum_{j=1}^{J} \sum_{m=0}^{k} q_m\left(k+1, \overline{L}_m, \overline{A}_k, a_m^{*j}\right) - \gamma_{k+1}^*\left(\overline{A}_k, V_0^*; \psi\right)$$

where the a_m^{*j} are independent draws from $f\left[a_m \mid \overline{L}_m, \overline{A}_{m-1}; \eta\right]$. A related algorithm is available when $\Phi(x) = e^x$.

REMARK 8.22. Note that our estimator of ψ under the model (8.80) did not require that we compute a "non-parametric smooth" (i.e., an estimate of conditional expectation or density whose functional form is left unrestricted by the model (8.80)). In contrast, it can be shown that to estimate model ψ in model (8.80) with $\Phi(x) = e^x / (1 + e^x)$, we would have to estimate such a "non-parametric smooth," which is not feasible in moderate sized samples due to the curse of dimensionality. Formally, this can be expressed by the fact that the curse of dimensionality-appropriate information bound is zero for ψ in model (8.80) when $\Phi(x) = e^x / (1 + e^x)$ but is positive when $\Phi(x) = x$ or e^x. The reason for this is that the expectation operator E is a linear operator and thus commutes with addition (i.e., $\Phi(x) = x$) and multiplication ($\Phi(x) = e^x$).

REMARK 8.23. A continuous time version of a marginal structural model in which the treatment process can jump in continuous time is as follows. For simplicity, we consider an outcome $Y = Y(\tau)$ with counterfactuals $Y_{\overline{a}}, \overline{a} = \{a(u); 0 \leq u \leq \tau\} \in \mathcal{A}$. Here, τ is a fixed, non-random end-of-follow-up time. We assume

$$\Phi^{-1}\left[E\left(Y_{\overline{a}} \mid V_0^*\right)\right] = \gamma^*\left(\overline{a}, V_0^*\right) \tag{8.85}$$

for a known continuous increasing function Φ. Further we assume

$$\gamma^*(\bar{a}, V_0^*) \in \{\gamma^*(\bar{a}, V_0^*; \psi); \psi \in \boldsymbol{\psi}\} . \tag{8.86}$$

We assume the processes $\overline{L}(u)$ and $\overline{A}(u)$ have CADLAG sample paths, and we let $L(t^-)$ and $A(t^-)$ be the left-hand limits of $A(u)$ and $L(u)$ as $u \uparrow t$. Further, for simplicity, we assume $A(t) \in \{0, 1)$ and that the hazard (intensity)

$$\lambda_A\left(t \mid \overline{L}(t^-), \overline{A}(t^-)\right) = \lim_{h \to 0} h^{-1} pr\left[A(t+h) \neq A(t^-) \mid \overline{L}(t^-), \overline{A}(t^-)\right]$$

is uniformly bounded and smooth as a function of t with probability 1. Let

$$\begin{aligned} q\left(t, \bar{\ell}(t^-), \bar{a}\right) = {} & \Phi^{-1}\left\{E\left(Y_{\bar{a}} \mid \bar{\ell}(t^-), \bar{a}(t)\right)\right\} \\ & - \Phi^{-1}\left\{E\left(Y_{\bar{a}} \mid \bar{\ell}(t^-), \bar{a}(t^-), A(t) \neq a(t)\right)\right\}. \end{aligned} \tag{8.87}$$

If $\Phi(x) = x$, let

$$\begin{aligned} H(\psi) \equiv {} & \Big\{Y - \sum_{\{u; A(u) \neq A(u^-)\}} q(u, \overline{L}(u^-), \overline{A}) \\ & - \int_0^\tau q(t, \overline{L}(t^-), \overline{A}) \lambda_A(t \mid \overline{L}(t^-), \overline{A}(t^-))\, dt - \gamma^*(\overline{A}, V_0^*; \psi)\Big\} \Big/ \\ & \Big\{\prod_{\{u; A(u) \neq A(u^-)\}} \lambda_A[u \mid \overline{L}(u^-), \overline{A}(u^-)] \exp\Big[-\int_0^\tau \lambda_A(t \mid \overline{L}(t^-), \overline{A}(t^-))\, dt\Big]\Big\}. \end{aligned} \tag{8.88}$$

If $\Phi(x) = e^x$, let

$$\begin{aligned} H(\psi) = {} & \\ & \Big\{Y \exp\Big[-\sum_{\{u; A(u) \neq A(u^-)\}} q\left(u, \overline{L}(u^-), \overline{A}\right) + z\left(\overline{L}, \overline{A}\right)\Big] - \gamma^*\left(\overline{A}, V_0^*; \psi\right)\Big\} \Big/ \\ & \Big\{\prod_{\{u; A(u) \neq A(u^-)\}} \lambda_A[u \mid \overline{L}(u^-), \overline{A}(u^-)] \exp\Big[-\int_0^\tau \lambda_A(t \mid \overline{L}(t^-), \overline{A}(t^-))\, dt\Big]\Big\}, \end{aligned} \tag{8.89}$$

where

$$z\left(\overline{L}, \overline{A}\right) \equiv \int_0^\tau \left\{\exp\left[-q\left(t, \overline{L}(t^-), \overline{A}\right)\right] - 1\right\} \lambda_A\left(t \mid \overline{L}(t^-), \overline{A}(t^-)\right) dt .$$

Let $W(\psi) \equiv W(\psi, g) = g\left(\overline{A}, V_0^*\right) H(\psi)$ where $g(\bar{a}, V_0^*)$ is a function chosen by the investigator, usually chosen to be of dimension of ψ when ψ is finite-dimensional. Our main result is the following.

THEOREM 8.15. $E[W(\psi^*)] = 0$ *where* ψ^* *is the true value of* ψ *in (8.86).*

Proof. It follows from Theorem (8.14a) by letting the time δt between measurements at k and $k+1$ go to zero. It also can be shown directly by the continuous time version of the proof of Theorem (8.14a) in Appendix B. □

In practice, in order to estimate ψ^*, we will in general specify a model such as the Cox proportional hazards model

$$\lambda_A\left(t \mid \overline{L}\left(t^-\right), \overline{A}\left(t^-\right)\right) = \lambda_0(t) \exp\left(\eta_0' H(t)\right)$$

where $H(t)$ is a known vector-valued function of $\left(\overline{L}\left(t^-\right), \overline{A}\left(t^-\right)\right)$ and $\lambda_0(t)$ is an unspecified positive function, and η_0 is an unknown parameter vector to be estimated. We then estimate ψ by solving the equation $\sum_i W_i(\psi) = 0$ with $\lambda_A\left(t \mid \overline{A}\left(t^-\right), \overline{L}\left(t^-\right)\right)$ replaced by its estimate based on the above Cox model.

8.7. Marginal structural distribution models. In this section, for ease of presentation, we only consider univariate marginal structural distribution models. The generalization to include multivariate marginal structural distribution models is straightforward. A univariate marginal structural distribution model specifies a model for a counterfactual continuous outcome $Y_{\overline{a}} \equiv Y_{\overline{a}(K+1)}$ measured at end of follow-up as a function of baseline variables V_0^*. In this setting, we have the observed data $O = \left(\overline{L}, \overline{A}, Y\right) = \left(\overline{L}_K, \overline{A}_K, Y_{K+1}\right)$. Then our model states

$$f_{Y_{\overline{a}}}\left(y \mid V_0^*\right) \in \left\{f\left(y \mid V_0^*; \psi\right); \psi \in \boldsymbol{\psi}\right\} \tag{8.90}$$

where $f\left(y \mid V_0^*; \psi\right)$ is a known density depending on an unknown parameter (possibly infinite dimensional) ψ.

8.7.1. Likelihood inference for marginal structural distribution models. We shall consider the likelihood based on the following parameterization. This parameterization is useful for the semiparametric sensitivity analysis estimators described in Sec. 8.7.2 below. However, for fully parametric likelihood-based inference, as we shall see, this parameterization results in essentially an intractable likelihood function.

Let $m\left(y, \overline{\ell}_m, \overline{a}\right)$ be the unique increasing function of y satisfying

$$pr\left[m\left(Y_{\overline{a}}, \overline{\ell}_m, \overline{a}\right) < y \mid \overline{\ell}_m, \overline{a}_m\right] = pr\left(Y_{\overline{a}} < y \mid \overline{\ell}_m, \overline{a}_{m-1}\right) . \tag{8.91}$$

Let $m^*\left(y, \overline{\ell}_m, \overline{a}\right)$ be the unique increasing function of y satisfying

$$pr\left[m^*(Y_{\overline{a}}, \overline{\ell}_m, \overline{a}) < y \mid \overline{\ell}_m, \overline{a}_{m-1}\right] = pr\left[Y_{\overline{a}} < y \mid \overline{\ell}_{m-1}, \overline{a}_{m-1}, v_0^*\right] . \tag{8.92}$$

Set

$$M_{K+1}^* = Y$$

for $k = K, K-1, \ldots, 0$, set

$$M_k = m\left(M_{k+1}^*, \overline{L}_m, \overline{A}\right) \tag{8.93}$$

and

$$M_k^* = m^* \left(M_k, \overline{L}_m, \overline{A}\right) \ . \tag{8.94}$$

By the proof of Theorem 11.1 in Robins (1999), we have

$$M_0^* \coprod \overline{L}_K \mid \overline{A}_K \tag{8.95}$$

$$f_{M_0^*}\left(y \mid \overline{A}_k, V_0^*\right) = f_{Y_{\overline{a}}}\left(y \mid V_0^*\right) \tag{8.96}$$

$$f\left(O\right) = \left\{\partial M_0^* / \partial Y\right\} f\left[M_0^* \mid \overline{A}_k, V_0^*\right] f\left(\overline{L}_K, \overline{A}_K\right) \ . \tag{8.97}$$

However, to obtain an unrestricted variation-independent parameterization, we cannot directly parameterize $m\left(y, \overline{\ell}_m, \overline{a}\right)$ and $m^*\left(y, \overline{\ell}_m, \overline{a}\right)$. To see the problem, we first consider the following failed parameterization motivated by our successful parameterization of marginal structural mean models. Let $q\left(y, \overline{\ell}_m, \overline{a}, a_m^*\right)$ be defined by

$$pr\left[q(Y_{\overline{a}}, \overline{\ell}_m, \overline{a}, a_m^*) < y \mid \overline{\ell}_m, \overline{a}_m\right] = pr\left[Y_{\overline{a}} < y \mid \overline{\ell}_m, \overline{a}_{m-1}, a_m^*\right] \ . \tag{8.98}$$

Let $\nu^*\left(y, \overline{\ell}_m, \overline{a}\right)$ be defined by

$$pr\left[\nu^*(Y_{\overline{a}}, \overline{\ell}_m, \overline{a}) > y \mid \overline{\ell}_m, \overline{a}_{m-1}\right] = pr\left[Y_{\overline{a}} > y \mid \overline{\ell}_{m-1}, \overline{a}_{m-1}, \ell_m \backslash v_0^* = 0\right], \tag{8.99}$$

where $\ell_m \backslash v_0^* = \ell_m$ for $m \neq 0$. Now consider sets of functions.

$$\left\{q\left(y, \overline{\ell}_m, \overline{a}, a_m^*; \mu_1\right); q\left(y, \overline{\ell}_m, \overline{a}, a_m; \mu_1\right) = y \ and \ \mu_1 \in \boldsymbol{\mu}_1\right\} \tag{8.100a}$$

$$\left\{\nu^*(y, \overline{\ell}_m, \overline{a}; \mu_2); \nu^*(y, \overline{\ell}_{m-1}, \ell_m \Big\backslash v_0^* = 0, \overline{a}; \mu_2) = y \ and \ \mu_2 \in \boldsymbol{\mu}_2\right\} \tag{8.100b}$$

and densities

$$\left\{f\left(\ell_k \mid \overline{\ell}_{k-1}, \overline{a}_{k-1}; \gamma\right); \gamma \in \boldsymbol{\gamma}, k = 0, \ldots, K\right\} \ . \tag{8.100c}$$

Then, using (8.100), (8.44), and (8.90), the likelihood function is, with $\rho = (\psi, \gamma, \eta, \mu_1, \mu_2)$,

$$\begin{aligned} f(O;\rho) &= \left\{\partial M_0^*\left(\rho\right) / \partial Y\right\} f\left[M_0^*\left(\rho\right) \mid V_0^*; \psi\right] \\ &\times \prod_{m=0}^{K} f\left[A_k \mid \overline{L}_k, \overline{A}_{k-1}; \eta\right] \prod_{m=0}^{K} f\left[L_k \mid \overline{L}_{k-1}, \overline{A}_{k-1}; \gamma\right] . \end{aligned} \tag{8.101}$$

As indicated in (8.101), there will almost always be at most one law of O and at most one random variable $M_0^*\left(\rho\right)$ associated with each choice of ρ. In particular, this will be so if $\nu^*\left(y, \overline{\ell}_m, \overline{a}; \mu_2\right)$ and $q\left(y, \overline{\ell}_m, \overline{a}, a_m; \mu_1\right)$

tend to ∞ as $y \to \infty$. However, this parameterization is not variation-independent. That is, there are parameters $\rho \in \boldsymbol{\rho} = \boldsymbol{\psi} \times \boldsymbol{\gamma} \times \boldsymbol{\eta} \times \boldsymbol{\mu}_1 \times \boldsymbol{\mu}_2$ that fail to correspond to any joint distribution. The problem is that in order to compute $m\left(y, \overline{\ell}_m, \overline{a}\right)$ and $m^*\left(y, \overline{\ell}_m, \overline{a}\right)$ in terms of the components of ρ, we need to solve integral equations that may not admit solutions. The basic problem is that the following conjecture is false.

CONJECTURE 8.1. *Given any function $q(y,x)$ satisfying $q(y,0) = y$ and increasing in y, a continuous distribution function $F(y)$, and a distribution $G(x)$ for X, there exists a joint law for (X,Y) with Y marginally distributed F, X with marginal G, and with $q(y,x)$ the quantile-quantile function linking F_x with F_0, i.e., $q(y,x) = F_x^{-1}\{F_0(y)\}$ where $F_x(y)$ is the law of Y given $X = x$ and 0 is in the support of X.*

Robins (1997b) had earlier proposed an alternative parameterization that he claimed was variation-independent. Unfortunately, this claim was incorrect. Specifically, on pg. 114 of Robins (1997b), there is suggested a parameterization, in the notation of that paper, in terms of $b(y, \overline{a})$ and $\nu^*(y, \overline{\ell}_m, \overline{a})$ which is used to obtain the quantile-quantile function $\nu(y, \overline{\ell}_m, \overline{a})$. This quantile-quantile function is analogous to our $m^*(y, \overline{\ell}_m, \overline{a})$. The difficulty is that Robins assumes that $\nu\left(y, \overline{\ell}_m, \overline{a}\right)$ so obtained is increasing in y and thus a valid quantile-quantile function. However, this is not proved and is in fact false in general.

Even though the above parameterization in terms of ρ is not variation-independent, it is nonetheless true that this submodel with q known [i.e., the set μ_1 in (8.100a) having but a single member] and the other components of ρ completely unrestricted is a non-parametric just-identified model for the law of F_O (even though certain values of ρ allowed by the model do not correspond to any joint distribution, which can create difficulties when fitting a fully parametric submodel by the method of maximum likelihood).

However, we can obtain a variation independent parametrization based on the following theorem.

THEOREM 8.16. *Given any non-negative function $q(y,x)$ satisfying $q(y,0) = 1$, a continuous distribution function $F(y)$, and a distribution $G(x)$ for X, there exists a joint law for (X,Y) with Y marginally distributed F, X with marginal G, and with $q(y,x)$ the relative risk (i.e., hazard ratio) function linking F_x with F_0, i.e., $q(y,x) = \lambda_x(y)/\lambda_0(y)$ where $\lambda_x(y)$ is the hazard of Y given $X = x$ and 0 is in the support of X.*

Proof. Define $\lambda_0(y)$ to be the unique solution to the Volterra-like integral equation

$$\lambda_0(y) = f(y) \Big/ \int \left\{ \exp\left[-\int_{-\infty}^{y} q(u,x)\lambda_0(u)\, du \right] \right\} q(y,x)\, dG(x) \ .$$

□

Then the joint law determined by $G(x)$, $q(y,x)$ and $\lambda_0(y)$ is such a joint law since upon multiplying both sides of the last display by the negative of the denominator and integrating w.r.t. to y we obtain, as required,

$$1 - F(y) = \int \left\{ \exp \left[- \int_{-\infty}^{y} q(u,x) \lambda_0 (u)\, du \right] \right\} dG(x) \; .$$

It follows that we could obtain a variation independent parametrization by redefining

$$q\left(y, \overline{\ell}_m, \overline{a}, a_m^*\right) = \lambda_{Y_{\overline{a}}} \left[y \mid \overline{\ell}_m, \overline{a}_{m-1}, a_m^*\right] \Big/ \lambda_{Y_{\overline{a}}} \left[y \mid \overline{\ell}_m, \overline{a}_m\right]$$

and

$$\nu^*\left(y, \overline{\ell}_m, \overline{a}\right) = \lambda_{Y_{\overline{a}}} \left[y \mid \overline{\ell}_m, \overline{a}_{m-1}\right] \Big/ \lambda_{Y_{\overline{a}}} \left[y \mid \overline{\ell}_{m-1}, \overline{a}_{m-1}, \ell_m \Big\backslash v_0^* = 0\right]$$

where $\lambda_{Y_{\overline{a}}}[y \mid \cdot]$ is the hazard of the random variable $Y_{\overline{a}}$. Then (8.100a) and (8.100b) need only be modified by replacing "$= y$" by "$= 1$." Note this parametrization contains the implicit assumption that the above hazard ratios are finite, which thus restricts the magnitude of selection bias that can be represented, since, for any choice of the rate ratio function $q\left(y, \overline{\ell}_m, \overline{a}, a_m^*\right)$, the support of $Y_{\overline{a}}$ among subjects with history $\overline{\ell}_m, \overline{a}_{m-1}$ is contained within that for subjects with history $\overline{\ell}_{m-1}, \overline{a}_{m-1}, \ell_m \backslash v_0^* = 0$. The previous parametrization where $q\left(y, \overline{\ell}_m, \overline{a}, a_m^*\right)$ is a quantile-quantile function does not imply a similar restriction. Furthermore in the model in which the rate ratio selection bias function $q\left(y, \overline{\ell}_m, \overline{a}, a_m^*\right)$ is specified and regarded as known, we could, in principle, reject the hypothesis that $\nu^*\left(y, \overline{\ell}_m, \overline{a}\right)$ is everywhere finite, as the hazards $\lambda_{Y_{\overline{a}}}\left[y \mid \overline{\ell}_m, \overline{a}_{m-1}\right]$ are identified from the law of the observed data, and the hazard ratio defining $\nu^*\left(y, \overline{\ell}_m, \overline{a}\right)$ may be infinite.

8.7.2. Semiparametric inference in marginal structural distribution models. Robins (1998b, Appendix 3) provides semiparametric estimators of the finite dimensional parameter β of a marginal structural distribution model in which

(8.102) $\quad q\left(y, \overline{\ell}_m, \overline{a}, a_m^*\right)$ *of Eq.(8.98) is known*

(8.103) $\quad \psi = (\beta, \theta)$ *in (8.90) is composed of a finite-dimensional parameter* of interestβ*and an infinite-dimensional nuisance parameter* θ

(8.104) $\quad \eta$ *in (8.44a) is a finite-dimensional vector.*

Specifically, Robins (1998b) gives a semiparametric estimation algorithm that provides regular, asymptotically linear estimators of β. However, in contrast to semiparametric estimation of marginal structural mean models, because the parameterization ρ described in the previous subsection is not variation-independent, it is possible that there will exist no joint distribution compatible with the estimates $\widehat{\beta}$, $\widehat{\eta}$ and the specified selection bias function q. We do not know of a simple way to check for mutual compatibility of resulting estimates and selection bias functions. Unfortunately, the variation independent parametrization described above in which the selection bias function $q\left(y, \overline{\ell}_m, \overline{a}, a^*_m\right)$ is a known hazard ratio function rather than the quantile-quantile function of Eq. (8.98) does not allow for estimation of the parameter β of this model without "high dimensional nonparametric smoothing," which is not feasible in the moderate size samples occurring in practice.

9. A General non-parametric identified (NPI) model with non-monotone non-ignorable missing data. In this section, we return to missing data models. The missing data models discussed in Secs. 2–5 assumed a monotone missing data pattern. In this section, we consider non-monotone missing data patterns. For the most part, we concentrate on settings in which there is a positive probability for each subject of observing a complete observation, without any missing data.

Robins (1997a) and Gill and Robins (1997) proposed a class of NPI models for non-monotone non-ignorable missing data called the Group Permutation Missingness (GPM) models by Robins (1997a) and Sequential Coarsening at Random models by Gill and Robins (1997). The GPM models are representable by a sequence of nested coarsening at random (CAR) models. Interestingly, a sequence of CAR models is, in general, not itself CAR. As noted by Robins (1997a), the class of GPM models has a serious drawback that prevents it from serving as an all-purpose class of missing data models with which to model non-monotone non-ignorable missing data. Specifically, GPM models do not allow for the probability that a particular variable is missing to depend on the value of that variable, although this probability can depend on the values of other missing variables. The NPI models described in Section 9.1 overcome the above deficiency of the GPM models. However, as we will see, new difficulties arise. These new difficulties are largely solved by introducing a new class of NPI models — The Selection Bias Permutation Missingness Models (PM) of Sec. 9.2.

9.1. A class of NPI models. The results in this subsection are based on joint unpublished work with Richard Gill.

Gill et al. (1997) provc in their Theorem 1 that CAR models are NPI. Our new models are based on the following generalization of their Theorem.

Let X be a discrete random variable with sample space E. We observe χ, a random subset of E. Let A denote a realization of χ. Consider the model

$$pr\,[\chi = A \mid X = x] = \pi_A q_A\,(x)\ ,\quad x \in A, \tag{9.1}$$
$$pr\,[\chi = A \mid X = x] = 0\ ,\quad x \notin A,$$

where $q_A\,(x)$ is a known function of x and A, π_A is a completely unknown function of A, and the sample space E is also unknown. Thus, for each A, $q_A\,(x)$ is a "known" selection bias function that we vary in a sensitivity analysis. Note if $q_A\,(x) = 1$ for all (A, x) (or more generally $q_A\,(x)$ does not depend on x), then model (9.1) is a NPI CAR model. Let $f_A = pr\,(\chi = A)$ denote the law of the observed data χ.

THEOREM 9.1. *Given model* (9.1) *and* f_A, *there exists* π_A *and a distribution* p_x *on some discrete sample space* E *such that* $f_A = p_A \pi_A$ *for all* A *in the power set of* E,*where* $p_A = \sum_{x \in A} q_A\,(x)\,p_x$, *for each* $x \in E$

$$\sum_{\{A;A \ni x\}} \pi_A q_A\,(x) = 1\ , \tag{9.2}$$

$\sum_{x \in E} p_x = 1$, $p_x > 0$, $\pi_A \geq 0$. *Furthermore,* π_A *and* p_A *are unique if* $f_A > 0$.

REMARK 9.1. As discussed below, there are two differences between Theorem 9.1 and Theorem 1 of Gill et al. (1997). The first and most obvious is that $q_A\,(x)$ may be a function of x for $x \in A$, in which case model (9.1) is non-ignorable (i.e., non-CAR). Secondly, the sample space E is not given beforehand. Rather it is determined by the requirement that $p_x > 0$. In contrast, in Theorem 1 of Gill et al., E was given beforehand and $p_x > 0$ was replaced by $p_x \geq 0$. As we will see below, Theorem (9.1) is false if E is given beforehand.

The proof of Theorem 9.1 follows exactly the proof of Theorem 1 in Gill et al. (1997). We obtain p_x and E by maximizing $\sum_A f_A \log p_A$ subject to the constraint that $\sum_{x \in E} p_x = 1, p_x > 0$ and then, defining $\pi_A = f_A/ p_A$ for $p_A \neq 0$. Theorem 9.1 implies that model (9.1) is a non-parametric model for the observed data χ. Furthermore, if, for all $x \in E$, $f_{\{x\}} \neq 0$ (i.e., there is a non-zero probability of observing any singleton), then the distribution p_x is identified. As we will show below, it is possible that p_x is identified even when there is not a positive probability of observing any singleton. An example will clarify the theorem.

EXAMPLE 1. Let $X = (X_0, X_1)$, where X_0 and X_1 are dichotomous $(0, 1)$ variables. Suppose there are four events A with positive probability. Specifically, observe X_0 only and it takes value 1; observe X_0 only and it is 0; observe X_1 only and it is 1; observe X_1 and it is 0. This example models a study where X_0 and X_1 are counterfactual dichotomous outcomes corresponding to a control treatment 0 and an active treatment 1,respectively, so you always observe one but not both of X_0 and X_1. If treatment has been randomly assigned, we have CAR. Otherwise, we have an observational study with non-ignorable missingness (i.e., confounding by unmeasured factors). The four possible events can be characterized as $X_0 = 1, X_0 = 0, X_1 = 1, X_1 = 0$, which we denote by $A = 1, 2, 3, 4$, respectively.

TABLE 1

		X			
		$(0,0)$	$(0,1)$	$(1,0)$	$(1,1)$
	$X_0 = 1$	0	0	$\pi_1 q_1(1,0)$	$\pi_1 q_1(1,1)$
A	$X_0 = 0$	$\pi_2 q_2(0,0)$	$\pi_2 q_2(0,1)$	0	0
	$X_1 = 1$	0	$\pi_3 q_3(0,1)$	0	$\pi_3 q_3(1,1)$
	$X_1 = 0$	$\pi_4 q_4(0,0)$	0	$\pi_4 q_4(1,0)$	0
	E	1	1	1	1

We assume the law f_A is given and model (9.1) holds, so $q_A(x)$ and thus, by Theorem 9.1, the π_A are known for $A \in \{1,2,3,4\}$. Now consider Table 1. The four events with non-zero probability are given in column 1. The entries in the first four rows are $pr[\chi = A \mid X = (x_0, x_1)] \equiv \pi_A q_A(x_0, x_1)$. The fifth row is all 1's. Let M denote the 5×4 matrix given by the interior of the table. Then, by the laws of probability,

$$M(p_{00}, p_{01}, p_{10}, p_{11})' = (f_1, f_2, f_3, f_4, 1)', \tag{9.3}$$

where, e.g., p_{00} is $p_{x_0=0,x_1=0}$ and $f_1 = f_{A=1}$. Under the CAR model in which treatment was randomly assigned [i.e., $g_A(x) \equiv 1$], M is of rank 3 so that the four unknowns $p = (p_{00}, p_{01}, p_{10}, p_{11})'$ are not identified by (9.3). This corresponds to the fact that it is not possible to identify the joint distribution of (X_0, X_1) in a randomized trial, although one can identify $pr(X_1 = 0) = p_{00} + p_{10}$ and $pr[X_0 = 0] = p_{01} + p_{00}$.

However, when the non-zero entries in some row are not equal (i.e., $q_A(x)$ depends on x for some $A \in \{1,2,3,4\}$), M can be of rank 4 in which case the joint law p_x of $X = (X_0, X_1)$ will be identified, even though the model (9.1) is non-parametric for χ, no restrictions are imposed on the joint distribution of (X_0, X_1), and X_0 and X_1 are never simultaneously observed.

As odd as this may seem, things may become even odder. For example, consider model (9.1) with $q_3(1,1) = b \neq 1$ and $q_A(x_0, x_1) = 1$ for all other A and x. Now, as conditional probabilities given X, the first four rows in each of the columns of M must sum to the value 1 in the fifth row, (i.e., Eq. (9.2) must hold). This implies that

$$\pi_2 + \pi_4 = 1, \quad \pi_2 + \pi_3 = 1, \quad \pi_1 + \pi_4 = 1, \quad \pi_1 + b\pi_3 = 1\,. \tag{9.4}$$

If, as we have assumed, $b \neq 1$, we conclude from (9.4) that $\pi_3 = \pi_4 = 0$ whatever be the law f_A. However, from the third and fourth rows of M, we see that $\pi_3 = \pi_4 = 0$ implies that the probability that we observe X_1

must be zero (i.e., $f_3 + f_4 = 0$), which may be contradicted by the given law f_A. Thus it appears that model (9.1) must be misspecified since the choice of $q_A(x)$ is incompatible with f_A. However, according to Theorem 9.1, model (9.1) is nonparametric. The resolution of the paradox is that the sample space E for which Theorem 9.1 is true will exclude at least one of the four possible values of $x = (x_0, x_1)$, i.e., for at least one of these values of x, $p_x = 0$. In that case, at most three of the four equations in (9.4) must hold which will not restrict the possible f_A, since Theorem 1 does not require Eq. (9.2) to hold for values of x that are not in the sample space E (i.e., for values of x for which $p_x = 0$). Note that Theorem 1 of Gill et al. proves that in the case in which model (9.1) is CAR, it is never necessary to delete any points from an *a priori* sample space E in order that Eq. (9.2) hold.

As odd as the above results may seem, model (9.1) has two even greater problems that will probably make it unsuitable for use in sensitivity analysis. First, it is quite unclear what the substantive meaning of $q_A(x)$ is in a given problem, thus making it hard to choose plausible functions $q_A(x)$ for sensitivity analysis. Second, suppose there is a positive probability of observing the full data X and our analytic strategy is to first model the non-response mechanism and then. to estimate the law of X by inverse probability weighting. If X is high dimensional, it is difficult to know how to do dimension reduction in model (9.1). Specifically, if we specify a model $\pi_A(\alpha)$ (depending on a finite dimensional parameter α) for the unknown π_A and then estimate α by maximizing $\sum_A f_A \log \pi_A(\alpha)$, it is unlikely that (9.2) will hold with our estimate replacing π_A. Indeed, there may be no parameter value α for which (9.2) holds with π_A replaced by $\pi_A(\alpha)$, which would imply that we could conclude that our model $\pi_A(\alpha)$ is misspecified even before seeing the data χ. This same difficulty arises even with CAR models.

9.2. Selection bias permutation missingness models. As in Robins and Gill (1997) and Robins (1997a), we assume data $L = \left(L_0, \ldots, L_K\right)'$ and let R_k be the indicator that variable L_k is observed. The observed data is $\left(R, L_{(R)}\right)$ where $L_{(r)}$ are the observed components of L when $R = r$. We assume that there is a positive probability of complete observations, i.e., $pr\left[R = \mathbf{1} \mid L\right] > 0$ with probability 1, where $\mathbf{1}$ is the vector of 1's. To be able to use the notation of Robins and Gill (1997), we assume, as they did, that $L = (Y, X')'$ where $Y = L_0$ is an always observed variable and X may have one or more components missing. We shall obtain a separate NPI model for each of the $K!$ permutations of the variables $(X_1, \ldots, X_K)$. Given a permutation, let $\left(X^{(1)}, \ldots, X^{(K)}\right)$ denote the first to last variables in our permutation. Let R^k denote the indicator of whether variable $X^{(k)}$ is observed. Define $W_k = \left\{R^{k+1}, \ldots, R^k, X^{(1)}, \ldots, X^{(k-1)}, R^{(k+1)} X^{(k+1)}, \ldots, R^K X^{(K)}, Y\right\}$. Then a NPI selection odds PM model specifies

$$\text{(9.5)} \qquad logit\ pr\left[R^k = 1 \mid W_k, X^{(k)}\right] = h_k\left(W_k\right) + q_k\left(X^{(k)}, W_k\right)$$

with

$$\text{(9.6)} \qquad q_k\left(X^{(k)}, W_k\right)\ known$$

and

$$\text{(9.7)} \qquad h_k\left(W_k\right)\ unrestricted\ .$$

Robins (1997a) shows that this model is a NPI model in the special case in which q_k is identically zero. In this case, he shows also how to carry out estimation in the restricted model characterized by (9.5), (9.6), and

$$\text{(9.8)} \qquad h_k\left(W_k\right) = h_k\left(W_k; \gamma_k^*\right), \quad k = 1, \ldots, K$$

where $h_k\left(W_k; \gamma_k\right)$ is a known function and γ_k^* is an unknown finite dimensional vector to be estimated. Specifically, Robins (1997a) shows how to estimate γ_k^* by sequential inverse-probability-weighted-estimators and then estimate the functionals of the joint distribution of the full data (Y, X) by inverse-probability-weighting as well.

We can use this same strategy for selection odds PM models under the additional restriction (9.8). Specifically, note that for $k = 1$, we have an ordinary selection odds model, since W_1 is completely observed. Thus, we can consistently estimate γ_1^* using the inverse-probability-of-censoring-weighted methods of Rotnitzky, Robins, and Scharfstein (1998) and Secs. 2–4. Now consider $k = 2$. This would also be a selection odds model of the type studied in Secs. 2–4, except that the component $X^{(1)}$ of W_2 is not completely observed. However, we can restrict attention to this subset of the population in which $X^{(1)}$ is completely observed by reweighting by our estimate of $pr\left[R^1 = 1 \mid W_1, X^{(1)}\right]$. We can then proceed this way recursively until all the γ_k^*'s have been estimated. The strategy is exactly that described on page 27 of Robins (1997a) for the special case in which q_k was zero.

10. A Non-ignorable Generalization of RMM Models. Robins and Gill (1997) when faced with the difficulty with CAR models described in the last paragraph of Sec. 9.1, proposed to solve it by introducing the class of randomized monotone missingness (RMM) models, a subclass of the class of CAR models. In this section, we introduce a non-CAR generalization of Markov RMM models — The non-ignorable selection odds Markov RMM models. We first review the definition of a Markov RMM model.

Consider Figure 3, taken from Robins and Gill (1997). In Figure 3, at stage m, $m = 1, 2, \ldots, M + 1$, there are $\binom{M}{m-1} = M! / \{m-1\}!\,[M-$

$(m-1)]!$ groups of $m-1$ variables $X^{mk}, k = 1, \ldots, \binom{M}{m-1}$. For example, at stage $m = 3$, we have $3!/(2!\,1!) = 3$ groups of $m-1 = 2$ variables. Each group $X^{mk}, m \le M$, is connected by arrows to the $M-(m-1)$ groups $\{X_j, X^{mk}\}$ at stage $(m+1)$ with $X_j \notin X^{mk}$. For example, if $X^{21} = \{X_1\}$, X^{21} is connected to the $3-(2-1) = 2$ groups $\{X_1, X_2\}$ and $\{X_1, X_3\}$. The probabilities $p_j(X^{mk}, Y)$ on Figure 3 are the conditional probabilities that the variable $X_j, X_j \notin X^{mk}$, will be observed in the next stage conditional on the observed values of Y and of the variables X^{mk} that have been observed through stage m. (The dependence of these probabilities on the always-observed variable Y is suppressed in the figure.) $p_-(X^{mk}, Y) \equiv 1 - \sum_{\{j; X_j \notin X^{mk}\}} p_j(X^{mk}, Y)$ is the conditional probability of quitting without proceeding to the next stage. A parametric Markov RMM models specifies a parametric form for the unknown $p_j(X^{mk}, Y)$.

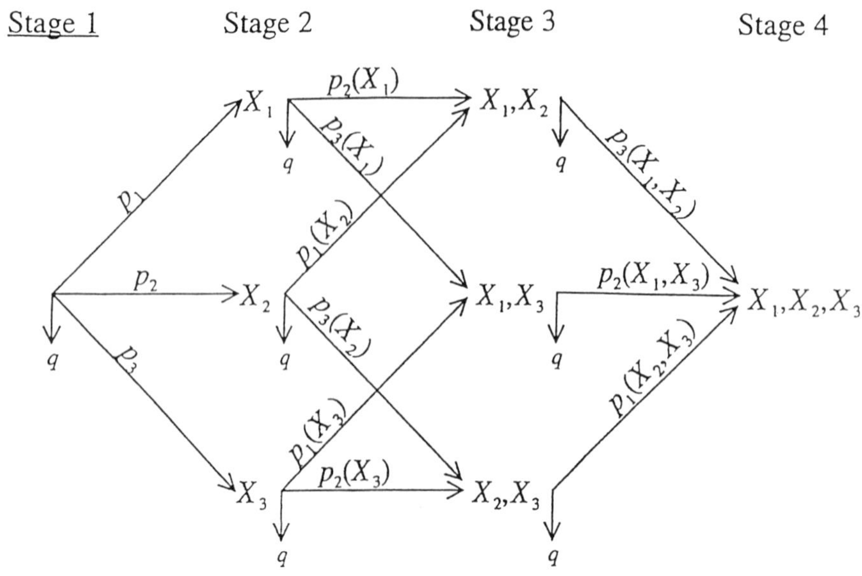

FIG. 3.

We can generalize this Markov RMM to a non-ignorable selection odds model. We now redefine $p_j(X^{mk}, Y)$ to be $p_j(X^{mk}, Y, \underline{X}^{mk})$ where $\underline{X}^{mk}$ are the components of X other than X^{mk}. Then an unrestricted (possibly) non-ignorable selection odds Markov RMM model assumes

$$(10.1) \qquad p_j\left(X^{mk}, Y, \underline{X}^{mk}\right) = \phi_{jmk} \Big/ \left\{1 + \sum_{\{j; X_j \notin X^{mk}\}} \phi_{jmk}\right\}$$

where

$$\phi_{jmk} = \exp\left[h_{jmk}\left(X^{mk}, Y\right) + q_{jmk}\left(X, Y\right)\right] \tag{10.2}$$

and the q_{jmk} are known functions and the functions h_{jmk} are completely unknown. Robins and Gill (1997) showed in the special case where $q_{jmk}(X, Y)$ does not depend on $\underline{X}^{mk}$ (so the model is CAR) an unrestricted RMM model is not a nonparametric model for the law of the observed data.

In practice, to overcome the curse of dimensionality, we specify that

$$h_{jmk}\left(X^{mk}, Y\right) = h_{jmk}\left(X^{mk}, Y; \gamma\right) \tag{10.3}$$

where γ is an unknown finite-dimensional parameter and $h_{jmk}(\cdot, \cdot; \gamma)$ is a known function. As in Robins and Gill (1997), our goal is to use our non-ignorable selection odds Markov RMM models to first estimate γ and then, under the assumption that

$$pr\left[R = \mathbf{1} \mid L\right] > \sigma > 0 \ w.p.1, \tag{10.4}$$

estimate the distribution of X by inverse probability weighting.

To estimate the law of L by inverse probability weighting, it is necessary that $pr[R = \mathbf{1} \mid L]$ be identified where $\mathbf{1}$ is a vector of ones. At present, it is an open question whether the unrestricted non-ignorable selection odds Markov RMM given by (10.1) and (10.2) is sufficient to identify $pr[R = \mathbf{1} \mid L]$ under assumption (10.4). Note that even with X and Y discrete, the functions h_{jmk} will not be identified. However, we conjecture that the probability $pr[R = r \mid L]$ will be identified under model (10.1)–(10.2).

We now discuss how one might estimate parameters γ of (10.3) of our dimension-reduced model. Note that (10.1)–(10.3) imply that $pr[R = r \mid L]$ is a known function $pr[R = r \mid L; \gamma]$ of L and γ. Thus we consider estimating γ by the

$$\sum_i B_i(\phi, \gamma) = 0 \tag{10.5}$$

where $B(\phi, \gamma) = \sum_r \left(I(R = r) - I(R = \mathbf{1})\, pr[R = r \mid L; \gamma] / pr\left[R = \mathbf{1} \mid L; \gamma\right]\right) \phi_r\left(L_{(r)}\right)$ where the $\phi_{(r)} \mid \cdot$ are functions chosen by the data analyst. In general, γ may not be identified, in which case Eq. (10.5) may have many solutions. However, we conjecture under regularity conditions, all such solutions $\widehat{\gamma}$ imply the same value for $pr[R = r \mid L; \widehat{\gamma}]$. When a dimension K of L is large, solving (10.5) will be computationally intractable because $B(\phi, \gamma)$ is a sum over 2^Kterms . It will be of interest to determine if computationally tractable simulation methods exist for approximately solving (10.5) can be derived.

11. Sensitivity Analysis and Bayesian Inference.

11.1. A parametric missing data example. If a decision is required, one may wish to consider a Bayesian analysis in place of a sensitivity analysis. We shall consider the following simple setting. We return to the missing data setting of Sec. 2. Let $K = 1$, $L_0 = Z$, $L_1 = W$, $L_2 = Y$, $L = \overline{L}_2 = (Z, W, Y)$. We assume the censoring-time C is either at times 1 or 2 with probability 1. The observed data are

$$O = (Z, W, \Delta, \Delta Y)$$

where $\Delta = 1 \iff C = 2$. We consider the model

$$pr\left[\Delta = 1 \mid L\right] = h\left(Z, W\right) + q\left(L\right) \tag{11.1}$$

where

$$h\left(\overline{\ell}_1\right) = h\left(z, w\right) \;\; is\; unknown \tag{11.2}$$

and

$$q\left(\ell\right) \;\; is\; known. \tag{11.3}$$

We know from Theorem 2.2 that the semiparametric model **a** determined by the restrictions (11.1)–(11.3) is a non-parametric model for the observed data O and that $F_{\Delta,L}$ is identified.

The setting we are thinking of here is a randomized clinical trial where *(i)* $Z \in (0,1)$ is the treatment arm randomization indicator, *(ii)* W is an always observed post-randomization variable that is discrete with d points of support, and *(iii)* Y is an outcome of interest which is not observed for some subjects who have dropped out. Thus, our parameter of interest is

$$\beta \equiv E\left(Y \mid Z = 1\right) - E\left(Y \mid Z = 0\right) \;,$$

the effect of treatment on the outcome Y.

Note, by assuming W is discrete, we are considering the case where we are not afflicted by the curse of dimensionality.

To perform a Bayesian analysis, rather than treating $q \equiv q\left(\ell\right)$ as known and varying it in a sensitivity analysis, we shall put a prior $\pi\left(q\right)$ on the function q in (11.1). Since $L = (W, Z, Y)$ has $4d$ points of support, a particular function q can be identified with a point in $\mathcal{R}^{4d}$. Similarly, $h = h\left(Z, W\right)$ can be identified with a point in $\mathcal{R}^{2d}$, so when we only impose (11.1), q and h can be viewed as unknown parameters in $\mathcal{R}^{4d}$ and $\mathcal{R}^{2d}$. Thus, our prior $\pi\left(q\right)$ on q is simply a probability distribution on $\mathcal{R}^{4d}$.

We now consider approximate Bayesian inference on β. Let $\beta\left(q\right)$ be the value of β defined by the law F_O of O and the known function q in the semiparametric model **a** characterized by (11.1)–(11.3). Let $\widehat{\beta}\left(q\right)$ be a semiparametric efficient estimator of β under model **a**. To compute $\widehat{\beta}\left(q\right)$, one could use the discrete version of the methods described in Sec. 4, or one could estimate $\widehat{\beta}(q)$ by non-parametric maximum likelihood. We shall suppose the sample size n is sufficiently large that, given q is known, the sampling distribution of $\widehat{\beta}(q)$ is approximately normal with mean $\beta(q)$ and standard error that can be consistently estimated by $\widehat{\sigma}(q)$, say, using the methods described in Sec. 4. Then *(i)*, since, given q, $\beta(q)$ is identified and *(ii)* for large n, the data should dominate the prior, any reasonable robust Bayesian procedure should by the Bernstein-von Mises theorem result in inferences such that, given both q known and the data [i.e., $\{O_i; i = 1, \ldots, n\}$], the posterior distribution of β will be approximately normal with mean $\widehat{\beta}(q)$ and variance $\widehat{\sigma}^2(q)$. Indeed, any prior for which the above approximation of the posterior is inadequate will be suspect, as the prior will have dominated the data.

Hence the following algorithm gives an asymptotic approximation $\widetilde{\pi}(\beta \mid data)$ to the posterior density $\pi(\beta \mid data)$ of β.

Algorithm: For $j = 1, \ldots, J$, *(i)* draw q_j from $\pi(q \mid data)$, where $\pi(q \mid data)$ is the posterior density of q given the data $\{O_i; i = 1, \ldots, n\}$, and *(ii)* compute $\widetilde{\pi}(\beta \mid data) = J^{-1}\sum_{j=1}^{J}\phi(\beta; \widehat{\beta}(q_j), \widehat{\sigma}^2(q_j))$ where $\phi(\beta; \mu, \sigma^2)$ is a $N(\mu, \sigma^2)$ density evaluated at β.

Thus it only remains to determine how to draw from the posterior distribution of q given the data. Since q is not identified in the model characterized by (11.1) with both h and q unknown, the posterior distribution $\pi(q \mid data)$ of q equals the prior distribution if and only if *a priori* q is independent of the distribution F_O of the observed data [i.e., $\pi(F_O, q) = \pi(F_O)\pi(q)$]. Given such independence, we can simply draw q from its prior $\pi(q)$. However, we now argue that it may be more natural and substantively plausible not to assume that F_O and q are *a priori* independent. Note that the joint distribution $F_{\Delta,L}$ of (Δ, L) can be written $F_{\Delta,L} = (h, \beta, \gamma, \theta, q) \equiv (\eta, q)$ where γ parameterizes the distribution $f(W \mid Y, Z)$ and can be represented as a point in $\mathcal{R}^{4(d-1)}$, $\theta = E[Y \mid Z = 0]$, and $\eta \equiv (h, \beta, \gamma, \theta)$. Now as a marginal law, the law F_O of O is a function, say s, of $F_{\Delta,L}$ i.e., $F_O = s(\eta, q)$. In general, $s(\cdot,\cdot)$ will be a smooth differentiable map between two Euclidean spaces. By Theorem 2.2, we know that, for fixed q, $s(\eta, q)$ is one-to-one in η, since Theorem 2.2 states that q and F_O determine $F_{\Delta,L} = (\eta, q)$. That is, $\eta = s^{-1}(F_O, q)$. Note that if, we for example, assume that η is *a priori* independent of q, i.e., $\pi(\eta, q) = \pi(\eta)\pi(q)$, then $F_O = s(\eta, q)$ and q will not be *a priori* independent and $\pi(q \mid data) \neq \pi(q)$. We believe it is more natural to specify a prior $\pi(\eta, q)$ for the distribution of $F_{\Delta,L}$ than to directly specify a prior distributions for F_O. Under such prior specification, we now develop an approach to sampling from $\pi[q \mid data]$. Given a prior $\pi(\eta, q)$, let

$$\omega(q) = \pi(q \mid data) / \pi(q)$$

be the posterior-prior importance weights. Let $\widehat{F}_O$ be the empirical distribution of the $O_i, i = 1, \ldots, n$.

THEOREM 11.1. *Suppose that* $\pi(\eta, q)$ *is continuous in* (η, q). *Then* $\widehat{\omega}(q) = c\omega(q) + o_p(1)$, *where*

$$\widehat{\omega}(q) = \pi_{\eta|q}[\widehat{\eta}(q) \mid q] \mid \partial s(\eta, q)/\partial\eta \mid^{-1}_{\eta=\widehat{\eta}(q)} \tag{11.4}$$

where c *is an unknown normalizing constant,* $\widehat{\eta}(q) = s^{-1}\left(\widehat{F}_O, q\right)$ *is the non-parametric maximum likelihood estimator of* η *when* q *is known,* $|A|$ *is the Jacobian determinant of* A, $\pi_{\eta|q}$ *is the conditional density of* η *given* q, *and* $o_p(1)$ *is a random variable converging to zero under* F_O.

It follows from Theorem 11.1 that we can consistently estimate $\omega(q)$ up to a normalizing constant. Thus, we can modify our previous algorithm and use the following approximation $\pi^*(\beta \mid data)$ to the posterior $\pi(\beta \mid data)$ suggested by L. Wasserman.

Modified algorithm: For $j = 1, \ldots, J$, *(i)* draw q_j from $\pi(q)$, and *(ii)* compute $\pi^*(\beta \mid data) = h(\beta) / \int h(\beta)\, d\beta$ where $h(\beta) = J^{-1}\sum_{j=1}^{J} \phi(\beta; \widehat{\beta}(q_j), \widehat{\sigma}^2(q_j))\widehat{\omega}(q_j)$ and $\int h(\beta)\, d\beta$ can be evaluated numerically.

Note $\pi^*(q \mid data)$ will converge to $\pi(q \mid data)$ as $n \to \infty$ and $J \to \infty$.

In practice, we use our large sample approximation $\widehat{\omega}(q)$ in place of $\omega(q)$.

REMARK 11.1. In usual Bayesian inference, we cannot sample from $\pi(q \mid data)$ by sampling from $\pi(q)$ and then using importance weights $\omega(q)$, since $\pi(q \mid data)$ is a much more peaked distribution than $\pi(q)$ when the sample size is large. However, in our setting, since q is not identified in the model characterized by (11.1a) alone, $\pi(q \mid data)$ will not be a highly peak function of q even as $n \to \infty$. Indeed, we can empirically check whether it is reasonable to importance sample from the prior by plotting the distribution of the $\widehat{\omega}(q_j^*)$. If this distribution is not too highly variable nor too skew, our importance sampling approach is adequate.

Proof of Theorem 11.1. $\pi(q \mid data) = \int \pi(q \mid F_O)\pi(F_O \mid data)\, d\mu(F_O) = \pi(q \mid \widehat{F}_O) + o_p(1)$ since *(i)* $q \coprod data \mid F_O$, and *(ii)* $\pi(F_O \mid data) = \delta_{\widehat{F}_O} + o_p(1)$ by the consistency of Bayes estimators, and, by assumption, $\pi(q \mid F_O)$ is smooth in F_O. Here $\delta_{\widehat{F}_O}$ is the distribution that puts all its mass $\widehat{F}_O$. Now $\pi(q \mid \widehat{F}_O) \propto \pi_{F_O|q}(\widehat{F}_O \mid q)\pi(q)$. So $\omega(q) = c\pi_{F_O|q}(\widehat{F}_O \mid q) + o_p(1)$. But, by the change of variables formula, $\pi_{F_O|q}(\widehat{F}_O \mid q) = \pi_{\eta|q}[s^{-1}(\widehat{F}_O, q) \mid q] \mid \partial s^{-1}(\widehat{F}_O, q)/\partial F_O \mid = \pi_{\eta|q}[\widehat{\eta}(q) \mid q] \mid \partial s(\eta, q)/\partial\eta \mid^{-1}_{\eta=\widehat{\eta}(q)}$. □

11.2. A parametric causal inference example.

11.2.1. Smooth priors. Consider the simple logistic SNMM of Sec. 8.4 with $K = 0$, $Y \equiv L_{K+1} = L_1$, $V \equiv L_0$, $A \equiv A_0$, with Y dichotomous, and V and A discrete with d_V and d_A points of support, respectively. Then (8.30) becomes

$$\gamma^*(v, a) = logit E(Y_a \mid a, v) - logit E(Y_0 \mid a, v) \ , \tag{11.5}$$

Eq. (8.11a) becomes

$$E(Y_0 \mid v, a) = expit\left[t(v) + q(v, a)\right] \tag{11.6}$$

where $q(v, 0) = 0$ and the logistic current treatment interaction function becomes

$$\begin{aligned} r(v, g) = & \left\{logitE\left[Y_g \mid v, A = g(v)\right] - logitE\left[Y_0 \mid v, A = g(v)\right]\right\} \\ & - \left\{logitE\left[Y_g \mid v, A \neq g(v)\right] - logitE\left[Y_0 \mid v, A \neq g(v)\right]\right\} . \end{aligned}$$

Note by the remarks following Eq. (8.29), the parameter space for $r(v, g)$ is precisely the set of all functions $r^*(v, a)$ satisfying $r^*(v, 0) = 0$. Hence, any function $r(v, g)$ can be represented as a point in $R^{d_V(d_A - 1)}$. Further, since $K = 0$ and thus A is time-independent, Theorem (8.13) is true with $r(v, g)$ the logistic current treatment interaction function for all regimes g both dynamic and non-dynamic.

Now let $\eta = \left(F_V, F_{A|V}, \gamma^*, t\right)$ with $\gamma^* = \gamma^*(v, a)$ and $t = t(\ell)$. Let F_O be the joint distribution of (V, A, Y) which can be identified as a point in $\mathcal{R}^{2d_V d_A - 1}$. It follows from Theorems 8.5 and 8.13 that $F_O = s(\eta, q, r) = s(\eta, q)$ is a function of (η, q) alone. Further, given q, this function is invertible, i.e., $\eta = s^{-1}(F_O, q)$. Furthermore, $E(Y_g)$ is a deterministic function of (η, q, r).

Let $\beta = \beta(\eta, q, r)$ be a possible vector-valued functional of interest such as $E(Y_g)$ or a function of γ^*. We want to derive an approximation to the posterior distribution of β. For fixed F_O, define $\eta(q) = s^{-1}(F_O, q)$ and let $\widehat{\eta}(q) = s^{-1}\left(\widehat{F}_O, q\right)$ be the NPMLE of $\eta(q)$ where $\widehat{F}_O$ is the NPMLE of F_O. Arguing as in the last subsection, in large samples, the posterior distribution of η given the data and (q, r) will be approximately normal with mean $\widehat{\eta}(q)$ and variance $\widehat{\Sigma}(q)$ where $\widehat{\Sigma}(q)$ is a consistent estimator of the asymptotic variance of $\widehat{\eta}(q)$. Now let $\omega(q, r) = \pi(q, r \mid data) / \pi(q, r)$. Analogously to Theorem 11.1, we have

THEOREM 11.2. *Suppose the prior $\pi(\eta, q, r)$ is continuous. Then $\widehat{\omega}(q, r) = c\omega(q, r) + o_p(1)$ where c is a constant and*

$$\widehat{\omega}(q, r) = \pi_{\eta|q,r}\left[\widehat{\eta}(q) \mid q, r\right] \left| \partial s(\eta, q) / \partial \eta \right|_{\eta = \widehat{\eta}(q)}^{-1} . \tag{11.7}$$

By the delta method and the Bernstein-von Mises theorem, the posterior distribution of $\beta = \beta(\eta, q, r)$ given (q, r) will be asymptotically normal with mean $\widehat{\beta}(q, r) \equiv \beta(\widehat{\eta}(q), q, r)$ and variance $\widehat{\Sigma}_\beta(q, r)$ where $\widehat{\Sigma}_\beta(q, r) = \widehat{\tau}(q, r) \widehat{\Sigma}(q) \widehat{\tau}(q, r), \widehat{\tau}(q, r) = \partial \beta(\eta, q, r) / \partial \eta \mid_{\eta = \widehat{\eta}(q)}$. Thus, we can consider the following approximation $\pi^*(\beta \mid data)$ for the posterior $\pi(\beta \mid data)$.

Algorithm: For $j = 1, \ldots, J$, *(i)* draw (q_j, r_j) from $\pi(q, r)$, and *(ii)* compute $\pi^*(\beta \mid data) = h(\beta) / \int h(\beta)\, d\beta$ where

$$h(\beta) = J^{-1} \sum_{j=1}^{J} \phi\left(\beta; \widehat{\beta}(q_j, r_j), \widehat{\Sigma}_\beta(q_j, r_j)\right) \widehat{\omega}(q_j, r_j) . \tag{11.8}$$

11.2.2. Allowing for a prior non-zero probability of non-causality. Heretofore, we have assumed our prior $\pi(\eta, q, r)$ was smooth. However, it is likely that one would wish to place positive prior mass on the causal null hypothesis that γ^* and r are zero, provided that treatment A was not already known to be a cause of Y. Therefore, define $M = 1$ to be the submodel in which γ^* and r are identically zero and let $M = 0$ denote the submodel in which neither is zero. For convenience, we shall assume a zero prior probability that only one of γ^* and r are precisely zero. Let $\pi(M = 1)$ be the prior probability that $M = 1$. We shall assume that the conditional prior $\pi(\eta, q, r \mid M = 0)$ is smooth except that we have deleted the point $\gamma^* = r = 0$. Let the parameter $\nu = (F_V, F_{A|V}, t, q)$ be the unknown parameter in model $M = 1$. We assume $\pi(\nu \mid M = 1)$ is a smooth prior. We now approximate the Bayes factor $\{\pi[M = 1 \mid data] / \pi[M = 0 \mid data]\} / \{\pi[M = 1] / \pi[M = 0] = f[data \mid M = 1] / f[data \mid M = 0]\}$. Since by Theorems 8.5 and 8.13, both models $M = 0$ and $M = 1$ are non-parametric models for the law F_O of the observed data, we know that, by Laplace's method,

$$\begin{aligned} &f[data \mid M = m] \\ &\quad \propto f\left[data \mid \widehat{F}_O\right] n^{-(2d_V d_A - 1)/2} \pi_{F_O|M=m}\left(\widehat{F}_O\right) \left(1 + O_p\left(n^{-1}\right)\right) . \end{aligned} \tag{11.9}$$

Hence, $\dfrac{f[data \mid M = 1]}{f[data \mid M = 0]}$ is approximately

$$\frac{\pi_{F_O|M=1}\left(\widehat{F}_O\right)}{\pi_{F_O|M=0}\left(\widehat{F}_O\right)} = \frac{\pi_{\nu|M=1}(\widehat{\nu}) \left|\partial s^*(\widehat{\nu}) / \partial \nu\right|^{-1}}{\int \pi\left[\widehat{\eta}(q), q, r \mid M = 0\right] \left|\partial s(\eta, q) / \partial \eta\right|^{-1}_{\eta = \widehat{\eta}(q)} dq dr}$$

where s^* is the one to one function mapping of ν into F_O under model $M = 1$ and $\widehat{\nu} = s^{*^{-1}}\left(\widehat{F}_O\right)$.

Our goal remains to compute $f[\beta \mid data]$ as in Sec. 11.2.1. Given the above approximate formulas for the Bayes factors, we need approximate formulas for $f[\beta \mid M = 0, data]$ and $f[\beta \mid M = 1, data]$. Now $f\left[\beta \mid data, M = 0\right]$ is calculated just like $f[\beta \mid data]$ in Sec. 11.2.1, except now all conditioning events include $M = 0$. In model $M = 1$, the posterior distribution of β will be a point mass at zero whenever β is a causal contrast such as $E\left[Y_g - Y_g^*\right]$ since, in model $M = 1$, $\gamma^* = r = 0$. In model 1, if β is not a contrast [e.g., $\beta = E(Y_g)$], then $\beta \equiv \beta(F_O)$ is identified. Thus, asymptotically, the posterior distribution of β given the data in model $M = 1$ will be normal with mean $\beta\left(\widehat{F}_O\right)$ and variance equal to a consistent estimator of the asymptotic variance of $\beta\left(\widehat{F}_O\right)$.

11.2.3. Allowing for non-zero probability of non-confounding and non-causality. It is argued in Robins (1997b) that practicing epidemiologists will assign a prior probability of zero to the event of no confounding [i.e., the event that q is precisely zero] as in models $M = 0$ and $M = 1$ above. However, as discussed in Robins (1997b) and Robins and Wasserman (1998), the "faithfulness" analyses of Spirtes, Glymour, and Scheines (1993) and Pearl and Verma (1991) that allow one to go from association to causation without subject matter-specific knowledge rely on the assumption that there is a non-zero probability of non-confounding. Thus, to help further understand the results of Sprites et al. and Pearl and Verma, it is of interest to study the effect on our inferences of allowing a non-zero prior probability of non-confounding. Thus, we let model $M = 2$ be the model in which $q = r = 0$ *a priori* and $\pi[\eta \mid M = 2]$ is smooth. Note here that we have assumed that if $q = 0$, then we should choose $r = 0$ as well. with prior probability 1 since, if conditional on V, different levels of treatment are comparable with respect to the counterfactual Y_0, then it is reasonable to assume that they are comparable with respect to the magnitude of the treatment effect on a logistic scale. We let model $M = 3$ be the model in which $q = r = \gamma^* = 0$ and $\pi[\nu_- \mid M = 3]$ is smooth, where $\nu_- = (F_V, F_{A|V}, t)$ is the parameter ν less the component q. Again, we stress that we believe practicing epidemiologists will assign a prior probability of zero to the models $M = 2$ and $M = 3$. However, we will not do so here to help understand the results of Spirtes et al. and Pearl and Verma.

Model 2 is a non-parametric just-identified model for the law F_O. Thus the approximate Bayes factor $f(data \mid M = 2)/f(data \mid M = 0)$ comparing model 2 to model 0 is

$$\begin{aligned} &\pi_{F_O|M=2}\left(\widehat{F}_O\right)/\pi_{F_O|M=0}\left(\widehat{F}_O\right) \\ &\quad = \frac{\pi\left[\widehat{\eta}(0) \mid M = 2\right]\left|\partial s\left(\widehat{\eta}(0), 0\right)/\partial\eta\right|^{-1}}{\int \pi\left[\widehat{\eta}(q), q, r \mid M = 0\right]\left|\partial s(\eta, q)/\partial\eta\right|^{-1}_{\eta=\widehat{\eta}(q)} dqdr}. \end{aligned} \tag{11.10}$$

In contrast to models 0–2, model 3 is no longer a non-parametric model for F_O. In fact, it imposes the sole restriction that Y is mean-independent of A given V. That is,

$$E[Y \mid A, V] = E[Y \mid V]. \tag{11.11}$$

Hence, under model 3, F_O lies in a space of dimension $d_A d_V + d_V - 1$ rather than a space of dimension $2d_A d_V - 1$. It follows, by Laplace's method. that

$$\begin{aligned} &f[data \mid M = 3] \propto \\ &\quad f\left[data \mid \widehat{F}_{res}\right] n^{-\left(d_V d_A + d_V - 1\right)/2} \pi_{F_O|M=3}\left(\widehat{F}_{res}\right)\left[1 + O_p\left(n^{-1}\right)\right] \end{aligned} \tag{11.12}$$

where $\widehat{F}_{res}$ is the maximum likelihood estimator of F_O when (11.11) is imposed. Thus the Bayes factor $f[data \mid M = 3]/f[data \mid M = 0]$ is, to

$O_p(n^{-1})$, given by the ratio of (11.12) to (11.9) evaluated at $m = 0$. If the model $M = 3$ is true, then this Bayes factor will tend to infinity at rate $O_p(n^{d_V(d_A-1)/2})$. If model $M = 0$, $M = 1$, or $M = 2$ is true, then this Bayes factor will tend to zero exponentially quickly. [Note that following Sprites et al. and Pearl and Verma, we have assigned probability zero to any model for which the function $q(v,a)$ is not identically zero for all (v,a) and *(ii)* $q(v,a)$ is zero for some v and some a other than $a = 0$. Extensions of our results that do not impose this latter prior can easily be obtained.] It follows that if the prior probability $\pi(M = 3)$ that model 3 holds exceeds $O_p\left(n^{d_V(d_A-1)/2}\right)$ and (11.11) is true, we will asymptotically conclude that $q = \gamma^* = r = 0$ and thus conclude both no confounding and no causal effect of treatment. That is, we will have gone from association to causation without strong background subject matter knowledge.

We have only considered simple examples. In practice, we will be interested in examples where K is large and L_k and A_k can be multivariate with continuous and discrete components. It is a major open research question how to generalize the approach described above to this more complicated and realistic setting.

APPENDIX

A. Proof of Theorem 8.2. We shall need the following lemma.

LEMMA A.1. *Suppose $Y = (Y_1, \ldots, Y_M)$ given A has a continuous density w.r.t. Lebesgue measure on R^M. Then given a function $q(y,a)$ satisfying $q(y,0) = 0$, and a joint distribution for (Y,A) specified via densities $f_{Y|A=a}(y) \equiv f_{Y|a}(y)$ and $f_A(a) \equiv f(a)$, there exists a unique function $\gamma(y,a)$ satisfying (i) $\gamma(y,0) = y$, (ii) for each a, $\gamma(y,a)$ is a one-one function of y, (iii) if $y_1 > y_2$, then $\gamma(y_1,a) > \gamma(y_2,a)$, (iv) $\gamma(y,a) \to \infty$ as $y \to \infty$ and $\gamma(y,a) \to -\infty$ as $y \to -\infty$, and (v) with $U \equiv \gamma(Y,A)$,*

$$f[a \mid U = y] = t(a)\exp[q(y,a)] \Big/ \left\{ \int t(a)\exp[q(y,a)]\, d\mu(a) \right\} \tag{A.1}$$

for some $t(a)$ satisfying $\int t(a)\,d\mu(a) = 1$. Specifically, with the function $\gamma^{-1}(u,a)$ defined by $\gamma^{-1}(u,a) = y$ if $\gamma(y,a) = u, \gamma^{-1}(u,a)$ is the unique solution to

$$F_{Y|a}\left(\gamma^{-1}(u,a)\right) = \tau(u,a)/\tau(\infty,a) \tag{A.2}$$

where

$$\tau(u,a) = \int_{-\infty}^{u} f_{Y|0}(y)\exp[q(y,a)]\,dy\ . \tag{A.3}$$

Furthermore,

$$t(a) = f(a)\,\tau(\infty, a)^{-1} / \left\{ \int f(a)\,\tau(\infty, a)^{-1}\, d\mu(a) \right\} \tag{A.4}$$

and

$$f_U(y) = f_{Y|0}(y) \int_{-\infty}^{\infty} f(a) \exp[q(y, a)] \{\tau(\infty, a)\}^{-1}\, d\mu(a) \ . \tag{A.5}$$

Proof. Note (A.1) implies

$$f_{U|a}(y) / f_{U|a}(0) = \exp[q(y, a)]\, f_{U|0}(y) / f_{U|0}(0) \tag{A.6}$$

where, without loss of generality, we assume 0 is in the support of U. We now show that if $\gamma(y, a)$ satisfying *(i)–(v)* exists, then (A.2) must be true. Since, by *(i)*, $f_{U|0}(y) = f_{Y|0}(y)$, it follows from the change of variables formula, that (A.6) implies

$$\left|\partial\gamma^{-1}(y, a) / \partial y\right|\, f_{Y|a}\left(\gamma^{-1}(y, a)\right) = \exp\{q(y, a)\}\, f_{Y|0}(y) / k(a) \tag{A.7}$$

where $k(a) \equiv f_{U|a}(0) / f_{Y|0}(0)$. Upon integrating both sides of (A.7) over y in the set $[-\infty, u]$, we obtain

$$F_{Y|a}\left[\gamma^{-1}(u, a)\right] = \int_{-\infty}^{u} \exp[q(y, a)]\, f_{Y|0}(y)\, dy / k(a) \ . \tag{A.8}$$

Evaluating (A.8) as $u \to \infty$ and thus, by *(iii)*, as $\gamma^{-1}(u, a) \to \infty$, we obtain $k(a) = \int_{-\infty}^{\infty} \exp[q(y, a)]\, f_{Y|0}(y)\, dy$. Hence, $\gamma^{-1}(u, a)$ is given by (A.2), which has a unique solution since the RHS of (A.8) is a continuous multivariate distribution.

We next obtain (A.5) assuming *(i)–(v)*. Multiply both sides of (A.6) by $f_{U|a}(0)$ and integrate with respect to y to obtain

$$1 = \int_{-\infty}^{\infty} f_{U|a}(y)\, dy = f_{U|a}(0)\, \tau(\infty, a) / f_{U|0}(0) \ . \tag{A.9}$$

Hence,

$$f_{U|a}(0) = f_{U|0}(0) / \tau(\infty, a) \ . \tag{A.10}$$

Substituting the RHS of (A.10) for $f_{U|a}(0)$ in (A.6) and solving for $f_{U|a}(y)$, we obtain

$$f_{U|a}(y) = \exp[q(y, a)]\, f_{Y|0}(y) / \tau(\infty, a) \ . \tag{A.11}$$

Hence, $f_U(y) = \int f_{U|a}(y)\, f(a)\, d\mu(a)$ is given by (A.5).

We next obtain (A.4) under *(i)–(v)*. By (A.1) and Bayes' Theorem, we have

$$t(a) = \left\{ f_{U|a}(y) f(a) / f_U(y) \right\} \exp\left[-q(y,a)\right] j(y) \tag{A.12}$$

with $j(y) = \int t(a) \exp[q(y,a)] \, d\mu(a)$. By $\int t(a) \, d\mu(a) = 1$, (A.12) implies $j(y) / f_U(y) = \left\{ \int f_{U|a}(y) f(a) \exp[-q(y,a)] \, d\mu(a) \right\}^{-1}$. Hence, by (A.12),

$$t(a) = \exp\left[-q(y,a)\right] f_{U|a}(y) f(a) \Big/ \left\{ \int \exp\left[-q(y,a)\right] f_{U|a}(y) f(a) d\mu(a) \right\}. \tag{A.13}$$

Upon substituting the RHS of (A.11) for $f_{U|a}(y)$ into the numerator and denominator of (A.13), we obtain (A.4).

We thus conclude that if *(i)–(v)* hold, then (A.2), (A.4), and (A.5) are true. Hence, the theorem is true if we can show that *(1.)* the density of U as given by (A.5) integrates to 1, *(2.)* $\gamma^{-1}(y,a)$ and $t(a)$ given by (A.2) and (A.4) satisfy *(i)–(v)*, and *(3.)* the change of variables formula

$$f_{Y|a}(y) f_A(a) = \{\partial \gamma(y,a) / \partial y\} f_U[\gamma(y,a)] f[a \mid U = \gamma(y,a)] \tag{A.14}$$

is satisfied with the RHS of (A.14) defined by (A.2), (A.4) and (A.5). It is straightforward to verify *(1.)–(3.)*. □

Proof of Theorem 8.2. We prove the theorem by a backward recursion beginning with K. Specifically, we apply Lemma A.1 conditional $\overline{L}_K = \overline{\ell}_K, \overline{A}_{K-1} = \overline{a}_{K-1}$. Then *(i)–(iv)* of Lemma A.1 are satisfied with $\gamma(y,a) \equiv \gamma_K(\underline{y}_K \overline{\ell}_K, \overline{a}_K), A \equiv A_K, Y \equiv \underline{Y}_{K+1}$. Further, it follows from model (8.3) and Theorem A.1 that conditional on $\overline{L}_K = \overline{\ell}_K, \overline{A}_{K-1} = \overline{a}_{K-1}$, *(v)* of Lemma A.1 holds with $U = U_K, q(y,a) \equiv q_K(\underline{y}_{K+1}, \overline{\ell}_K, \overline{a}_K)$ and $t(a) = t(a_K \mid \overline{\ell}_K, \overline{a}_{K-1})$. Hence, we conclude from Lemma A.1 that model (8.3) is a non-parametric model for the law of the observed data given $\overline{L}_K = \overline{\ell}_K, \overline{A}_{k-1} = \overline{a}_{K-1}$ and, furthermore, that (8.4)–(8.6) are correct with $m = K$. To proceed we then reapply Lemma A.1 but now conditional on $\overline{L}_{K-1} = \overline{\ell}_{K-1}, \overline{A}_{K-2} = \overline{a}_{K-2}$. Specifically with $\gamma(y,a) \equiv \gamma_{K-1}(\underline{y}_K, \overline{\ell}_{K-1}, \overline{a}_{K-1}), A = A_{K-1}, Y = (Y_K, U_K')'$, *(i)–(iv)* of Lemma A.1 hold. Further, again by Theorem 8.1, *(v)* of Lemma A.1 holds with $q(y,a) = q_{K-1}(y, \overline{\ell}_{K-1}, \overline{a}_{K-1}), U = U_{K-1}, t(a) = t(a_{K-1} \mid \overline{\ell}_{K-1}, \overline{A}_{K-2})$. We thus obtain (8.4)–(8.6) for $m = K-1$ by applying Lemma A.1. We continue by backward recursion until $K = 0$. □

Proof of Theorem 8.3. To prove Theorem 8.3, we may use the following lemma.

LEMMA A.2. *Suppose $Y = (Y_1, \ldots, Y_M)$ given A has a continuous density with respect to Lebesgue measure on R^M. Given a function $\gamma(y,a)$ satisfying (i)–(iv) of Lemma A.1, and a joint density for (Y, A) specified by* *the densities* $f_{Y|a}(y), f_A(a) = f(a)$, *there exists a unique function* $q(y,a)$ *satisfying* $q(y,0) = 0$ *such that A.1 holds with* $U = \gamma(Y,A)$. *Specifically,*

$$\exp[q(y,a)] = \{f_{U|a}(y) / f_{U|a}(0)\}\{f_{U|0}(0) / f_{U|0}(y)\}.$$

Proof. It follows immediately from the fact that A.1 implies A.6. □

Proof of Theorem 8.3. Theorem 8.3 follows by recursive application of Lemma A.2. The details are similar to that of the proof of Theorem 8.2 and are omitted. □

B. Proof of Theorem 8.14a. We shall prove the theorem for $\Phi(x) = x$. The proof for $\Phi(x) = e^x$ is similar. It is sufficient to show

$$E\left[g_k\left(\overline{A}_k, V_0^*\right) H_k\left(\psi^*, \eta^*\right) \mid V_0^*\right] = 0 . \tag{B.1}$$

By (8.53), (B.1) is equivalent to

$$\begin{aligned}
0 &= E\left[\left\{\sum_{j=0}^{k} m_{k+1}^*\left(\overline{L}_k, \overline{A}_k\right)\right\} g_k\left(\overline{A}_k, V_0^*\right) \Big/ \prod_{m=0}^{k} f\left(A_m \mid \overline{A}_{m-1}, L_m\right) \mid V_0^*\right] \\
&= \iint \prod_{m=0}^{k} d\mu\left(A_m\right) g_k\left(\overline{A}_k, V_0^*\right)\left[\sum_{j=0}^{k} \iint m_{k+1}^*\left(\overline{L}_j, \overline{A}_k\right)\right. \\
&\qquad \left. \times \prod_{m=0}^{j} dF\left[L_m \mid \overline{L}_{m-1}\overline{A}_{m-1}, V_0^*\right]\right] .
\end{aligned}$$

However, by (8.55), $\int m_{k+1}^*\left(\overline{L}_j, \overline{A}_k\right) dF\left[L_j \mid \overline{L}_{j-1}, \overline{A}_{j-1}, V_0^*\right] = 0$.

REFERENCES

BAKER, S.G., ROSENBERGER, W.F., AND DERSIMONIAN, R. (1992). Closed-form estimates for missing counts in two-way contingency tables. *Statistics in Medicine*, **11**:643–657.

BALKE, A. & PEARL, J. (1997). Bounds on Treatment from Studies with Imperfect Compliance. *Journal of the American Statistical Association*, **92**:1171–1176.

BICKEL, P.J., KLAASSEN, C.A.J., RITOV, Y., AND WELLNER, J.A. (1993). **Efficient and Adaptive Inference in Semiparametric Models**. Baltimore, MD: Johns Hopkins University Press.

CHAMBERLAIN, G. (1987). Asymptotic Efficiency in Estimation with Conditional Moment Restrictions. *Journal of Econometrics,* **34**:305–324.

CORNFIELD, J., HAENSZEL, W., HAMMOND, E.C., LILIENFELD, A.M., SHIMKIN, M.B., AND WYNDER, E.L. (1959). Smoking and lung cancer: Recent evidence and a discussion of some questions. *Journal of the National Cancer Institute,* **22**:173–203.

DABROWSKA, D. (1988). Kaplan-Meier estimate on the plane. *Annals of Statistics,* **16**:1475–1489.

GILL, R.D. AND ROBINS, J.M. (1996). Sequential Models for Coarsening and missingness. **Proceedings of the First Seattle Symposium on Survival Analysis**, Springer-Verlag Lecture Notes in Statistics, pp. 295–305.

GILL, R.D., VAN DER LAAN, M.J., AND ROBINS, J.M. (1996). Coarsening at random: Characterizations, conjectures and counterexamples. **Proceedings of the First Seattle Symposium on Survival Analysis**, Springer-Verlag Lecture Notes in Statistics, pp. 255–294.

HECKMAN, J.J. (1976). The common structure of statistical models of truncation, sample selection and limited dependent variables, and a simple estimator for such models. *Ann. Econ. Socl. Measurement.*, **5**:475–492.

HEITJAN, D.F., AND RUBIN, D.B. (1991). Ignorability and Coarse Data. *The Annals of Statistics*, **19**:2244–2253.

KLEIN, J.P. AND MOESCHBERGER, M.L. (1988). Bounds on net survival probabilities for dependent competing risks. *Biometrics*, **44**:528–538.

LIN, D.Y., PSATY, B.M., AND KRONMAL, R.A. (1998). Assessing the sensitivity of regression results to unmeasured confounders in observational studies. *Biometrics*, **54**:948–963.

LITTLE, R.J., AND RUBIN, D.B. (1987). **Statistical Analysis with Missing Data**. New York: John Wiley.

LITTLE, R.J.A. (1994), A Class of Pattern-Mixture Models for Normal Missing Data. *Biometrika*, **81**:471–483.

MANSKI, C.F. (1990). Nonparametric bounds on treatment effects. *American Economic Reviews, Papers, and Proceedings*, **80**:319–323.

MOESCHBERGER, M.L. AND KLEIN, J.P. (1995). Statistical models for dependent competing risks. *Lifetime Data Analysis,* **1**:195–204.

NEWEY, W.K. (1990). Semiparametric Efficiency Bounds. *Journal of Applied Econometrics*, **5**:99–135.

NEWEY, W.K., AND MCFADDEN, D. (1993). Estimation in Large Samples. **Handbook of Econometrics** (Vol. 4), D. McFadden and R. Engler, eds., Amsterdam: North Holland.

NORDHEIM, E.V. (1984). Inference from Nonrandomly Missing Categorical Data: An Example from a Genetic Study on Turner's Syndrome. *Journal of the American Statistical Association*, **7**:772–780.

PEARL, J., AND VERMA, T. (1991). A theory of inferred causation. In **Principles of Knowledge Representation and Reasoning: Proceedings of the 2nd International Conference**. J.A. Allen, R. Fikes, and E. Sandewall, eds., pp. 441–452. San Mateo, CA: Morgan Kaufmann.

RITOV, Y., AND WELLNER, J.A. (1988). Censoring, Martingales, and the Cox Model. *Contemporary Mathematical Statistics Inf. Stochastic Procedures*, N.U. Prabhu, editor, American Mathematical Society, **80**:191–220.

ROBINS, J.M. (1986). A new approach to causal inference in mortality studies with sustained exposure periods — Application to control of the healthy worker survivor effect. *Mathematical Modelling*, **7**:1393–1512.

ROBINS, J.M. (1987). Addendum to "A new approach to causal inference in mortality studies with sustained exposure periods — Application to control of the healthy worker survivor effect." *Computers and Mathematics with Applications*, **14**:923–945.

ROBINS, J.M. (1989). The analysis of randomized and non-randomized AIDS treatment trials using a new approach to causal inference in longitudinal studies. **Health Service Research Methodology: A Focus on AIDS**. Sechrest L., Freeman H., and Mulley A., eds., NCHSR, U.S. Public Health Service. pp. 113–159.

ROBINS, J.M. (1992). Estimation of the time-dependent accelerated failure time model in the presence of confounding factors. *Biometrika*, **79**:321–34.

ROBINS, J.M., BLEVINS D, RITTER G, AND WULFSOHN M. (1992). *G*-estimation of the effect of prophylaxis therapy for pneumocystis carinii pneumonia on the survival of AIDS patients. *Epidemiology*, **3**:319–336.

ROBINS, J.M., BLEVINS D, RITTER G, AND WULFSOHN M. (1993). Errata to *G*-estimation of the effect of prophylaxis therapy for pneumocystis carinii pneumonia on the survival of AIDS patients. *Epidemiology*, **4**:189.

ROBINS, J.M. (1994). Correcting for non-compliance in randomized trials using structural nested mean models. *Communications in Statistics*, **23**:2379–2412.

ROBINS, J.M. (1996). Locally efficient median regression with random censoring and surrogate markers. **Proceedings of the 1994 Conference on Lifetime Data Models in Reliability and Survival Analysis**, Boston, MA. In: **Lifetime Data: Models in Reliability and Survival Analysis**, N.P. Jewell et al., eds., Kluwer Academic Publishers, 263–274.

ROBINS, J.M. (1997a). Non-response models for the analysis of non-monotone non-ignorable missing data. *Statistics in Medicine,* **16**:21–37.

ROBINS, J.M. (1997b). Causal inference from complex longitudinal data. In: **Latent Variable Modeling and Applications to Causality. Lecture Notes in Statistics (120)**, M. Berkane, editor. NY: Springer Verlag, pp. 69–117.

ROBINS, J.M. (1998a). Marginal structural models. In: *1997 Proceedings of the American Statistical Association, Section on Bayesian Statistical Science*, pp. 1–10.

ROBINS, J.M. (1999b). Marginal Structural Models versus Structural Nested Models as Tools for Causal Inference. **Statistical Models in Epidemiology, the Environment and Clinical Trials** , M. Elizabeth Halloran and Donald Berry, editors, NY: Springer-Verlag, pp. 95–134.

ROBINS, J.M. (1998c). Correction for non-compliance in equivalence trials. *Statistics in Medicine*, **17**:269–302.

ROBINS, J.M. AND GILL, R. (1997). Non-response models for the analysis of non-monotone ignorable missing data. *Statistics in Medicine*, **16**:39–56.

ROBINS, J.M. AND RITOV, Y. (1997). A curse of dimensionality appropriate (CODA) asymptotic theory for semiparametric models. *Statistics in Medicine,* **16**:285–319.

ROBINS, J.M., AND ROTNITZKY, A. (1992). Recovery of information and adjustment for dependent censoring using surrogate markers. In: **AIDS Epidemiology — Methodological Issues**. Jewell N., Dietz K. and Farewell V., eds., Boston, MA: Birkhäuser, pp. 297–331.

ROBINS, J.M., ROTNITZKY, A., ZHAO LP. (1994). Estimation of regression coefficients when some regressors are not always observed. *Journal of the American Statistical Association,* **89**:846–866.

ROBINS, J.M. AND WASSERMAN, L. (1999). On the impossibility of inferring causation from association without background knowledge. **Computation, Causation, and Discovery**. C. Glymour and G. Cooper., eds., Cambridge, MA: The MIT Press (to appear).

ROSENBAUM, P.R. (1995). **Observational Studies**. New York: Springer-Verlag.

ROSENBAUM, P.R., AND RUBIN, D.B. (1983). Assessing sensitivity to an unobserved binary covariate in an observational study with binary outcome. *Journal of the Royal Statistical Society, Series B,* **11**:212–218.

ROTNITZKY, A., AND ROBINS, J.M. (1997). Analysis of semiparametric regression models with non-ignorable non-response. *Statistics in Medicine,* **16**:81–102.

ROTNITZKY, A., ROBINS, J.M. AND SCHARFSTEIN, D. (1998). Semiparametric regression for repeated outcomes with non-ignorable non-response. *Journal of the American Statistical Association,*. **93**:1321–1339.

RUBIN, D.B. (1976). Inference and Missing Data. *Biometrika*, **63**:581–592.

SCHARFSTEIN, D., ROTNITZKY, AND A., ROBINS, J.M. (1999). Adjusting for non-ignorable drop-out with semiparametric non-response models (to appear, *Journal of the American Statistical Association*).

SCHLESSELMAN J.J. (1978). Assessing effects of confounding variables. American Journal of *Epidemiology*, **108**:3–8.

SLUD, E.V. AND RUBENSTEIN, L.V. (1983). Dependent competing risks and summary survival curves. *Biometrika,* **70**:643–649.

SPIRTES, P., GLYMOUR, C., AND SCHEINES, R. (1993). **Causation, Prediction, and Search**. New York: Springer Verlag.

VAN DER LAAN, M.J. AND ROBINS, J.M. (1998). Locally efficient estimation with current status data and time-dependent covariates. *Journal of the American Statistical*

Association, **93**:693–701.
VAN DER VAART, A. (1991). On differentiable functionals. *Annals of Statistics*, **19**:178–204.
ZHENG, M. AND KLEIN, J.P. (1994). A self-consistent estimator of marginal survival functions based on dependent competing risks and an assumed copula. *Communication in Statistics — Theory and Methods*, **23**:2299–2311.
ZHENG, M. AND KLEIN, J.P. (1995). Estimates of marginal survival for dependent competing risks based on an assumed copula. *Biometrika*, **82**:127–138.

MARGINAL STRUCTURAL MODELS VERSUS STRUCTURAL NESTED MODELS AS TOOLS FOR CAUSAL INFERENCE

JAMES M. ROBINS*

Abstract. Robins (1993, 1994, 1997, 1998ab) has developed a set of causal or counterfactual models, the structural nested models (SNMs). This paper describes an alternative new class of causal models – the (non-nested) marginal structural models (MSMs). We will then describe a class of semiparametric estimators for the parameters of these new models under a sequential randomization (i.e., ignorability) assumption. We then compare the strengths and weaknesses of MSMs versus SNMs for causal inference from complex longitudinal data with time-dependent treatments and confounders. Our results provide an extension to continuous treatments of propensity score estimators of an average treatment effect.

1. Introduction. Robins (1993, 1994, 1997, 1998ab) has developed a set of causal or counterfactual models, the structural nested models (SNMs). Robins (1998abcd) has recently described an alternative new class of causal models – the (non-nested) marginal structural models (MSMs). We describe a class of semiparametric estimators for the parameters of these new models under a sequential randomization (i.e., ignorability) assumption. We then compare the strengths and weaknesses of MSMs versus SNMs for causal inference from complex longitudinal data with time-dependent treatments and confounders. Two major strengths of MSMs compared to SNMs are as follows.

- MSMs can be used to provide semiparametric estimates of the causal effect of a time-dependent treatment on a binary outcome using models (e.g. logistic models) which naturally respect the fact that probabilities lie in the interval $[0, 1]$.
- MSMs cohere much more closely than do SNMs with models for the analysis of time-dependent treatments that are standardly used in the absence of time-dependent confounders. For example, in the absence of time-dependent confounders, a time-dependent Cox proportional hazards model for the effect of time-dependent treatment on a time-to-event (survival time) outcome is commonly employed. The MSMs provide a natural extension of the time-dependent proportional hazards model. Unlike the usual time-dependent Cox model, the marginal structural time-dependent Cox model can be used to obtain valid causal inferences for the effect of a time-varying treatment in the presence of time-varying confounding factors. [We remind the reader that, as discussed in Robins (1986), one cannot estimate the effect of a time-dependent treatment on

*Epidemiology and Biostatistics, Harvard School of Public Health, 677 Huntington Avenue, Boston, MA 02115; Email: robins@hsph.harvard.edu.

survival in the presence of time-dependent confounding factors by using an ordinary time-dependent Cox model that adjusts for the time-dependent confounding factors since, in general, these time-dependent confounding factors will be both determinants of later treatment and affected by earlier treatment. Marginal structural Cox models overcome this deficiency.] Disadvantages of MSMs are discussed later. The relationship of our approach to the propensity score approach of Rosenbaum and Rubin (1983) is considered in section 4.1.

We now give a somewhat informal introduction to marginal structural models, and we report the results of a preliminary data analysis of AIDS Clinical Trial Group (ACTG) Trial 002 using MSMs. We begin with the following simple setting. Consider a study of AIDS patients. Let $A(t)$ be the dose of a treatment of interest, say AZT, at time t with time measured as days since start of follow-up. Let Y be an outcome of interest measured at end-of-follow-up at time $K+1$. Our goal is to estimate the causal effect of the time-dependent treatment $A(t)$ on the mean of Y. Let $\overline{A}(t) = \{A(u); 0 \leq u \leq t\}$ be treatment history through t and let $\overline{L}(t) = \{L(u); 0 \leq u \leq t\}$ be the history through t of a vector of relevant prognostic factors $L(u)$ for (i.e., predictors of) Y, such as CD4 lymphocyte count, white blood count (WBC), hematocrit, age, gender, etc. Suppose Y is a dichotomous outcome (e.g., $Y = 1$ if HIV RNA is detectable in the blood and zero otherwise), and we entertain a model that says the mean of Y given AZT history, $\overline{A} \equiv \overline{A}(K+1)$, is a linear logistic function of a subject's cumulative AZT dose. We write the model

$$E\left[Y \mid \overline{A}\right] = g\left(\overline{A}; \gamma\right)$$

where

$$g\left(\overline{A}; \gamma\right) = \left[1 + \exp\left\{-\gamma_1 - \gamma_2 cum\left(\overline{A}\right)\right\}\right]^{-1}$$

and $cum\left(\overline{A}\right) = \int_0^{K+1} A(t)\,dt$ is the subject's cumulative treatment. The maximum likelihood estimator (MLE) of γ can then be computed from the observed data $O_i = \left(\overline{L}_i, \overline{A}_i, Y_i\right), i = 1, \ldots, n$, on the n study subjects using standard logistic regression software with Y as the Bernoulli outcome variable and $cum\left(\overline{A}\right)$ as the regressor. That is, the MLE of $\gamma = (\gamma_1, \gamma_2)'$ maximizes $\prod_{i=1}^{n} Lik_i(\gamma)$ with $Lik_i(\gamma) = g\left(\overline{A}_i; \gamma\right)^{Y_i}\left[1 - g\left(\overline{A}_i; \gamma\right)\right]^{1-Y_i}$ being the likelihood contribution for a single subject. [Note $Lik_i(\gamma)$ does not depend on the patient's prognostic factor history $\overline{L}_i \equiv \overline{L}_i(K+1)$.] Alternatively, we could have used Bayesian methods by specifying a prior distribution for γ and then estimating γ by its posterior mean given the data. In reasonable large samples, the MLE and Bayes estimate will closely approximate one another.

Causal interpretation of regression parameters. The question then is when does γ_2 have an interpretation as the causal effect of treatment history on the mean of Y? To approach this question, imagine that the decision to administer treatment at each time t were made totally at random by the treating physician. In that hypothetical case, giving treatment at time t is not expected to be associated with any measured or unmeasured prognostic factors (i.e., there would be no "confounding") and therefore γ_2 would intuitively have a causal interpretation. Similarly, γ_2 would keep its causal interpretation if the physician's decision were based only on the history of treatment prior to t. Whenever the conditional probability of receiving treatment on day t given past treatment and prognostic factors history (measured and unmeasured) depends only on past treatment history, we say the process is a "causally exogenous or ancillary treatment process". (A more formal mathematical definition is provided below.) It is well-recognized in the social sciences, econometrics, epidemiologic, and biostatistical literature that γ_2 will have a causal interpretation if $A(t)$ is a causally exogenous (or ancillary) covariate process. Randomized treatments like the one described above are causally exogenous treatments.

We say that a treatment $A(t)$ is a "statistically exogenous or ancillary process" if the probability of receiving treatment at time t does not depend on the history of measured time-dependent prognostic factors $\overline{L}(t)$ up to t conditional on treatment history prior to t, i.e.,

$$\overline{L}(t) \amalg A(t) \mid \overline{A}(t-1),$$

where $A \coprod B \mid C$ *means that* A *is independent of* B *given* C.

Note that a necessary condition for $A(t)$ to be "causally exogenous" is for it to be "statistically exogenous." However, that a process is "statistically exogenous" does not imply it is "causally exogenous," because there may be unmeasured prognostic factors (i.e., confounders) that predict the probability of treatment $A(t)$ at time t given past treatment history. We can test from the data whether $A(t)$ is statistically exogenous but are unable to test whether a statistically exogenous process is causally exogenous.

Suppose $A(t)$ is discrete and we can correctly model the probability $f\left[a(t) \mid \overline{\ell}(t), \overline{a}(t-1)\right]$ of receiving treatment $a(t)$ on day t as a function of past treatment $\overline{a}(t-1)$ and measured prognostic factor history $\overline{\ell}(t)$. We could then measure the degree to which the treatment process is statistically non-exogenous through day t by the random quantity

$$\mathcal{W}(t) = \prod_{k=0}^{t} f\left[A(k) \mid \overline{A}(k-1), \overline{L}(k)\right] / f\left[A(k) \mid \overline{A}(k-1)\right].$$

The numerator in each term in $\mathcal{W}(t)$ is the probability that a subject received his own observed treatment at time k, $A(k)$, given his past treatment and prognostic factor history. The denominator is the probability that a subject received his observed treatment conditional on his past treatment history but not further adjusting for his past prognostic factor history. Note that the treatment process is statistically exogenous just in the case that $\mathcal{W}(t) = 1$ for all t. Of course, $\mathcal{W}(t)$ is unknown and will have to be estimated from the data but, for pedagogic purposes, assume for the moment that it were known.

When $A(t)$ is a statistically endogenous process, we shall consider estimating γ by a weighted logistic regression in which a subject is given the weight $\mathcal{W}^{-1} \equiv [\mathcal{W}(K)]^{-1}$. The weighted logistic regression estimator maximizes $\prod_{i=1}^{n} [Lik_i(\gamma)]^{\mathcal{W}_i^{-1}}$. This weighted logistic regression would agree with the usual unweighted analysis described above just in the case in which $A(t)$ were exogenous. The somewhat surprising result described in detail below is that, if the vector of prognostic factors recorded in $L(t)$ constitutes all relevant time-dependent prognostic factors (i.e., confounders), then, whether or not the treatment process is statistically exogenous, the weighted logistic regression estimator of γ_2 will converge to a quantity β_2 that can be appropriately interpreted as the causal effect of treatment history on the mean of Y. In contrast, when $A(t)$ is statistically endogenous, the usual logistic regression estimator will still converge to the parameter γ_2, but now γ_2 will have no causal interpretation.

To prove such a claim, we need to give a formal mathematical meaning to the informal concept of the causal effect of treatment history on the mean of Y. To do so, we first introduce some notational conventions. We use capital letters to represent random variables and lower case letters to represent possible realizations (values) of random variables. For example, O_i is the random observed data for the ith study subject and o is a possible realization (value) of O_i. Further, we assume that the random vector O_i for each subject is drawn independently from a distribution common to all subjects. Because the O_i have the same distribution, we often suppress the i subscript.

Counterfactual outcomes. Now we introduce counterfactual or potential outcomes. For any fixed non-random treatment history $\overline{a} = \{a(u); 0 \leq u \leq K+1\}$, let $Y_{\overline{a}}$ be the random variable representing a subject's outcome had, possibly contrary to fact, the subject been treated with history $\overline{a}$ rather than his observed history $\overline{A}$. Note the $\overline{a}$'s are possible realizations of the random variable $\overline{A}$. For each possible history $\overline{a}$, we are assuming a subject's response $Y_{\overline{a}}$ is well defined (although generally unobserved). Indeed we only observe $Y_{\overline{a}}$ for that treatment history $\overline{a}$ equal to a subject's actual treatment history $\overline{A}$, i.e., $Y = Y_{\overline{A}}$. Then formally our statement that the effect of treatment history on the mean of Y is a linear logistic function of cumulative treatment is the statement that, for each $\overline{a}$,

$$E[Y_{\overline{a}}] = g(\overline{a}; \beta) \text{ where } g(\overline{a}; \beta) = [1 + \exp\{-\beta_1 - \beta_2 \, cum(\overline{a})\}]^{-1},$$

which we refer to as a MSM for the effect of treatment on the mean of Y. The model for $E[Y_{\overline{a}}]$ is a marginal structural model since it is a model for the marginal distribution of counterfactual variables and, in the econometric and social science literature, causal models (i.e., models for counterfactual variables) are often referred to as structural.

The parameter β_2 of our MSM is of important policy interest. To see why, consider a new subject exchangeable with (i.e., drawn from the same distribution as) the n study subjects. We must decide which treatment history $\overline{a}$ to administer to the new subject. We would like to provide the treatment that minimizes the subject's probability of having HIV RNA in his blood at end of follow-up. That is, we want to find $\overline{a}$ that minimizes $E[Y_{\overline{a}}]$. Thus, for example, if the parameter β_2 of our causal model is positive, we will withhold AZT treatment from our subject (i.e., we will give him the treatment history $\overline{a} \equiv 0$), since positive β_2 indicates that the probability of having HIV RNA in one's blood at the end of follow-up increases with increasing cumulative AZT dose. In contrast to β_2, the parameter γ_2 of our association model $E\left[Y \mid \overline{A}\right] = g\left(\overline{A};\gamma\right)$ may have no causal interpretation. For example, suppose physicians preferentially started AZT on subjects who, as indicated by their prognostic factor history, were doing poorly and that AZT has no causal effect on the mean of Y (i.e., $\beta_2 = 0$). Nonetheless, the mean of Y will increase with cumulative AZT doses and thus γ_2 will be positive. In this setting, we say that the parameter γ_2 of the association model lacks a causal interpretation because it is confounded by the association of the prognostic factors $\overline{L}(u)$ with the treatment $A(u)$.

Formally, in terms of counterfactuals, we say that the $A(t)$ process is "causally exogenous" if, for all histories $\overline{a}$,

$$Y_{\overline{a}} \amalg A(t) \mid \overline{A}(t-1)$$

which is equivalent to

$$Y_{\overline{a}} \coprod \overline{A}\,.$$

Given the covariates recorded in $L(t)$, we say there are no unmeasured confounders if for each $\overline{a}$

$$Y_{\overline{a}} \amalg A(t) \mid \overline{L}(t), \overline{A}(t-1)\,.$$

With these formalizations, it can then be shown mathematically, that when there are no unmeasured confounders, *(i)* statistical exogeneity [i.e., $\overline{L}(t) \amalg A(t) \mid \overline{A}(t-1)$] implies that the $A(t)$ process is "causally exogenous," *(ii)* the weighted logistic estimator converges to the parameter β_2 of the marginal structural model for $E[Y_{\overline{a}}]$, and *(iii)* the limit γ_2 of the usual logistic estimator generally differs from the causal parameter β_2 of the MSM unless the treatment process is statistically exogenous.

We shall also refer to the assumption of no unmeasured confounders as the assumption that treatment $A(t)$ is sequentially ignorable or randomized given the past. The assumption states that, conditional on AZT history and the history of all recorded covariates prior to t, increments in AZT dosage rate at t are independent of the counterfactual random variables $Y_{\overline{a}}$. This assumption will be true if all prognostic factors for, i.e., predictors of, $Y_{\overline{a}}$ that are used by patients and physicians to determine the dosage of AZT at t are recorded in $\overline{L}(t)$ and $\overline{A}(t-1)$. For example, since physicians tend to withhold AZT from subjects with low white blood count, and in untreated subjects, low white blood count is a predictor of HIV RNA, the assumption of no unmeasured confounders would be false if $\overline{L}(t)$ does not contain WBC history. It is the primary goal of the epidemiologists conducting an observational study to collect data on a sufficient number of covariates to ensure that the assumption of no unmeasured confounders will be at least approximately true.

The assumption of no unmeasured confounders is the fundamental condition that will allow us to draw causal inferences from observational data. It is precisely because it cannot be guaranteed to hold in an observational study and is not empirically testable that it is so very hazardous to draw causal inferences from observational data. Note that if, as in a sequentially randomized trial, at each time t, the dose of AZT was chosen at random by the flip of a coin, then the assumption of no unmeasured confounders would be true even if the probability that the coin landed heads depended on past measured covariate and AZT-history. It is because physical randomization guarantees the assumption that most people accept that valid causal inferences can be obtained from a randomized trial. See Rubin (1978), Robins (1986) and Holland (1986) for further discussion. Robins (1997, 1998b) and Robins et al. (1999) discuss how the consequences of violations of the assumption of no unmeasured confounders can be explored through sensitivity analysis. Also see Appendix C below.

Given the assumption of no unmeasured confounders, Robins (1987) shows the mean of the dichotomous variable $Y_{\overline{a}}$ is non-parametrically identified from the joint distribution F_O of the observed data O by the g-computation algorithm formula of Robins (1986). Specifically, $E(Y_{\overline{a}}) = b(\overline{a})$ where

$$(*) \qquad b(\overline{a}) \equiv \int \cdots \int E\left(Y \mid \overline{\ell}_K, \overline{a}_K\right) \prod_{k=0}^{K} f\left(\ell_k \mid \overline{\ell}_{k-1}, \overline{a}_{k-1}\right) d\mu\left(\ell_k\right)$$

and for notational convenience we have written $\overline{z}(k)$ as $\overline{z}_k$ and $z(k)$ as z_k.

The g-computation algorithm functional $b(\overline{a})$ is the marginal mean of Y in the manipulated subgraph of the directed acyclic graph (DAG) G representing the observed data O in which all arrows into the treatment variables $\overline{A} = \left(A_1, \ldots, \overline{A}_K\right)$ have been removed and $\overline{A}$ is set to $\overline{a}$ with probability 1 (Spirtes et al., 1993). More specifically, let DAG G be the complete DAG with temporally ordered vertex set $O = \{L_0, A_0, L_1, A_1, \ldots, A_K, Y\}$ and let DAG $G_{\overline{a}}$ be the subgraph of G in which all arrows into the $A_k, k =$

$0, \ldots, K$ have been cut. Then $b(\overline{a})$ is the marginal mean of Y based on a distribution for O represented by DAG $G_{\overline{a}}$ in which $f\left(A_k \mid \overline{A}_{k-1}, \overline{L}_k\right)$ is replaced by a degenerate density that takes the value a_k with probability 1 while the conditional density of each other variable in the set O given its parents remains as in F_O.

We say that the distribution of $O = \{L_0, A_0, L_1, A_1, \ldots, A_K, Y\}$ is standardly parameterized if, for each variable in O, we have specified a parametric or semiparametric model for the conditional distribution of that variable given its temporal predecessors (the past) and the parameters of each conditional model are variation-independent of those of any other conditional model. When our goal is to estimate the effect of a sequential (time-dependent) treatment $\overline{A}$ on an outcome Y, Lemma 1 and Theorem 2 of Robins and Wasserman (1997) imply that inference procedures based on the standard parameterization will fail. Specifically, they prove that common choices for the parametric families in a standard parameterization often lead to joint densities such that the g-computation formula for $E\left(Y_{\overline{a}}\right)$ can never satisfy the causal null hypothesis that $E\left(Y_{\overline{a}}\right)$ is the same for all $\overline{a}$. In particular, the causal null hypothesis does not imply that $Y \coprod \overline{A}_K \mid \overline{L}_K$. As a consequence, in large samples, the causal null hypothesis, even when true, will be falsely rejected regardless of the data. Robins and Wasserman propose reparameterizing the distribution of O using structural nested models. MSMs represent an alternative reparameterization that also overcomes the fatal deficiencies of the standard parameterization.

Theory of Inverse-Probability-of-Treatment-Weighting. We now explain why weighting by $\mathcal{W}^{-1}$ corrects our logistic regression estimator for the "confounding" due to the prognostic factors in $L(t)$. The first point to note is that in the definition of $\mathcal{W}(t)$ we could have replaced the denominator $f[A(t) \mid A(t-1)]$ by any other function of $\overline{A}(t)$ without influencing the consistency of our weighted logistic estimator of the parameter β_2 of the MSM; only the efficiency (variance) of our estimator would be influenced. However, our estimator would be inconsistent if we replaced the numerator by any other function of $\overline{A}(t)$ and $\overline{L}(t)$. Thus one can view weighting by $\mathcal{W}^{-1}$ as weighting by the inverse of a subject's probability of having his own observed treatment history. Now view each person as a member of a pseudo- or ghost population consisting of themselves and $\mathcal{W}^{-1} - 1$ ghosts (copies) of themselves who have been added by weighting. In this new ghost or pseudo population, it is easy to show that $\overline{L}(t)$ does not predict treatment at t given past treatment history, and thus we have created a pseudo-population in which treatment is exogenous. Furthermore, the causal effect of $\overline{A}$ on Y in the ghost population is the same as in the original population. That is, if $E\left[Y_{\overline{a}}\right] = g(\overline{a}; \beta)$ in the true population, the same will be true of the ghost population. Hence, we would like to do ordinary logistic regression in the pseudo-population. That is essentially what our weighted logistic regression estimator is doing, since the weights create, as required, $\mathcal{W}^{-1} - 1$ additional copies of each subject.

A formal, mathematical explanation of why weighting by W^{-1} corrects our logistic regression estimator for "confounding" is given in the following lemma characterizing the g-computation algorithm functional $b(\overline{a})$ defined in (*) above.

LEMMA 1.1. *$b(\overline{a})$ defined in (*) is the unique function $c(\overline{a})$ of $\overline{a}$ such that $E\left[q\left(\overline{A}\right)\left(Y - c\left(\overline{A}\right)\right)/\mathcal{W}\right] = 0$ for all functions $q\left(\overline{A}\right)$ for which the expectation exists.*

Lemma 1.1 has the following corollary.

LEMMA 1.2. *Under sequential randomization, $E\left(Y_{\overline{a}}\right)$ is unique function $c(\overline{a})$ of $\overline{a}$ such that $E\left[q\left(\overline{A}\right)\left(Y - c\left(\overline{A}\right)\right)/\mathcal{W}\right] = 0$ for all functions $q\left(\overline{A}\right)$ where the expectation exists.*

Consistency of our weighted estimator then follows from the fact that the probability limit of our weighted score equation is $E[q\left(\overline{A}\right)\left(Y - c\left(\overline{A}\right)\right)/\mathcal{W}] = 0$ with $q\left(\overline{A}\right) = (1, cum(\overline{A}))'$ and $c\left(\overline{A}\right) = g(\overline{A}, \beta)$.

Under a mild strengthening of our assumption of sequential randomization (no unmeasured confounders), a simple, quite revealing, purely "causal" proof of Lemma 1.2 can be obtained that does not use the fact that $E\left(Y_{\overline{a}}\right)$ is given by the g-computation algorithm formula $b(\overline{a})$ of Eq. (*). Let $Y_{\overline{\mathcal{A}}} = \left\{Y_{\overline{a}}; \overline{a} \in \overline{\mathcal{A}}\right\}$ where $\overline{\mathcal{A}}$ is the support of the random variable $\overline{A}$. Suppose we strengthen our assumption of no unmeasured confounders to

$$Y_{\overline{\mathcal{A}}} \coprod A_k \mid \overline{L}_k, \overline{A}_{k-1} \ .$$

Denote the factual and counterfactual data by $Z = \left(Y_{\overline{\mathcal{A}}}, \overline{A}, \overline{L}\right)$ and the observed data by $O = \left(Y \equiv Y_{\overline{A}}, \overline{A}, \overline{L}\right)$. We can factor the true joint density of Z that generated the data as

$$f(Z) = f\left(Y_{\overline{\mathcal{A}}}\right) \prod_{k=0}^{K} f\left(L_k \mid \overline{L}_{k-1}, \overline{A}_{k-1}, Y_{\overline{\mathcal{A}}}\right) \prod_{k=0}^{K} f\left(A_k \mid \overline{L}_k, \overline{A}_{k-1}\right).$$

Now let $f^*\left(A_k \mid \overline{A}_{k-1}\right)$ be a density for A_k given $\overline{A}_{k-1}$. It need not equal the true density $f\left(A_k \mid \overline{A}_{k-1}\right)$. Let $f^*(Z)$ be a joint density for Z that differs from the true joint density $f(Z)$ only in that $f^*\left(A_k \mid \overline{L}_k, \overline{A}_{k-1}\right) = f^*\left(A_k \mid \overline{A}_{k-1}\right)$ so that A_k is strictly exogenous. Thus,

$$f^*(Z) = f\left(Y_{\overline{\mathcal{A}}}\right) \prod_{k=0}^{K} f\left(L_k \mid \overline{L}_{k-1}, \overline{A}_{k-1}, Y_{\overline{\mathcal{A}}}\right) \prod_{k=0}^{K} f^*\left(A_k \mid \overline{A}_{k-1}\right).$$

Now $E\left(Y_{\overline{a}}\right) = E^*\left(Y_{\overline{a}}\right)$ since $f(Z)$ and $f^*(Z)$ have the same marginal law for $Y_{\overline{a}}$. Second, since $\overline{A}$ is causally exogenous under $f^*(z)$ [i.e., $Y_{\overline{a}} \coprod^* \overline{A}$], we have that $E^*\left[Y_{\overline{a}}\right] = E^*\left[Y_{\overline{a}} \mid \overline{A} = \overline{a}\right] = E^*\left[Y_{\overline{A}} \mid \overline{A} = \overline{a}\right] = E^*\left[Y \mid \overline{A} = \overline{a}\right]$. That is, by $\overline{A}$ causally exogenous, the mean of $Y_{\overline{a}}$ is given by the regression function $E^*\left[Y \mid \overline{A} = \overline{a}\right]$ of Y on $\overline{A} = \overline{a}$. Now it is a standard result that the regression function $E^*\left(Y \mid \overline{A} = \overline{a}\right)$ is characterized as the unique function

$c(\overline{a})$ solving $E^{*}\left\{q\left(\overline{A}\right)\left[Y-c\left(\overline{A}\right)\right]\right\} \equiv \int q\left(\overline{A}\right)\left(Y-b\left(\overline{A}\right)\right) f^{*}(Z)\, d\mu(Z)=0$ for all $q\left(\overline{A}\right)$ where μ is a dominating measure. But, $\int q\,(A)(Y-c(\overline{A}))\, f^{*}(Z) d\mu(Z)=\int q\,(A)\left(Y-c\left(\overline{A}\right)\right) \frac{f^{*}(Z)}{f(Z)} f(Z) d\mu(Z)=E[q(A)(Y-c(\overline{A})) \frac{f^{*}(Z)}{f(Z)}]$. But, by definition, $\frac{f^{*}(Z)}{f(Z)}=\mathcal{W}^{-1}$ when $f^{*}\left(A_{k} \mid \overline{A}_{k-1}\right)=f\left(A_{k} \mid \overline{A}_{k-1}\right)$. Lemma 1.2 then follows, since $E^{*}(Y \mid A=\overline{a})=E\left(Y_{\overline{a}}\right)$. The proof also makes clear that consistency of our weighted estimator does not require that we choose $f^{*}\left(A_{k} \mid \overline{A}_{k-1}\right)=f\left(A_{k} \mid \overline{A}_{k-1}\right)$.

Data analyses: Marginal structural mean model for a repeated measures outcome. To give a better picture of the meaning and use of MSMs, we report preliminary results of two data analyses. Full details will be published elsewhere. We estimate the joint effect in ACTG Randomized Trial 002 of AZT treatment arm and aerosolized pentamidine (AP) on the evolution of CD4 count in the first analysis and on mortality in the second analysis. This trial was designed to compare the effect of high-dose AZT with low-dose AZT on survival. However, over fifty percent of the subjects failed to comply with the assigned treatment protocol and initiated treatment with a non-randomized therapy, AP, during the course of the trial. The joint effects of AP and AZT treatment arm on survival have been previously estimated using structural nested failure time models by Robins and Greenland (1994). We first consider a MSM model for the effect of AP therapy on the mean of the log transformed CD4 count history while adjusting for baseline variables. CD4 count measurements were obtained at weeks 8, 16, 24, and 32 measured in days. Specifically, we consider the MSM

$$E\left[Y_{\overline{a}}(m) \mid V^{\dagger}\right]=g_{m}\left[\overline{a}(m), V^{\dagger}, \beta\right]$$

where $Y(m)=\log [CD4(m)+2]$, $CD4(m)$ is the CD4 count on day m, $Y_{\overline{a}}(m)$ is the counterfactual version of $Y(m)$ under the AP history $\overline{a}$, $V^{\dagger}=(1, m, R, Y(0), \log WBC(0))'$ is the vector of baseline regressors with $R=1$ denoting the high AZT treatment arm and $R=0$ the low AZT treatment arm, $Y(0)$ is defined above, and $WBC(0)$ is baseline white blood count. We modeled the regression function as $g_{m}\left[\overline{a}(m), V^{\dagger}, \beta\right]=\beta_{1}' V^{\dagger}+\beta_{2} cum(m, \overline{a})$ with $cum(m, \overline{a})=\int_{0}^{m} a(t)\, dt$ being cumulative AP treatment up to day m. We make the assumption of no unmeasured confounders with $L(t)$ being white blood count, the number of episodes of pneumocystis pneumonia (PCP), an AIDS-related pneumonia, up to day t, and CD4 count on day t. Furthermore, the baseline covariates $V^{\dagger}$ are included in $L(0)$. Arguing as above, it can be shown a consistent estimator of β is obtained by fitting the model $E\left[Y(m) \mid V^{\dagger}, \overline{A}\right]=g_{m}\left[\overline{A}(m), V^{\dagger}, \beta\right]$ using the generalized estimating equation (GEE) option of Proc genmode in the SAS software package under a working independence matrix and weighting the observation $Y(m)$ for a subject by $\{\mathcal{W}(m)\}^{-1}$. The GEE option of Proc genmode is simply a program that fits the above model by weighted least squares to obtain an estimate of β. In estimating β, the program treats each individual at each of the four times m as four separate observations when computing the least squares estimator. However, the program outputs a robust variance estimator that appropriately accounts for the fact that the four observations on a given subject are correlated.

Since $\mathcal{W}(m)$ was unknown, it was estimated from the data by fitting logistic models for $pr\left[A(k) \mid \overline{L}(k), \overline{A}(k-1)\right]$ and $pr\left[A(k) \mid \overline{A}(k-1), V^{\dagger}\right]$. [Note that when our MSM conditions on baseline variables $V^{\dagger}$, they should be included in the denominator of $\mathcal{W}(m)$.] Specifically, we fit the model

$$logit\, pr\left[A(k) = 0 \mid \overline{L}(k), \overline{A}(k-1) \equiv 0\right] = \alpha' Q(k)$$

where $Q(k) = (1, \log k, \log[WBC(k-1)], Y(k-1), PCP\, bouts(k-1), Y(0), \log[WBC(0)], R)$. Here, PCP bouts $(k-1)$ is the number of episodes (bouts) of pneumocystis pneumonia through $k-1$. In fitting the model, we treated each subject at each day $k, k = 0, 1, \ldots, 224$ as an independent observation (which is justified by the conditional martingale structure of the model). We note that since in the 002 data file, any subject starting AP remained on it thereafter, it was only necessary to fit a model for $A(k)$ for subjects who had yet to begin AP [i.e., $\overline{A}(k-1) \equiv 0$]. We estimated $pr\left[A(k) \mid \overline{A}(k-1) \equiv 0, V^{\dagger}\right]$ by fitting the above model after eliminating the random time-dependent terms that were functions of $(k-1)$. The 95 percent Wald intervals computed using the robust variance outputted by the GEE program are conservative (i.e., they are guaranteed to cover the true β at least 95 percent of the time in large samples) because they do not account for estimation of the weights $\mathcal{W}(m)$. It is interesting that estimating the weights shrinks the variance of our estimator of β, so that our intervals (which do not account for the fact that the weights are estimated) are conservative. Note that the elements of the vectors α multiplying the time-dependent covariates $\log[WBC(k-1)]$, $Y(k-1)$ and PCP bouts $(k-1)$ will all be zero if and only if the AP treatment process is statistically ancillary. A three degree of freedom likelihood ratio test of the hypothesis that all three components of α were zero rejected at the $p < .01$ level. As a consequence, we rejected the hypothesis of statistical exogeneity.

The analysis just described assumes that there is no drop-out or censoring by end of follow-up. To correct for this, we defined a subject as censored (i.e., permanently missing) the first time he missed one of his scheduled visits or was censored by end of follow-up. Under the assumption of ignorable drop-out given the time-dependent factors $L(t)$ and treatment $A(t)$, we still obtain consistent estimators of β in the presence of drop-out if we weight a subject uncensored at day m by $\left\{\mathcal{W}(m)\mathcal{W}^{\dagger}(m)\right\}^{-1}$ where $\mathcal{W}^{\dagger}(m) = \prod_{k=0}^{m} \{p\left[R(k) = 0 \mid \overline{R}(k-1) = 0, \overline{L}(k-1), \overline{A}(k-1)\right] / pr\left[R(k) = 0 \mid \overline{R}(k-1) = 0, \overline{A}(k-1), V^{\dagger}\right]\}$ is the ratio of a subject's probability of remaining uncensored up to day m divided by that probability calculated as if there had been no time-dependent determinants of drop-out except past treatment history. Here, $R(m) = 0$ if a subject has not dropped out or reached end to follow-up by day m. Since $\mathcal{W}^{\dagger}(m)$ is unknown, it was estimated from the data in a manner completely analogous to the estimation of $\mathcal{W}(m)$ except with $A(k)$ replaced by $R(k)$ as the outcome variable and with $A(k-1)$ added as an additional regressor. Furthermore, in the presence of censoring, it is necessary when estimating $pr[A(k) = 0 \mid \cdot]$ to add the event $R(k) = 0$ to the conditioning event.

We fit the above models and obtained an estimate $\widehat{\beta}_2 = .001$ and conservative 95 percent confidence interval $(-.026, .028)$ for the parameter β_2 representing the causal effect of cumulative AP dose on CD4 count. Furthermore, since in trial 002 the assignment to AZT treatment arm was at random with probability 1/2, the AZT treatment arm indicator is exogenous. It follows that the component β_{1R} of β_1 multiplying the AZT treatment indicator R has the interpretation as the direct effect of AZT treatment arm on the evolution of mean CD4 count that is not through AP history. We obtained an estimate of .0196 with a conservative 95 percent confidence interval of $(-.123, .163)$ for β_{1R}.

Marginal Structural Cox Proportional Hazards Model. We next estimated the joint effects of AP therapy and AZT treatment arm on survival by specifying a marginal structural Cox proportional hazards model

$$\lambda_{T_{\overline{a}}}\left(t \mid V^{\dagger}\right) = \lambda_0(t)\exp\left[\beta_1' V^{\dagger} + \beta_2 a(t)\right]$$

where $T_{\overline{a}}$ is the subject's time to death if he had followed AP history $\overline{a}$, $\lambda_{T_{\overline{a}}}\left(t \mid V^{\dagger}\right)$ is the hazard of $T_{\overline{a}}$ at t given $V^{\dagger}$, $\lambda_0(t)$ is an unspecified baseline hazard function, and $V^{\dagger} = (R, Y(0), \log WBC(0))$. Note this model specifies that the hazard of failure at time t depends on current AP status rather than on cumulative AP history. Arguing as in the previous subsection, we can obtain consistent estimates of the unknown parameter $\beta = (\beta_1', \beta_2)'$ by fitting the ordinary time-dependent Cox model $\lambda_T\left(t \mid \overline{A}(t), V^{\dagger}\right) = \lambda_0(t)\exp\left[\beta_1' V^{\dagger} + \beta_2 A(t)\right]$ except that the contribution of subject to a calculation performed on subjects at risk at time t is weighted by $\widehat{\mathcal{W}}(t)^{-1}\widehat{\mathcal{W}}^{\dagger}(t)^{-1}$. Note that now when we model $pr[R_k = 0 \mid \cdot]$ and $pr[A_k = 0 \mid \cdot]$ we must include the event $T > k$ among the conditioning events. Here we have adopted the convention that on any day k censoring occurs at the end of the day. Note since the subject-specific weights change with time, one either needs to write a special program or trick a standard time-dependent Cox model that allows weights into allowing for time-varying weights by a clever use of the time-varying stratum option available in many off-the-shelf Cox programs. To obtain conservative 95 percent confidence intervals for β, one needs to compute the so-called robust variance of Lin et al. (1989). Implementing the above procedure, we obtained an estimate $\widehat{\beta}_2 = -.1362$ with 95 percent conservative confidence interval $(-.35, .09)$ for β_2. For the component β_{1R} of β_1 representing the direct effect of AZT treatment arm on survival, we obtained an estimate of .1890 with a 95 percent confidence interval of $(-.01,.21)$ indicating borderline statistically significant evidence for a beneficial effect of the low-dose AZT arm. Both the results obtained for the prophylaxis effect and for the AZT effect were consistent with those obtained by Robins and Greenland (1994) using SNFTMs.

Philosophical interlude. We pause to comment briefly on the definition and nature of the counterfactual random variables $T_{\overline{a}}$. Following Lewis (1973), we consider $T_{\overline{a}}$ to be a subject's death time in the closest possible world to this in which, possibly contrary to fact, the subject was treated with the AP history $\overline{a}$. Consider a subject i who, in the 002 trial, was assigned to the high-dose AZT arm, received AP from week 10 to 40, took the assigned 1500 mg. of AZT daily until week 12 but then stopped all further AZT therapy, and finally died in week 40. If AP had been withheld, it is quite conceivable that subject i would have continued to be assigned 1500 mg. of AZT daily past week 12 if either *(1)* AP potentiated the toxic effects of AZT, precipitating a life-threatening toxic episode in week 12, or *(2)* the subject, although not toxic, had stopped AZT at week 12 because he felt himself to be adequately protected by the AP treatment. To be concrete, say, in the closest possible world, subject i would have continued to take 1500 mg. of AZT daily through week 14 and none thereafter if AP had been withheld. We now consider the meaning of the counterfactual $T_0 \equiv T_{\overline{a}\equiv 0}$ in which AP was always withheld. Then, by its definition, T_0 would be equal to subject i's failure time when the subject was assigned to the high-dose arm, never received AP, and took AZT daily through week 14 (rather than through week 12). Thus, T_0 might well differ from the counterfactual variable, say T_0^*, representing a subject's survival time in the closest possible world in which AP was withheld but, as in this world, AZT was stopped after week 12. Several comments are in order.

First, T_{0i} is conceptually rather well-defined, even if we do not observe what the particular subject i would have done about his AZT dose after week 10 in the absence of AP therapy, as T_{0i} is just subject i's outcome in the closest possible world to this one in which all AP therapy is withheld and all consequences which flow from that (including possibly taking AZT in week 12–14) are all allowed to occur. Second, it may be quite reasonable to make (at least to a good approximation) the assumption of no unmeasured confounders for T_0, in which case its distribution is non-parametrically identified by inverse-probability-of-treatment-weighting, (equivalently, by the g-computation algorithm formula) from the distribution of the observed data. The intuitive reason for this successful identification is that for a subset of the population (i.e., those who never did take AP), we do observe T_0, and under the assumption of no unmeasured confounders, we can appropriately reweight them by $\mathcal{W}^{-1}$ to construct a ghost population whose distribution of $T_0 = T$ is the same as that of T_0 in the true study population. Third, from a public health point of view, it is much more important to identify the distribution of T_0 than T_0^* since it is the distribution of T_0 that would result if we made the public policy decision to withhold AP therapy. Fourth, T_0^* may be more relevant than T_0 in a legal case against the manufacturers of AP. For example, the manufacturers would argue that they should not be held responsible for any damages if a subject's observed death time T equalled their counterfactual death time T_0^* (even if T differed from T_0 due to differences in the amount of AZT taken). Fifth, the distribution of T_0^* is not identified even in an experiment in which both AP and AZT are randomly assigned. Thus, no amount of data evidence will ever determine the distribution of T_0^*, even in a randomized experiment (Robins and Greenland, 1989).

Comparison with SNMs. Marginal structural models are an alternative to structural nested models. A SNM is model for the magnitude of the causal effect of a final brief blip of a time-dependent treatment at time t as a function of past time-dependent treatment and prognostic factor history. The causal parameter of a structural nested model is identified under the assumption of no unmeasured confounders. The essential difference between MSMs and SNMs is that SNMs model the magnitude of the effect of a treatment given at t as a function of the prognostic factor history up to t. In contrast, MSMs model the causal effect of treatment given at t only as a function of baseline prognostic factors. Sec. 5 below is devoted to describing what is known about the advantages and disadvantages of MSMs versus SNMs. Some of the advantages of MSMs were discussed above. Possible disadvantages include the following. *(i)* Inability to easily estimate the effects of dynamic treatment regimes (i.e., treatment plans where a subject's covariate history up to time k determines the treatment to be taken at k). Actual medical treatments are usually dynamic, since if a subject becomes toxic to a drug, the drug must be stopped. *(ii)* The inability to directly test the null hypothesis of no effect of any treatment regime (dynamic or non-dynamic) on outcome. *(iii)* The difficulty in performing likelihood-based inference for MSMs, since the likelihood is a computational nightmare. *(iv)* Lack of identifiability of the MSM model parameters when sequential ignorability holds for a so-called "instrumental variable" but not for the actual treatment of interest. *(v)* MSMs, in contrast to SNMs, cannot be used if there exists a value of ℓ_k, say $\ell_k = 0$, such that for all but one value of a_k, $f\left[a_k \mid \overline{\ell}_{k-1}, \ell_k = 0, \overline{a}_{k-1}\right] = 0$. An example would be a study of the effect of an occupational exposure on mortality with $\ell_k = 0$ if a subject is off work at time k, $\ell_k = 1$ otherwise, and subjects off work can only receive exposure level $a_k = 0$. We note that SNMs do not suffer from any of these five deficiencies.

2. A formal definition of MSMs.

2.1. The data. Consider a study where we observe n i.i.d. copies of data $O = \left(\overline{A}(C), \overline{L}(C)\right)$, where C is an administrative end of follow-up time, $\overline{A}(C)$ is a treatment process, $\overline{L}(C)$ is an outcome or response process and, for any $Z(u), \overline{Z}(t) \equiv \{Z(u); 0 \le u \le t\}$. We assume C is an element of $L(0)$ since it is assumed known at time 0.

For purposes of causal inference, we assume the existence of an underlying treatment process $\overline{A} = \{A(u); 0 \le u < \infty\}$ with $A(u)$ taking values in a set $\mathcal{A}(u)$ and the existence of underlying counterfactual random variables

$$\{\overline{L}_{\overline{a}}; \overline{a} \in \overline{\mathcal{A}}\} \tag{1}$$

where $\overline{L}_{\overline{a}} = \{L_{\overline{a}}(u); 0 \le u < \infty\}$, $\overline{a} = a(\cdot) = \{a(t); 0 \le t < \infty$ and $a(t) \in \mathcal{A}(t)\}$ is a treatment plan (equivalently, regime or function) lying in a set of functions $\overline{\mathcal{A}}$. Given a regime $\overline{a}$, let $\overline{L}_{\overline{a}(u),\mathbf{0}}$ be counterfactual history under a regime $\overline{a}^*$ that agrees with $\overline{a}$ through time u and is 0 thereafter, where 0 is the baseline value of $a(t)$. Then we assume that the $\overline{L}_{\overline{a}}$ satisfy the following consistency assumption with probability 1:

$$\overline{L}_{\overline{a}(u),\mathbf{0}}(u) = \overline{L}_{\overline{a}(t),\mathbf{0}}(u) = \overline{L}_{\overline{a}}(u) = \overline{L}_{\overline{a}^\dagger}(u) \tag{2}$$

for all $t > u$ and all $\overline{a}^\dagger$ with $\overline{a}^\dagger(u) = \overline{a}(u)$. This assumption essentially says that the future does not determine the past. The observed data are linked to the counterfactual data by

$$\overline{L}(C) = \overline{L}_{\overline{A}(C),0}(C). \tag{3}$$

Eq. (3) states that a subject's observed outcome history through end of follow-up is equal to their counterfactual outcome history corresponding to the treatment they did indeed receive. We assume $\overline{L}_{\overline{a}} = \left(\overline{Y}_{\overline{a}}, \overline{V}_{\overline{a}}\right)$ where $\overline{Y}_{\overline{a}}$ is an outcome process of interest and $\overline{V}_{\overline{a}}$ is the process of other recorded variables. Further, we shall make the sequential randomization (i.e., ignorable treatment assignment) assumption that for all t and $\overline{a} \in \overline{\mathcal{A}}$,

$$\underline{Y}_{\overline{a}}(t) \coprod A(t) \mid \overline{L}(t^-), \overline{A}(t^-) \tag{4}$$

where for any variable $\underline{Z}(t) = \{Z(u); u \ge t\}$ is the history of that variable from t onwards. We also refer to (4) as the assumption of no unmeasured confounders given prognostic factors $L(t)$. Because of measurability issues, (4) is not well-defined. If the $A(t)$ process can only jump at discrete non-random times $t_1, t_2, \ldots$ and the $\overline{L}(t)$ process has left-hand limits, i.e., $\overline{L}(t^-) \equiv \lim_{u \uparrow t} \overline{L}(u)$, (4) is formally, for each t_k,

$$f\left[A(t_k) \mid \overline{L}(t_k^-), \overline{A}(t_k^-), \underline{Y}_{\overline{a}}(t_k)\right] = f\left[A(t_k) \mid \overline{L}(t_k^-), \overline{A}(t_k^-)\right]. \tag{5}$$

where $f(\cdot \mid \cdot)$ is the conditional density of $A(t_k)$ with respect to a dominating measure. If $A(t)$ is a marked point process that can jump in continuous time with CADLAG (continuous from the right with left-hand limits) step-function sample paths, then Eq. (4) is formally that

$$\lambda_A\left[t \mid \overline{L}(t^-), \overline{A}(t^-), \underline{Y}_{\overline{a}}(t)\right] = \lambda_A\left[t \mid \overline{L}(t^-), \overline{A}(t^-)\right] \tag{6a}$$

and

$$f\Big[A(t) \mid \overline{L}(t^-), \overline{A}(t^-), A(t) \neq A(t^-), \underline{Y}_{\overline{a}}(t)\Big] = f\Big[A(t) \mid \overline{L}(t^-), \overline{A}(t^-), A(t) \neq A(t^-)\Big]. \tag{6b}$$

Here, the intensity process $\lambda_A(t \mid \cdot)$ is $\lim_{\delta t \to 0} pr[A(t+\delta t) \neq A(t^-) \mid A(t^-), \cdot]/\delta t$. Eq. (6a) says that given past treatment and confounder history, the probability that the A process jumps at t does not depend on the future counterfactual history of the outcome of interest. Eq. (6b) says that given that the covariate process did jump at t, the probability it jumped to a particular value of $A(t)$ does not depend on the future counterfactual history of the outcome of interest.

Following Heitjan and Rubin (1991), we say the data are coarsened at random (CAR) if

$$f\left[\overline{A}(C) \mid \{\overline{L}_{\overline{a}}; \overline{a} \in \overline{\mathcal{A}}\}\right] \textit{ depends only on } O = \left(\overline{A}(C), \overline{L}(C)\right). \tag{7}$$

Note that we can use ideas from the "missing data" literature because one's treatment history $\overline{A}(C)$ determines which components of one's counterfactual history $\{\overline{L}_{\overline{a}}; \overline{a} \in \overline{\mathcal{A}}\}$ one observes. Thus we can view causal inference as a missing data problem (Rubin, 1976). If, as in all the models we shall consider in this paper, for each $\overline{\mathcal{A}}^{\dagger} \subseteq \overline{\mathcal{A}}$ satisfying $\overline{a}_1(u) \neq \overline{a}_2(u)$ for all $\overline{a}_1, \overline{a}_2 \in \overline{\mathcal{A}}^{\dagger}$, the $\left\{L_{\overline{a}}(u); \overline{a} \in \overline{\mathcal{A}}^{\dagger}\right\}$ may have a non-degenerate joint distribution, then CAR implies sequential randomization (4) but the converse is not true (Robins et al., 1999). Robins (1997, pg. 83) gives examples where one would expect (4) to be true even when (7) is false. In this paper, we shall only need (4). However, even if (7) is also imposed this, by itself, essentially places no restrictions on the joint distribution of the observable random variables (Gill, van der Laan, Robins, 1997) and, thus, is not subject to empirical test.

2.2. MSMs. A MSM for $\{\overline{Y}_{\overline{a}}; \overline{a} \in \overline{\mathcal{A}}\}$ places restrictions on the marginal distribution of the $\overline{Y}_{\overline{a}}$ possibly conditional on a baseline variable $V^{\dagger}$ in $V(0)$ (with $C \in V^{\dagger}$ if C is random). Examples of MSMs follow. Each of these examples will be important in our comparison of MSMs with structural nested models below.

Model 1: Suppose $C = K+1$ w.p.1., the $\overline{A}(C)$ process jumps only at times $0, 1, 2, \ldots, K$ and the $\overline{L}_{\overline{a}}$ process jumps only at times $0^-, 1^-, 2^-, \ldots,$

$K^-, K+1^-$. In models 1a-1c, we are only concerned with an outcome measured at end of follow-up. Hence, we set $Y_{\overline{a}}(m) \equiv 0$ with probability 1 $for\ m \leq K$ and define $Y_{\overline{a}} = Y_{\overline{a}}(K+1)$. Then we have

Model 1a – non-linear least squares: $E\left[Y_{\overline{a}} \mid V^\dagger\right] = g[\,\overline{a}(K), V^\dagger, \beta_0\,]$ where $g(\cdot,\cdot,\cdot)$ is a known function. This is the logistic regression MSM we discussed in the Introduction.

Model 1b – semiparametric regression: $\eta\left\{E\left[Y_{\overline{a}} \mid V^\dagger\right]\right\} = g\left[\overline{a}(K), V^\dagger, \beta_0\right] + g^\dagger\left(V^\dagger\right)$ where $\eta(\cdot)$ is a known monotone link function, $g^\dagger(\cdot)$ is unknown and unrestricted and $g(\cdot,\cdot,\cdot)$ is a known function satisfying $g\left(\mathbf{0}, V^\dagger, \beta\right) = 0$. The requirement that $g\left(\mathbf{0}, V^\dagger, \beta\right) = 0$ implies that $g^\dagger\left(V^\dagger\right)$ is the "main effect of $V^\dagger$." Such models are also referred to as partial spline models. They are semiparametric because the main effect of $V^\dagger$ is modelled non-parametrically.

Model 1c – stratified transformation model: $pr[R(\overline{a}, \beta_0) < t \mid V^\dagger] = F_0\left(t \mid V^\dagger\right), F_0\left(t \mid V^\dagger\right)$ an unknown distribution function, $R(\overline{a}, \beta) = r\left(Y_{\overline{a}}, \overline{a}, V^\dagger, \beta\right)$ is a known increasing function of $Y_{\overline{a}}$ satisfying $r\ (y, \overline{a}, V^\dagger, \beta) = y$ if $\overline{a} \equiv \mathbf{0}$ or $\beta = 0$. This model says that we know the conditional quantile-quantile function linking the $Y_{\overline{a}}$'s given $V^\dagger$ up to an unknown parameter β. It is the natural generalization of model 1b for mean functions to quantile-quantile functions.

In the following model, we are interested in the outcome at each $m \geq 1$ so we no longer assume that $Y_{\overline{a}}(m) \equiv 0$ with probability 1.

Model 1d – multivariate non-linear least squares: $E\left[Y_{\overline{a}}(m) \mid V^\dagger\right] = g_m\left[\overline{a}(m-1), V^\dagger, \beta_0\right]$, $m = 1, \ldots, K+1$ where the $g_m(\cdot,\cdot,\cdot)$ are known. This is the natural MSM version of longitudinal generalized estimating equation models for marginal means (Liang and Zeger, 1986). It is the model we use to analyze the 002 CD4 count data in the Introduction.

Model 2: $C = \infty$, $Y_{\overline{a}}$ is a failure time process, i.e., $Y_{\overline{a}}$ jumps from 0 to 1 at some particular time and stays at 1. Then define the failure time $T_{\overline{a}}$ by the equation $Y_{\overline{a}}(T_{\overline{a}}) = 1$ and $Y_{\overline{a}}\left(T_{\overline{a}}^-\right) = 0$. Let $\lambda_0(t)$ and $\lambda_0\left(t \mid V^\dagger\right)$ be unknown non-negative functions of t and $\left(t, V^\dagger\right)$ respectively and, for any $Z, \lambda_Z(u)$ is the hazard of Z.

Model 2a – Cox proportional hazards model: $\lambda_{T_{\overline{a}}}\left[t \mid V^\dagger\right] = \lambda_0(t) \exp\left[r\left(\overline{a}(t^-), t, V^\dagger; \beta_0\right)\right]$ where $r()$ is a known function satisfying $r(\mathbf{0}, t, 0; \beta) = 0$. This is the model we use to analyze the 002 mortality data in the Introduction.

Model 2b – stratified Cox proportional hazards model: $\lambda_{T_{\overline{a}}}(t \mid V^\dagger) = \lambda_0\left(t \mid V^\dagger\right) \exp\left[r\left(\overline{a}(t^-)\, t, V^\dagger; \beta_0\right)\right]$ where, now, $r(\mathbf{0}, t, V^\dagger; \beta) = 0$.

Model 2c – stratified time-dependent accelerated failure time model: $pr[r\left(T_{\overline{a}}, \overline{a}, V^\dagger, \beta_0\right) < t \mid V^\dagger] = F_0\left(t \mid V^\dagger\right)$ where $r\left(u, \overline{a}, V^\dagger, \beta\right) = r\ (u, \overline{a}\ (u), V^\dagger, \beta)$ is a known function increasing in its first argument satisfying $r\left(u, \mathbf{0}, V^\dagger, \beta\right) = u$. This model can also be written as

$$\lambda_{R(\overline{a}, \beta_0)}\left(t \mid V^\dagger\right) = \lambda_0\left(t \mid V^\dagger\right)$$

for $\overline{a} \in \overline{\mathcal{A}}$, where $R(\overline{a},\beta) = r\left(T_{\overline{a}},\overline{a},V^{\dagger},\beta\right)$. This is the extension of model 1c to a failure time variable. It is the model studied by Robins and Tsiatis (1992).

3. Estimation.

3.1. Ancillary treatment process. In this section, we consider estimation of the parameter β_0 of our marginal structural models. In this subsection, we will suppose that $\overline{A}$ is a causally ancillary (i.e., exogenous) covariate process, i.e.,

$$\overline{A} \coprod \{\overline{L}_{\overline{a}};\ \overline{a} \in \overline{\mathcal{A}}\} \,|V^{\dagger}\ . \tag{8}$$

The often unrealistic assumption (8) implies CAR but, in contrast to CAR, places restrictions on the joint distribution of the data. Specifically (8) implies statistical ancillarity

$$A(t) \coprod \overline{L}\left(t^{-}\right) \mid \overline{A}\left(t^{-}\right), V^{\dagger} \tag{9}$$

and thus (8) is subject to an empirical test.

Given (8), the restrictions on the observables O implied by any MSM are (9) and that the restrictions on the distribution of $\overline{Y}_{\overline{a}}$ given $V^{\dagger}$ specified by the MSM hold for the conditional distribution of the observable $\overline{Y}(C)$ conditional on $\left(\overline{A}(C), V^{\dagger}\right)$.

For reasons that will become clear below, we indicate with a "*" any expectations, probabilities or hazard functions computed under the assumption that (8) and (9) hold. For convenience, denote $\overline{A}(C)$ as $\overline{A}$. Thus, for our MSM models (1a)–(2c), (8) implies the association models

Model 1a: $E^{*}\left[Y \mid V^{\dagger},\overline{A}\right] = g\left(\overline{A},V^{\dagger},\beta_0\right)$

Model 1b: $\eta\left\{E^{*}\left[Y \mid V^{\dagger},\overline{A}\right]\right\} = g\left(\overline{A},V^{\dagger},\beta_0\right) + g^{\dagger}\left(V^{\dagger}\right)$.

Model 1c: $R(\beta_0) \coprod^{*} \overline{A} \mid V^{\dagger}$ where $R(\beta_0) \equiv R\left(\overline{A},\beta_0\right)$.

Model 1d: $E^{*}\left[Y(m) \mid V^{\dagger},\overline{A}\right] = g_m\left[\overline{A}(m-1), V^{\dagger};\beta_0\right]$, $m = 1,\ldots,K+1$.

Model 2a: $\lambda_T^{*}\left[t \mid V^{\dagger},\overline{A}\right] = \lambda_T^{*}\left[t \mid V^{\dagger},\overline{A}\left(t^{-}\right)\right]$
$= \lambda_0(t)\exp\left[r\left(\overline{A}\left(t^{-}\right),t,V^{\dagger},\beta_0\right)\right]$.

Model 2b: $\lambda_T^{*}\left[t \mid V^{\dagger},\overline{A}\right] = \lambda_T^{*}\left[t \mid V^{\dagger},\overline{A}\left(t^{-}\right)\right]$
$= \lambda_0\left(t \mid V^{\dagger}\right)\exp\left[r\left(\overline{A}\left(t^{-}\right),t,V^{\dagger},\beta_0\right)\right]$.

Model 2c: $\lambda_{R(\beta_0)}^{*}\left[u \mid V^{\dagger},\overline{A}\right] = \lambda_{R(\beta_0)}^{*}\left[u \mid \overline{A}\left[r^{-1}\left(u,\overline{A},V^{\dagger},\beta_0\right)\right],V^{\dagger}\right]$
$= \lambda_0\left(u \mid V^{\dagger}\right)$ where $R(\beta_0) \equiv R\left(\overline{A},\beta_0\right)$ and $r^{-1}\left(u,\overline{a},V^{\dagger},\beta\right) \equiv t$ if $r\left(t,\overline{a},V^{\dagger},\beta\right) = u$.

We shall now consider estimation of these models for the observables, under assumption (9), and the further assumption that

(10) $\overline{A}(C)$ *has a known conditional distribution given* $V^{\dagger}$.

Semiparametric inference in the association models 1a–2c without (10) imposed has been examined previously by many authors. Below we use their results to solve the estimation problem in our semiparametric model.

We will show that associated with each MSM model with (9) and (10) imposed is a class of regular asymptotically linear (RAL) estimators $\left\{\widehat{\beta}^* (h, \phi)\right\}$ for β_0, indexed by vector functions $h \in \mathcal{H}$ and $\phi \in \Phi$ such that the set $\mathcal{IF}^* = \{IF^* (h, \phi)\}$ of influence functions of the $\widehat{\beta}^* (h, \phi)$ constitute all the influence functions for the model, in the sense that if $\widetilde{\beta}^*$ is any other RAL estimator, then the influence function of $\widetilde{\beta}^*$ equals $IF^* (h, \phi)$ for some functions $h \in \mathcal{H}, \phi \in \Phi$. Recall that an estimator $\widetilde{\beta}$ of β_0 is RAL with influence function IF if $n^{\frac{1}{2}} \left(\widetilde{\beta} - \beta_0\right) = n^{-\frac{1}{2}} \sum\limits_i IF_i + o_p (1)$, the IF_i are i.i.d, and the convergence of $\widetilde{\beta}$ to β_0 is locally uniform. Here $o_p (1)$ denotes a random variable converging in probability to zero. Thus a RAL estimator is asymptotically equivalent to a sum of the i.i.d random variables IF_i. We obtain $\widehat{\beta}^* (h, \phi)$ by solving the estimating equations $n^{-\frac{1}{2}} \sum_i \widehat{D}_i^* (\beta, h, \phi) = o_p (1)$ described below. [We put $o_p (1)$ on the right side of the estimating equation to take care of cases (e.g., rank estimators) in which the estimating function $\widehat{D}^* (\beta, h, \phi)$ is not continuous in β and, thus, the left-hand side of the previous equality may never be exactly zero.] The solution $\widehat{\beta}^* (h, \phi)$ has influence function $IF^* (h, \phi) = \{\kappa^* (h)\}^{-1} U^* (\beta_0, h, \phi)$ where $U_i^* (\beta_0, h, \phi)$ depends only on subject i's data, $\kappa^* (h) = -\partial E^* [U^* (\beta, h, \phi)] / \partial \beta_{|\beta = \beta_0}$ does not depend on ϕ, and $n^{-\frac{1}{2}} \sum_i \widehat{D}_i^* (\beta_0, h, \phi) = n^{-\frac{1}{2}} \sum_i U_i^* (\beta_0, h, \phi) + o_p (1)$. Furthermore, $\Lambda^{\perp} = \{U^* (\beta_0, h, \phi)\}$ with $h \in \mathcal{H}, \phi \in \Phi$ is the linear span of $\mathcal{IF}^*$ and thus is the orthogonal complement to the nuisance tangent space for the model in the Hilbert space induced by the covariance norm. (Here we are quoting a well known result from the theory of semiparametric models. See Robins and Ritov (1997) for discussion.) We refer to $U^* (\beta_0, h, \phi)$ as the influence function for the estimating function $\widehat{D} (\beta_0, h, \phi)$. More specifically, $U^* (\beta, h, \phi)$ and $\widehat{D}^* (\beta, h, \phi)$ are each expressed as the sum of the two components, one of which $U_{tp}^* (\phi) = D_{tp}^* (\phi)$ is independent of the choice of the MSM and follows from the fact that, for the "treatment process (tp)," (9) and (10) are assumed. Specifically, if the $A (t)$ can jump only at times $0, 1, 2, \ldots, U_{tp}^* (\phi) = \sum_{k=0}^{int(C)} \phi \left(k, \overline{A} (k), \overline{L} (k^-)\right) - E^* \left[\phi \left(k, \overline{A} (k), \overline{L} (k^-)\right) \mid \overline{L} (k^-), \overline{A} (k^-)\right]$ where $int (C)$ is the greatest integer less that or equal to C. It is easy to see that $\left\{U_{tp}^* (\phi)\right\}$ is, as ϕ varies, the sum over k of functions of the observed data $\left(\overline{A} (k), \overline{L} (k^-)\right)$ with mean zero given $\left(\overline{A} (k^-), \overline{L} (k^-)\right)$. If $A (t)$ is a continuous time marked point process, then $U_{tp}^*(\phi) = \int dM_A^*(u) \phi_1 (u, \overline{A}(u^-), \overline{L}(u^-)) + \int dN_A(u) \{\phi_2 (u, \overline{A}(u), \overline{L}(u^-)) - E^* [\phi_2 \left(u, \overline{A} (u), \overline{L} (u^-)\right) \mid A (u) \neq A (u^-), \overline{L} (u^-), \overline{A} (u^-)]\}$ where $dM_A^* (u) = dN_A (u) - \lambda_A^* \left[u \mid \overline{A} (u^-), \overline{L} (u^-)\right] du$ and $dN_A (u) = I \{A (u) \neq A (u^-)\}$ counts jumps in the $\overline{A}$ process. [In the examples of the Introduction, we chose the function ϕ to be identically zero so that $\widehat{D}_{tp}^* (\phi)$ was also zero. As we shall see later, the choice ϕ identically zero, although computationally convenient because we can then use standard software, is somewhat inefficient.]

The other structural model-specific component $\widehat{D}^*_{sm}(\beta, h)$ and $U^*_{sm}(\beta, h)$ of $\widehat{D}^*(\beta, h, \phi)$ and $U^*(\beta, h, \phi)$ are the well-known estimating functions and their associated influence functions for the association models 1a–2c with neither (9) nor (10) imposed.

Model 1a: $\widehat{D}^*_{sm}(\beta, h) = U^*_{sm}(\beta, h) = h(\overline{A}, V^\dagger)\,\varepsilon(\beta)$ with $\varepsilon(\beta) = Y - g(\overline{A}, V^\dagger, \beta)$ and $h(\overline{A}, V^\dagger)$ is any $\dim(\beta)$ vector function. In the linear logistic cumulative treatment model of the Introduction, $\widehat{D}^*_{sm}(\beta, h)$ was the score equation from the logistic model and thus $h(\overline{A}, V^\dagger)$ was the vector $(1, cum(\overline{a}))'$.

Model 1b: $\eta(x) = x : \widehat{D}^*_{sm}(\beta, h) = U^*_{sm}(\beta, h) = \{\varepsilon(\beta) - h_1(\overline{A}, V^\dagger)\}\{h_2(\overline{A}, V^\dagger) - E^*[h_2(\overline{A}, V^\dagger) \mid V^\dagger]\}$ where h_1 is any real valued function, $\varepsilon(\beta)$ is as just defined and the range of h_2 is of $\dim(\beta)$. $\eta(x) = \ln[x/(1-x)] : U^*_{sm}(\beta, h) = U^\dagger(h, P(\beta))$ and $\widehat{D}^*_{sm}(\beta, h) \equiv U^\dagger\left(h, \widehat{P}(\beta)\right)$, where $P(\beta) = expit\left[g(\overline{A}, V^\dagger, \beta) + g^\dagger(V^\dagger)\right], \widehat{P}(\beta) = expit\left[g(\overline{A}, V^\dagger, \beta) + \widehat{g}^\dagger(V^\dagger)\right], expit(x) = e^x/(1+e^x), \widehat{g}^\dagger(V^\dagger)$ is a $n^{\frac{1}{4}}$ - consistent estimate of $g^\dagger(V^\dagger)$, and $U^\dagger(h, P(\beta)) \equiv \{Y - P(\beta)\}\{\{h(\overline{A}, V^\dagger) - E^*[h(\overline{A}, V^\dagger) P(\beta)\{1 - P(\beta)\} \mid V^\dagger]/E^*[P(\beta)\{1-P(\beta)\} \mid V^\dagger]\}$.

Model 1c: $\widehat{D}^*_{sm}(\beta, h) = U^*(\beta, h) = h[R(\beta), \overline{A}, V^\dagger] - \int h[R(\beta), \overline{a}, V^\dagger]dF^*[\overline{a} \mid V^\dagger]$.

Model 1d: Let $\varepsilon(\beta) = \{\varepsilon_1(\beta), \ldots \varepsilon_{K+1}(\beta)\}'$, $\varepsilon_m(\beta) = Y(m) - g_m[\overline{A}(m-1), V^\dagger; \beta]$. Then $\widehat{D}^*_{sm}(\beta, h) = U^*_{sm}(\beta, h) = h(\overline{A}, V^\dagger)\,\varepsilon(\beta)$ where $h(\overline{A}, V^\dagger)$ is now any $\dim(\beta) \times (K+1)$ matrix of real valued functions.

Model 2a: $\widehat{D}^*_{sm}(\beta, h) = \int_0^\infty dN_T(u)\left\{h(u, \overline{A}(u), V^\dagger) - \widetilde{\mathcal{L}}(h, u, \beta)\right\}$, where $\widetilde{\mathcal{L}}(h, u, \beta) = \widetilde{J}[h, \beta]/\widetilde{J}[\mathbf{1}, \beta]$; for any $h(u, \overline{A}(u), V^\dagger), \widetilde{J}(h, \beta) = \widetilde{E}[h(u, \overline{A}(u), V^\dagger) I(T > u)\exp\{r[\overline{A}(u), u, V^\dagger, \beta]\}]$; for any H_i, $\widetilde{E}(H) = \sum_{i=1}^n H_i/n$; $\mathbf{1}$ is the constant function equal to one; and $N_T(u) = I(T \le u)$. $U^*_{sm}(\beta, h) = \int_0^\infty dM_T(u)\{h(u, \overline{A}(u), V^\dagger) - \mathcal{L}^*(h, u, V^\dagger, \beta)\}$ where $\mathcal{L}^*(h, u, \beta) = J^*[h, \beta]/J^*[\mathbf{1}, \beta]$; $J^*[h, \beta]$ is defined like $\widetilde{J}(h, \beta)$ but with E^* replacing $\widetilde{E}$; and $dM_T(u) = dN_T(u) - \lambda_T(u \mid \overline{A}, V^\dagger)\, I(T > u)\, du$.

Model 2b: $U^*_{sm}(\beta, h)$ and $\widehat{D}^*_{sm}(\beta, h)$ are as above except $J^*(h, \beta) \equiv E^*[h(u, \overline{A}(u), V^\dagger) I(T > u)\exp\{r[\overline{A}(u), u, V^\dagger, \beta]\} \mid V^\dagger]$ *and* $\widetilde{J}(h, \beta)$ replaces $E^*(\cdot \mid V^\dagger)$ in $J^*(h, \beta)$ by a $n^{\frac{1}{4}}$ - consistent estimator $\widehat{E}(\cdot \mid V^\dagger)$.

Model 2c: $\widehat{D}^*_{sm}(\beta, h) = \int_0^\infty du I[R(\beta) > u]\{H_2(u, \beta) - E^*[H_2(u, \beta) \mid V^\dagger]\} + \int_0^\infty dN_{R(\beta)}(u)\left[H_1(u, \beta) - E^*\left[H_1(u, \beta) \mid V^\dagger\right]\right]$ and, for $j = 1, 2$, $H_j(u, \beta) = h_j\left[u, \overline{A}\{r^{-1}(u, \overline{A}, V^\dagger, \beta)\}, V^\dagger\right]$. $U^*_{sm}(\beta, h) = \widehat{D}^*_{sm}(\beta, h)$.

REMARK 3.1. Note that in model 2b and in model 1b with $\eta(x) = \ln[x/(1-x)]$, smooths are necessary to estimate $g^\dagger(V^\dagger)$ and $E^*(\cdot \mid V^\dagger)$

if $V^\dagger$ has continuous components. In particular, due to the curse of dimensionality, it is not possible to obtain a reasonable $n^{\frac{1}{2}}$ – consistent estimator of β_0 in these models when $V^\dagger$ has multiple continuous components. This can be formalized using the concept of curse of dimensionality appropriate (CODA) semiparametric information bounds introduced by Robins and Ritov (1997). Specifically, models 2b and 1b have CODA information bounds of zero, although they have positive ordinary semiparametric information bounds.

3.2. Non-ancillary treatment process. In this section, we no longer assume (8) is true. The essential idea of this section (requiring some minor modification) is to reweight $\widehat{D}^*_{sm}(\beta, h)$ by the inverse of a subject's probability of having had his observed treatment history. We continue to assume that

$$f\left[a(t) \mid \overline{L}(t^-), \overline{A}(t^-), V^\dagger\right] \quad \text{is known for } t \le C \tag{11}$$

which implies that if $A(t)$ jumps at non-random times $0, \ldots, K$, $W(k) = f\left[A(k) \mid \overline{L}(k^-), \overline{A}(k^-)\right]$ and $\overline{W}(k) = \prod_{m=0}^{k} W(k)$ are known. If $A(t)$ jumps in continuous time, $\overline{W}(t) = \exp\left[-\int_0^t \lambda_A\left[u \mid \overline{L}(u^-), \overline{A}(u^-)\right] du\right] \prod_{\{u; A(u) \neq A(u^-), u<t\}} \lambda_A[u \mid \overline{L}(u^-), \overline{A}(u^-)]\ f[A(u) \mid \overline{A}(u^-), \overline{L}(u^-), A(u) \neq A(u^-)]$ is known.

We now come to a subtle but crucial idea. We need to artificially censor a subject at the first time $C^\dagger$ that the density of receiving his observed treatment $A(C^\dagger)$ at $C^\dagger$ was zero for some prognostic factor history $\overline{\ell}\left(C^{\dagger -}\right)$ in order to insure that the reweighted $\widehat{D}^*_{sm}(\beta_0, h)$ still has asymptotic mean zero. We formalize this idea as follows. If $A(t)$ jumps at non-random times, let $\overset{\circ}{\mathcal{A}}\left(k, \overline{a}(k^-), v^\dagger\right) = \{a(k); f\left[a(k) \mid \overline{L}(k^-), \overline{A}(k^-) = \overline{a}(k^-), V^\dagger = v^\dagger\right] \neq 0 \ w.p.1\}$ and set $C^\dagger = \min\{k; A(k) \notin \overset{\circ}{\mathcal{A}}\left(k, \overline{A}(k^-), V^\dagger\right)\}$. If $A(t)$ jumps in continuous time, let $\overset{\circ}{\mathcal{A}}\left(t, \overline{a}(t^-), v^\dagger\right) = \{a(t); f[a(t) \mid \overline{L}(t^-), \overline{A}(t^-) = \overline{a}(t^-), A(t) \neq a(t^-), V^\dagger = v^\dagger] \neq 0 \ w.p.1 \text{ or } a(t) = A(t^-)\}$ and set $C^\dagger = \inf\{t; A(t) \notin \overset{\circ}{\mathcal{A}}\left(t, \overline{A}(t^-), V^\dagger\right)\}$. The variable $C^\dagger$ is crucial because, as indicated in the remark following Lemma 3.1 below, one can only unbiasedly reweight a function of $A(t)$ for $A(t) \in \overset{\circ}{\mathcal{A}}\left(t, \overline{a}(t^-), v^\dagger\right)$.

Let $f^*\left(\overline{a} \mid V^\dagger\right)$ be a density (chosen by the analyst). Let F^* denote the joint distribution which differs from the true distribution F of O only in that $f\left[a(t) \mid \overline{L}(t^-), \overline{A}(t^-), V^\dagger\right]$ is replaced by the ancillary density $f^*\left[a(t) \mid \overline{A}(t^-), V^\dagger\right]$. Further, define $\mathcal{W}(t) \equiv \overline{W}(t) / f^*\left[\overline{A}(t) \mid V^\dagger\right]$ and

$O^{\dagger} = \left(\overline{L}\left(C^{\dagger}\right), \overline{A}\left(C^{\dagger}\right)\right)$. Note that in the examples of the Introduction, we chose $f^{*}\left[a(t) \mid \overline{A}(t^{-}), V^{\dagger}\right]$ to be $f\left[a(t) \mid \overline{A}(t^{-}), V^{\dagger}\right]$. Note even with this choice, the distribution F of O differs from the distribution F^{*} if (9) is false. A key result, which follows from direct calculation, is

LEMMA 3.1. *For any* $z\left(O^{\dagger}\right), E\left[z\left(O^{\dagger}\right)/\mathcal{W}\left(C^{\dagger}\right) \mid V^{\dagger}\right] = E^{*}\left[z\left(O^{\dagger}\right) \mid V^{\dagger}\right]$.

REMARK 3.2. It is false that $E\left[z(O)/\mathcal{W}(C) \mid V^{\dagger}\right] = E^{*}\left[z(O) \mid V^{\dagger}\right]$.

Let $D^{*}_{sm}(\beta, h)$ be the probability limit under F^{*} of $\widehat{D}^{*}_{sm}(\beta, h)$ and let $\{U_{sm}(\beta, h)\}$ and $\{D_{sm}(\beta, h)\}$ be the subsets of $\{U^{*}_{sm}(\beta, h)\}$ and $\{D^{*}_{sm}(\beta, h)\}$, respectively, that depend on the data only through $O^{\dagger}$. Set $\mathcal{W} = \mathcal{W}\left(C^{\dagger}\right)$ and note $D_{sm}(\beta, h)$ and $U_{sm}(\beta, h)$ often depend on $E^{*}\left[\cdot \mid V^{\dagger}\right] = E\left[\cdot/\mathcal{W} \mid V^{\dagger}\right]$ or $E^{*}[\cdot] = E[\cdot/\mathcal{W}]$. Define $\widehat{D}_{sm}(\beta, h)$ and $\widehat{U}_{sm}(\beta, h)$ like $D_{sm}(\beta, h)$ and $U_{sm}(\beta, h)$ except replace any unknown expectations $E[\cdot/\mathcal{W} \mid V^{\dagger}]$ and $E[\cdot/\mathcal{W}]$ with appropriate estimates $\widehat{E}\left[\cdot/\mathcal{W} \mid V^{\dagger}\right]$ and $\widehat{E}\left[\cdot/\mathcal{W}\right]$·.

EXAMPLE 1. In model 1b, with $\eta(x) = x$, $U_{sm}(\beta, h) = \widehat{D}_{sm}(\beta, h) = U^{*}_{sm}(\beta, h)$ has $h_1\left(\overline{A}, V^{\dagger}\right)$ and $h_2\left(\overline{A}, V^{\dagger}\right)$ being functions only of $\{\overline{A}(C^{\dagger}), V^{\dagger}\}$. Note $E^{*}\left[h_2\left(\overline{A}, V^{\dagger}\right) \mid V^{\dagger}\right]$ is known and need not be estimated.

In contrast, in models 2a and 2b, $\widehat{D}_{sm}(\beta, h)$ will be defined like $\widehat{D}^{*}_{sm}(\beta, h)$ except in defining $\widetilde{J}(h, \beta)$ we replace $I(T > u)$ by $I(T > u)/\mathcal{W}$ in order to estimate the unknown expectations. Alternatively, we can replace $I(T > u)$ by $I(T > u)/\mathcal{W}(u)$. This latter choice *(i)* will in general have better finite sample properties, *(ii)* tend to increase efficiency unless the estimator with $I(T > u)/\mathcal{W}$ was already semiparametric efficient, and *(iii)* was the approach we took in the Introduction. The issues are exactly those discussed in Robins (1993), which the reader may consult for further clarification.

In model 1b with $\eta(x) = \ln[x/(1-x)]$, $\widehat{g}\left(V^{\dagger}\right) \equiv \widehat{g}\left(V^{\dagger}, \beta\right)$ could be chosen to minimize $\widetilde{E}\left[\left(Y - expit\left\{g\left(\overline{A}, V^{\dagger}, \beta\right) + g^{\dagger}\left(V^{\dagger}\right)\right\}\right)^{2}/\mathcal{W}\right]$ over $g^{\dagger}\left(V^{\dagger}\right)$ in some class (e.g., splines), whose dimension may increase with sample size.

In the appendix we briefly sketch a proof of the following.

THEOREM 3.1. *Subject to regularity conditions, in the semiparametric model (i) characterized by (4), (11), the data O, and a MSM, the class* $\left\{\widehat{\beta}(h, \phi)\right\}$ *with* $h \in \mathcal{H}$ *and* $\phi \in \Phi$ *of estimators which solve* $0 = \sum_i \widehat{D}_i(\beta, h, \phi)$ *with* $\left\{\widehat{D}(\beta, h, \phi)\right\} = \left\{\widehat{D}_{sm}(\beta, h)/\mathcal{W} + D_{tp}(\phi)\right\}$ *is a class of RAL estimators with influence functions* $\mathcal{IF} = \{IF(h, \phi)\}$, $IF(h, \phi) = \{\kappa(h)\}^{-1} U(\beta_0, h, \phi)$, $\kappa(h) = -\partial E[U(\beta, h, \phi)]/\partial\beta_{|\beta=\beta_0}$, $U(\beta_0, h, \phi) = U_{sm}(\beta_0, h)/\mathcal{W} + U_{tp}(\phi)$, *where* $U_{tp}(\phi) = D_{tp}(\phi)$ *is defined like* $U^{*}_{tp}(\phi)$ *except with the true law F replacing* F^{*}. *Furthermore,* $\mathcal{IF}$ *is the set of all influence functions.*

3.3. Efficiency for fixed h. We now begin to explore efficiency issues. By a projection argument similar to that given in Robins et al. (1994), we have

THEOREM 3.2. *For a given h, among all estimators $\widehat{\beta}(h,\phi)$, the most efficient has ϕ equal to $\phi_{opt} \equiv \phi_{opt}(h)$: if $A(t)$ only jumps at non-random times $0,1,2,\ldots$ then $\phi_{opt} \equiv 0$ if $k > C^{\dagger}$, and if $k \le C^{\dagger}$, $\phi_{opt}\left[k,\overline{a}(k),\overline{\ell}(k^-)\right] = E[U_{sm}(h)/\mathcal{W} \mid \overline{A}(k) = \overline{a}(k), \overline{L}(k^-) = \overline{\ell}(k^-)] = \left\{\overline{W}(k)\right\}^{-1} \iint d\mu\left(\underline{a}_{k+1}\right)\ f^*\left(\overline{a} \mid v^{\dagger}\right)\ E\left[u_{sm}\left\{\overline{a}\left(C^{\dagger}\right), \overline{Y}_{\overline{a}}\left(C^{\dagger}\right), V^{\dagger}, h\right\} \mid \overline{L_{\overline{a}}}(k^-) = \overline{\ell}(k^-), \overline{A}(k) = \overline{a}(k)\right]$ and $U_{sm}(h) \equiv U_{sm}(\beta_0, h)$. Furthermore, if CAR holds, $\overline{A}(k) = \overline{a}(k)$ can be removed from the last conditioning event above. If $A(t)$ jumps in continuous time, $\phi_{1,opt} = E[U_{sm}(h)/\mathcal{W} \mid \overline{L}(u^-), \overline{A}(u^-), A(u) \neq A(u^-)] - E\left[U_{sm}(h)/\mathcal{W} \mid \overline{L}(u^-), \overline{A}(u^-)\right]$ since $E\left[U_{sm}(h)/\mathcal{W} \mid \overline{L}(u^-), \overline{A}(u^-)\right] = E\left[U_{sm}(h)/\mathcal{W} \mid \overline{L}(u^-), \overline{A}(u^-), A(u) = \overline{A}(u^-)\right]$, and $\phi_{2,opt} = E\left[U_{sm}(h)/\mathcal{W} \mid \overline{A}(u), \overline{L}(u^-)\right]$.*

We now relax unrealistic assumption (11) that the conditional density of $A(t)$ is known. We consider two cases. In the first case the density is completely unknown and in the second the density follows a parametric model.

THEOREM 3.3. ***a)*** *The semiparametric model (ii) characterized by (4), data O, and a MSM (with (11) not imposed), has the set of influence functions $\left\{IF\left(h,\phi_{opt}(h)\right)\right\}$ with $h \in \mathcal{H}$.*
b) *In model (iii) characterized by (4), data O, a MSM, and a parametric model indexed by parameter α for $f\left[a(t) \mid \overline{L}(t^-), \overline{A}(t^-)\right]$, the set of influence functions for the model is the set $\left\{\kappa(h)^{-1}\left[U(h,\phi) - E\left[U(h,\phi)S'_{\alpha}\right]\left\{E\left[S_{\alpha}S'_{\alpha}\right]\right\}^{-1}S_{\alpha}\right]\right\}$ of influence functions of $\left\{\widehat{\beta}(h,\phi,\widehat{\alpha})\right\}$ solving $o_p(1) = n^{-\frac{1}{2}}\sum_i \widehat{D}_i(\beta,h,\phi,\widehat{\alpha})$ where $\widehat{\alpha}$ is the MLE of α, $S_{\alpha} = \partial\log\left\{f\left[A(t) \mid \overline{L}(t^-), \overline{A}(t^-), \alpha\right]/\partial\alpha\right\}$ is the subject-specific score for α, and $D(\beta,h,\phi,\widehat{\alpha})$ is $D(\beta,h,\phi)$ evaluated at $\widehat{\alpha}$.*

Theorem 3.3b can be extended to semiparametric models for $f\left(a(t) \mid \overline{L}(t^-), \overline{A}(t^-)\right)$ such as a Cox proportional hazard model as in Robins (1993; 1998b, App. 2). In the non- and semi-parametric case, we have to plug an estimator of $f\left[a(t) \mid \overline{L}(t^-), \overline{A}(t^-)\right]$ into the estimating function $\widehat{D}_i(\beta,h,\phi)$. In general, the estimator needs to converge to the true density at a rate greater than $n^{\frac{1}{4}}$ to obtain a RAL estimator of β.

3.4. Censoring. No new idea is required to account for and adjust for right censoring. Specifically, let Q be censoring time in MSMs. Define a censoring process $A_2(u)$ by $A_2(u) = 0$ if $Q > u$ and $A_2(u) = 1$ otherwise. Let the treatment of interest be $a_1(u)$ and define $a(u) = (a_1(u), a_2(u))$ and write $T_{\overline{a}}$ as $T_{\overline{a}_1,\overline{a}_2}$. To want to adjust for censoring is only to say that interest is in the direct effect of $\overline{a}_1$ when $\overline{a}_2 \equiv 0$, i.e., when censoring is abolished. As a concrete example, the Cox model MSM 2a in the presence of censoring would become

$$\lambda_{T_{\overline{a}_1,\overline{a}_2\equiv 0}}\left(t \mid V^{\dagger}\right)=\lambda_0(t)\exp\left\{r\left[\overline{a}_1\left(t^{-}\right),t,V^{\dagger};\beta_0\right]\right\}.$$

If $\overline{A}$ is ancillary (now including the censoring process), $\widehat{D}^*_{sm}(\beta,h)$ and $U^*_{sm}(\beta,h)$ are as above except that now $N_T(u)=I[T\le u]\,I[T<Q]$ and $I[T>u]$ is everywhere replaced by $I[T>u]\,I[Q>u]$. Of course $\overline{W}(t)$ is now the probability that a subject would have his observed treatment and censoring history. This is exactly the approach we took in analyzing the 002 trial data in the Introduction.

4. Semiparametric efficiency.

4.1. The efficient score. In any semiparametric model, the semiparametric variance bound is the inverse of the variance of the efficient score S_{eff}. The efficient score in models *(i)–(iii)* of Theorems 3.1 and 3.2 are the same and, by Theorem 5.3 in Newey and McFadden (1993), equal $S_{eff}=U\left(\beta_0,h_{eff},\phi_{eff}\right)$ where $\phi_{eff}=\phi_{opt}\left(h_{eff}\right)$ and h_{eff} is uniquely characterized by the requirement that for all $U(\beta_0,h,\phi)$

$$E\left[U(\beta_0,h,\phi)\,U\left(\beta_0,h_{eff},\phi_{opt}\left(h_{eff}\right)\right)'\right]=\kappa(h)$$

which is equal to

$$E\left[U_{sm}(\beta_0,h)\,U\left(\beta_0,h_{eff},\phi_{opt}\left(h_{eff}\right)\right)'\right]=\kappa(h)\ . \qquad (12)$$

To show how to use (12) to calculate h_{eff}, we consider the following simple example.

Model 1a: Consider MSM 1a with $C^{\dagger}=C=K+1=1$ w.p.1 so $K=0$ and the $\overline{A}(C)$ process only jumps at time zero. So $\overline{A}=A(0)$ and $\mathcal{W}^{-1}=f^*\left[\overline{A}\mid V^{\dagger}\right]/f\left[\overline{A}\mid L(0)\right]$ where $V^{\dagger}\subset L(0)=V(0)$. For the purposes of computing the efficient score, we can choose $f^*\left(\overline{A}\mid V^{\dagger}\right)=1$ w.p.1 without worrying that it is not a density, because it can be absorbed into $h_{eff}\left(\overline{A},V^{\dagger}\right)$. In Appendix B, we prove the following.

THEOREM 4.1. *With $f^*\left(\overline{A}\mid V^{\dagger}\right)=1$ w.p.1, Eq. 12 implies $h_{eff}(\overline{A},V^{\dagger})$ is the unique solution to the type two Fredholm equation $h_{eff}(\overline{A},V^{\dagger})\left[\int var\left[\varepsilon\mid\overline{A},L(0)\right]\left\{f\left(\overline{A}\mid L(0)\right)\right\}^{-1}f\left(V^{\bullet}\mid V^{\dagger}\right)d\mu\left(V^{\bullet}\right)\right]+\int h_{eff}(\overline{a},V^{\dagger})\omega\left(\overline{a},\overline{A},V^{\dagger}\right)d\mu(\overline{a})=\partial g\left(\overline{A},V^{\dagger},\beta_0\right)/\partial\beta$ where $V^{\bullet}=L(0)\backslash V^{\dagger}$ and $\omega(\overline{a},\overline{A},V^{\dagger})=\left[\int E\left[\varepsilon\mid\overline{a},L(0)\right]E\left[\varepsilon\mid\overline{A},L(0)\right]f\left(V^{\bullet}\mid V^{\dagger}\right)d\mu\left(V^{\bullet}\right)\right]$. Note that if $\overline{A}$ has finite support, this is a finite dimensional matrix equation. Our estimators, specialized to this example, are continuous treatment extensions of efficient propensity score estimators of an average treatment effect. By dividing by the propensity score, we eliminate the bias due to within stratum confounding that can occur with subclassification on the propensity score as recommended by Rosenbaum and Rubin (1983).*

4.2. Efficiency calculations using missing data theory. Given (4), imposing CAR cannot change the efficient score. Thus, it is of interest to rederive the efficient score using the Hilbert space results of van der Vaart (1991) and of Robins et al. (1994) for missing data models under CAR. For convenience, assume C is non-random and write $\overline{A} \equiv \overline{A}(C)$. The full data are $\overline{L}^F = \{\overline{L}_{\overline{a}}; \overline{a} \in \overline{\mathcal{A}}\}$. Given any $B = b\left(\overline{L}^F\right)$, the score operator $\mathbf{s}(B) = E[B \mid O], O = \left(\overline{A}, \overline{L}_{\overline{A}}\right)$. For any $Q = q(O)$, the non-parametric adjoint operator $\mathbf{s}^{\dagger}$ under CAR is $\mathbf{s}^{\dagger}(Q) = E\left[Q \mid \overline{L}^F\right] = \int d\mu(\overline{a})\, q\left(\overline{a}, \overline{L}_{\overline{a}}\right) f\left[\overline{a} \mid \overline{L}_{\overline{a}}\right]$. Suppose for the remainder of this subsection that the $\overline{A}$ jumps only at times $0, 1, \ldots, K$ and $\overline{L}$ jumps at $0^-, \ldots, K+1^-$ and $C = K+1$. We then have by CAR

$$f\left[\overline{a}(k) \mid \overline{L}_{\overline{a}}\right] = \prod_{m=0}^{k} f\left[a(m) \mid \overline{a}(m-1), \overline{L}_{\overline{a}}(m)\right] \tag{13}$$

and $f\left[\overline{a} \mid \overline{L}_{\overline{a}}\right] = f\left[\overline{a}(K) \mid \overline{L}_{\overline{a}}\right]$. It is then easy to check the null space of $\mathbf{s}^{\dagger}$, $N\left(\mathbf{s}^{\dagger}\right) = \{U_{tp}(\phi)\}$. Now define the non-parametric information operator, $\mathbf{m} = \mathbf{s}^{\dagger}\mathbf{s} : \overline{L}^F \to R\left(\mathbf{s}^{\dagger}\right)$ where $R\left(\mathbf{s}^{\dagger}\right)$ is the range of $\mathbf{s}^{\dagger}$. Note that $R\left(\mathbf{s}^{\dagger}\right) = \left\{B = \int d\mu(\overline{a})\, b\left(\overline{a}, \overline{L}_{\overline{a}}\right)\right\}$. Let $\mathbf{m}^{-1} : R\left(\mathbf{s}^{\dagger}\right) \to R\left(\mathbf{s}^{\dagger}\right)$ be the inverse of $\mathbf{m}$ on $R\left(\mathbf{s}^{\dagger}\right)$. Given $\overline{a}_1, \overline{a}_2$, let u_{12} be the smallest u with $a_1(u) \neq a_2(u)$. We then have by a direct calculation

THEOREM 4.2. *If for all* $\overline{a}_1, \overline{a}_2$

$$\overline{L}_{\overline{a}_1} \coprod \overline{L}_{\overline{a}_2} \mid \overline{L}_{\overline{a}_1}\left(u_{12}^-\right) \tag{14}$$

then

$$\begin{aligned}\mathbf{m}^{-1}\left[\int d\mu(\overline{a})\, b\left(\overline{a}, \overline{L}_{\overline{a}}\right)\right] &= \int d\mu(\overline{a}) \left\{ \sum_{m=1}^{K+1} \left\{f\left[\overline{a}(m-1) \mid \overline{L}_{\overline{a}}\right]\right\}^{-1} \right. \\ &\left. \left\{E\left[b\left(\overline{a}, \overline{L}_{\overline{a}}\right) \mid \overline{L}_{\overline{a}}(m)\right] - E\left[b\left(\overline{a}, \overline{L}_{\overline{a}}\right) \mid \overline{L}_{\overline{a}}(m-1)\right]\right\} + E\left[b\left(\overline{a}, \overline{L}_{\overline{a}}\right) \mid \overline{L}_{\overline{a}}(0)\right] \right\}.\end{aligned} \tag{15}$$

REMARK 4.1. Gill and Robins (1999) show that (14) places no restriction on the law of the observed data O even when sequential randomization and a MSM are imposed. We can and do always assume that (14) holds.

Now let S_{eff}^F and $\Lambda^{F,\perp}$ be the efficient score and the orthogonal complement to the nuisance tangent space for the parameter β of our marginal structural model when we have data on $\overline{L}^F$. Then the efficient score S_{eff} based on data O under CAR is $g\left[m^{-1}\left(D_{eff}\right)\right]$ where D_{eff} is the unique member of $\Lambda^{F,\perp} \cap R\left(\mathbf{s}^{\dagger}\right)$ satisfying

$$\Pi\left[\mathbf{m}^{-1}\left(D_{eff}\right) \mid \Lambda^{F,\perp}\right] = S_{eff}^F\ , \tag{16}$$

where Π is the Hilbert space projection operator. To show how to use this result to calculate S_{eff}, we revisit the example given in the last subsection.

EXAMPLE 2. **Model 1a:** Consider MSM 1a as in Sec. 4.1. Then, by an extension of Theorem 8.3 of Robins et al. (1994)

$$\Lambda^{F,\perp} = \left\{ \int d\mu\left(\overline{a}\right) h\left(\overline{a}\right) \varepsilon\left(\overline{a}\right) \right\} \tag{17}$$

where *(i)* $\varepsilon\left(\overline{a}\right) = \varepsilon\left(\overline{a}, \beta_0\right)$, *(ii)* $h\left(\overline{a}\right)$ is a vector valued function of the dimension of β_0. Note that $\Lambda^{F,\perp}$ is contained in $R\left(\mathbf{s}^{\dagger}\right)$ as will be the case for MSMs with positive information.

REMARK 4.2.

$$\textit{If } \overline{\mathcal{A}} = \{\overline{a}_1, \ldots, \overline{a}_S\} \textit{ is finite,} \tag{18}$$

then $\varepsilon\left(\overline{a}\right)$ can be identified with the S vector that has components $\varepsilon_s\left(\overline{a}_s\right) = Y_{\overline{a}_s} - g\left(\overline{a}_s, V^{\dagger}, \beta_0\right)$. For arbitrary $\overline{\mathcal{A}}$, $\varepsilon\left(\overline{a}\right)$ is a stochastic process with index set $\overline{\mathcal{A}}$. For $\overline{a}, \overline{a}^* \in \overline{\mathcal{A}}$, let $\mathbf{cv}\left(\overline{a}, \overline{a}^*\right) = cov\left(\varepsilon\left(\overline{a}\right), \varepsilon\left(\overline{a}^*\right)\right)$. If $\overline{\mathcal{A}}$ is given by (18), $\mathbf{cv}\left(\overline{a}, \overline{a}^*\right)$ corresponds to the $S \times S$ matrix with j, k entry $\mathbf{cv}\left(\overline{a}_j, \overline{a}_k\right)$. Let $\mathbf{cv}^{-1}\left(\overline{a}^{**}, \overline{a}^*\right)$ be a (generalized) inverse of $\mathbf{cv}\left(\overline{a}, \overline{a}^*\right)$, i.e., by definition, for any function $q\left(\overline{a}^*\right)$, $\int \left[\int \mathbf{cv}^{-1}\left(\overline{a}^{**}, \overline{a}\right) \mathbf{cv}\left(\overline{a}, \overline{a}^*\right) d\mu\left(\overline{a}\right)\right] q\left(\overline{a}^*\right) d\mu\left(\overline{a}^*\right) = q\left(\overline{a}^{**}\right)$. In particular, if (18) holds, $\mathbf{cv}^{-1}\left(\overline{a}^*, \overline{a}\right)$ is just the inverse of the matrix identified with $\mathbf{cv}\left(\overline{a}, \overline{a}^*\right)$. Then, generalizing Chamberlain (1987),

$$S^F_{eff} = \int d\mu\left(\overline{a}\right) \left\{ \partial g\left(\overline{a}, V^{\dagger}; \beta_0\right) / \partial \beta \right\} \left[\int \mathbf{cv}^{-1}\left(\overline{a}, \overline{a}^*\right) \varepsilon\left(\overline{a}^*\right) d\mu\left(\overline{a}^*\right) \right]. \tag{19}$$

If $\overline{\mathcal{A}}$ is given by (18), $\partial g\left(\overline{a}, V^{\dagger}; \beta_0\right) / \partial \beta$ can be identified with the $\dim \beta \times S$ matrix with j, k entry $\partial g\left(\overline{a}_k, V^{\dagger}; \beta_0\right) / \partial \beta_j$. Again, generalizing Theorem 8.3 in Robins et al. (1994),

$$\begin{gathered} \Pi\left[\int d\mu\left(\overline{a}\right) b\left(\overline{a}, \overline{L}_{\overline{a}}\right) \mid \Lambda^{F,\perp} \right] = \\ \int d\mu\left(\overline{a}\right) E\left[b\left(\overline{a}, \overline{L}_{\overline{a}}\right) \varepsilon\left(\overline{a}\right) \mid V^{\dagger} \right] \left[\int \mathbf{cv}^{-1}\left(\overline{a}, \overline{a}^*\right) \varepsilon\left(\overline{a}^*\right) d\mu\left(\overline{a}^*\right) \right]. \end{gathered} \tag{20}$$

Hence to solve (16), we need to find the solution $h_{eff}\left(\overline{a}, V^{\dagger}\right)$ to the equation

$$E\left[\mathbf{m}^{-1} \left\{ \int d\mu\left(\overline{a}^*\right) h\left(\overline{a}^*, V^{\dagger}\right) \varepsilon\left(\overline{a}^*\right) \right\} \varepsilon\left(\overline{a}\right) \mid V^{\dagger} \right] = \partial g\left(\overline{a}, V^{\dagger}; \beta_0\right) / \partial \beta. \tag{21}$$

By (15) with $K = 0$ and the fact that, by CAR, $f\left(\overline{a} \mid \overline{L}_{\overline{a}}\right) = f\left(\overline{a} \mid L(0)\right)$, the LHS of (21) can be written

$$E\left\{\int d\mu(\overline{a}^*)\, h(\overline{a}^*, V^\dagger)\left\{[\varepsilon(\overline{a}^*) - E[\varepsilon(\overline{a}^*) \mid L(0)]]\{f(\overline{a}^* \mid L(0))\}^{-1} + E[\varepsilon(\overline{a}^*) \mid L(0)]\right\}\varepsilon(\overline{a}) \mid V^\dagger\right\} = E\left\{\int d\mu(\overline{a}^*)\, h(\overline{a}^*, V^\dagger) \times \left[cov[\varepsilon(\overline{a}^*), \varepsilon(\overline{a}) \mid L(0)]\{f(\overline{a}^* \mid L(0))\}^{-1} + E[\varepsilon(\overline{a}^*) \mid L(0)]\, E[\varepsilon(\overline{a}) \mid L(0)]\right] \Big| V^\dagger\right\}.$$

However, since by assumption (14), $Y_{\overline{a}_j} \coprod Y_{\overline{a}_k} \mid \bar{L}(0)$ for $k \neq j$, (21) reduces to

$$h(\bar{a}, V^\dagger)\, E\left\{var[\varepsilon(\overline{a}) \mid L(0)]\, f(\overline{a} \mid L(0))^{-1} \mid V^\dagger\right\} + \int d\mu(\overline{a}^*)\, h(\overline{a}^*, V^\dagger)\, E\left\{E[\varepsilon(\overline{a}^*) \mid L(0)]\, E[\varepsilon(\overline{a}) \mid L(0)] \mid V^\dagger\right\} = \partial g(\overline{a}, V^\dagger, \beta_0)/\partial\beta\,.$$

Upon noting that, by CAR, $f\left[\varepsilon \mid \overline{A} = \overline{a}, L(0)\right] = f[\varepsilon(\overline{a}) \mid L(0)], w$. We see that this is the same expression for $h_{eff}(\overline{a}, V^\dagger)$ as obtained in Theorem 4.1.

4.3. A practical approach to obtaining reasonable efficiency. Estimation of h_{eff} is computationally difficult because of the need to solve integral equations without closed form solutions. A practical approach to choosing h and $f^*(\overline{a} \mid V^\dagger)$ is important. Given a model for $f\left[a(t) \mid \overline{a}(t^-), \overline{\ell}(t^-)\right]$ depending on parameter $\alpha' = (\alpha_1', \alpha_2')$ such that $\alpha_1 = 0 \Leftrightarrow f\left[a(t) \mid \overline{a}(t^-), \overline{\ell}(t^-)\right] = f\left[a(t) \mid \overline{a}(t^-), v^\dagger\right]$, rather than choosing $f^*\left[\overline{a} \mid V^\dagger\right]$, we use $f^*\left[\overline{a} \mid V^\dagger; \widetilde{\alpha}_2\right]$ where $\widetilde{\alpha}_2$ is the MLE of α_2 with α_1 set to zero. This is exactly the approach we took in analyzing the 002 data in the Introduction. [The fact that $f^*\left[\overline{a} \mid V^\dagger\right]$ is estimated does not influence the asymptotic distribution of $\widehat{\beta}(h, \phi)$.] It follows that if (8) holds [i.e., $\overline{A}$ is an ancillary process], $\mathcal{W}$ will converge to 1. Further, in each of the models 1a–2c of Sec. 3.1, the efficient choice of h, say, h_{opt}, for solving $\sum_i \widehat{D}^*_{sm,i}(h) = 0$ when (9) is not imposed is well known. We suggest choosing h to be h_{opt} or an estimate $\widehat{h}_{opt}$ thereof, and choosing ϕ to be an estimate of $\phi_{opt}\left(\widehat{h}_{opt}\right)$. Such a choice guarantees that if $\overline{A}$ is an ancillary process, our estimate of β_0 will be more efficient than the estimate based on solving $0 = \sum_i \widehat{D}_{sm,i}(h_{opt})$. Specifically, in MSM 1a, $h_{opt} = \{\partial\varepsilon(\beta_0)/\partial\beta\}\left\{var\left(\varepsilon(\beta_0) \mid \overline{A}, V^\dagger\right)\right\}^{-1}$. For model 1b, Chamberlain (1988) gives $h_{1,opt}$ and $h_{2,opt}$. In model 1c, $h_{opt} = [\partial/\partial\beta]\left[ln\ \left\{[\partial R(\beta_0)/\partial Y]\, f\left[R(\beta_0) \mid V^\dagger\right]\right\}\right]$. In model 1d, h_{opt} is as in model 1a with $\varepsilon(\beta_0)$ now a vector. In model 2a, $h_{opt} = \partial ln\ r\left[\overline{A}(u^-), u, V^\dagger,\right.$

$\beta_0] / \partial\beta$. For model 2b, h_{opt} is given by Sasieni (1992). In model 2c, $h_{opt,2} = h_{opt,1}\lambda_0 \left(u \mid V^\dagger\right)$ and $h_{opt,1} = \partial \ln \lambda_{R(\beta)} \left(u \mid V^\dagger\right) / \partial\beta_{|\beta=\beta_0}$.

5. Comparison of MSMs and SNMs. We begin by recalling the definition of a structural nested distribution model.

5.1. Structural nested distribution models. For concreteness, we consider the setting of the MSM model 1a–1c with $Y_{\overline{a}} = Y_{\overline{a}}(K+1)$ and the A process and L process jumping at non-random times $0, \ldots, K$ and $0^-, \ldots, K+1^-$ respectively. Henceforth, we take $V^\dagger = \emptyset$. Suppose Y is a continuous variable with a continuous distribution function $F_Y(y) = pr[Y < y]$. Let $(\overline{a}(m), 0)$ denote the treatment history given by $\overline{a}(m)$ through time m and zero at times $m+1, \ldots, K$. Then let $\gamma\left(y, \overline{\ell}(m), \overline{a}(m)\right)$ be the unique function mapping quantiles of $Y_{\overline{a}(m),0}$ into those of $Y_{\overline{a}(m-1),0}$ conditional on $\overline{L}(m) = \overline{\ell}(m), \overline{A}(m) = \overline{a}(m)$ so that $\gamma\left(y, \overline{\ell}(m), \overline{a}(m)\right)$ measures the magnitude of the effect of a final blip of treatment $a(m)$ on quantiles of Y among subjects with observed history $\left\{\overline{\ell}(m), \overline{a}(m)\right\}$. A structural nested distribution model (SNDM) is a parametric model for this function. That is, it specifies that $\gamma(y, \overline{\ell}(m), \overline{a}(m)) = \gamma(y, \overline{\ell}(m), \overline{a}(m), \beta_0)$ where $\gamma\left(y, \overline{\ell}(m), \overline{a}(m), \beta\right)$ is a known increasing function of y satisfying $\gamma\left(y, \overline{\ell}(m), \overline{a}(m), \beta\right) = y$ if $a(m) = 0$ or $\beta = 0$. Recursively define random variables $\overset{\bullet}{R}_K(\beta), \ldots, \overset{\bullet}{R}_0(\beta)$ by $\overset{\bullet}{R}_K(\beta) = \gamma\left(Y, \overline{L}(K), \overline{A}(K), \beta\right)$ and $\overset{\bullet}{R}_m(\beta) = \overset{\bullet}{r}_m\left(Y, \overline{L}(K), \overline{A}(K), \beta\right) = \gamma\left(\overset{\bullet}{R}_{m+1}(\beta), \overline{L}(m), \overline{A}(m), \beta\right)$ and set $\overset{\bullet}{R}(\beta) = \overset{\bullet}{r}\left(Y, \overline{L}(K), \overline{A}(K), \beta\right) \equiv \overset{\bullet}{R}_0(\beta)$. [Heuristically, $\overset{\bullet}{R}_m(\beta_0)$ is $Y_{\overline{A}(m-1),0}$ and $\overline{R}(\beta_0)$ is Y_0, where Y_0 is the outcome when treatment is always withheld. This is heuristic because in fact it is only the conditional distributions through time m that are guaranteed to be the same.] Also let $\overset{\bullet}{r}^{-1}\left(y, \overline{\ell}(K), \overline{a}(K), \beta\right)$ be the inverse of the function $\overset{\bullet}{r}$ with respect to its first argument. If $\gamma\left(y, \overline{\ell}(m), \overline{a}(m), \beta\right) = \gamma\left(y, \overline{a}(m), \beta\right)$ does not depend on $\overline{\ell}(m)$ for each m, we say that the SNDM model has no interaction.

THEOREM 5.1. *Under (4), a no interaction SNDM model is a stratified transformation model (STM), i.e., MSM 1c, with* $R(\overline{a}, \beta) = \overset{\bullet}{r}(Y, \overline{a}, \beta)$ *and* $R(\beta) = \overset{\bullet}{R}(\beta)$. *However, the converse is not true.*

That is, a no-interaction SNDM is a MSM. The semiparametric information bound for β is greater if we correctly impose a no-interaction SNDM than if we only imposed the corresponding STM. An SNDM will be a MSM only if (as a fact of nature) there is no interaction. Theorem 5.1 indicates that a STM is the natural MSM analog of a SNDM in this case. If $\gamma\left(y, \overline{\ell}(m), \overline{a}(m)\right)$ depends on $\overline{\ell}(m)$, we must choose between analyzing the data under a SNDM versus a STM. To understand the advantages and disadvantages of each, we need some additional background. Define a regime $g = (g_0, \ldots, g_K) \in \mathcal{G}$ to be a collection of functions $g_m : \overline{\mathcal{L}}_m \to \mathcal{A}_m$. Define $g\left(\overline{\ell}(m)\right) = \left\{g_0\left(\overline{\ell}_0\right), \ldots, g_m\left(\overline{\ell}(m)\right)\right\}$. Let Y_g be the counterfactual value of Y if regime g were followed. If $g\left(\bar{\ell}_K\right)=\bar{a}_K\equiv\bar{a}$ does not depend on $\bar{\ell}_K$, then $Y_g=Y_{\bar{a}}$ and we say g is non-dynamic; otherwise, g is dynamic. Let $g\left[\bar{\ell}\left(k\right)\right]$ denote a realization of $\overline{A}\left(k\right)$. If we have sequential ignorability for regime g, i.e.,

$$Y_g \coprod A\left(t\right) \mid \overline{L}\left(t^-\right), \overline{A}\left(t^-\right)\ , \tag{22}$$

then, by Theorem 3.2 of Robins (1997), the law of Y_g is given by the G-computation algorithm formula

$$\begin{aligned} F_{Y_g}\left(y \mid \bar{\ell}\left(k\right), g\left[\bar{\ell}\left(k-1\right)\right]\right) &= \int\!\!\int F_Y\left(y \mid \bar{\ell}\left(K\right), g\left(\bar{\ell}\left(K\right)\right)\right) \\ &\times \prod_{m=k+1}^{K} dF\left[\ell\left(m\right) \mid \bar{\ell}\left(m-1\right), g\left(\bar{\ell}\left(m-1\right)\right)\right]. \end{aligned} \tag{23}$$

We obtain $F_{Y_g}\left(y\right)$ from (23) by substituting in $k=-1$. Using the fact that, for continuous Y, Y is $\dot{r}^{-1}\left(\overset{\bullet}{R}\left(\beta_0\right), \overline{L}\left(K\right), \overline{A}\left(K\right), \beta_0\right)$, it can be shown that (23) implies

$$\begin{aligned} F_{Y_g}\left(y\right) &= \int\!\!\int I\left[\overset{\bullet}{r}^{-1}\left\{u, \bar{\ell}\left(K\right), g\left(\bar{\ell}\left(K\right)\right), \beta_0\right\} > y\right] \\ &\times \prod_{m=0}^{K} dF\left[\ell\left(m\right) \mid \bar{\ell}\left(m-1\right), g\left(\bar{\ell}\left(m-1\right)\right), \overset{\bullet}{R}\left(\beta_0\right)=u\right] dF_{\overset{\bullet}{R}\left(\beta_0\right)}\left(u\right). \end{aligned} \tag{24}$$

In many settings, the g-null hypothesis that

$$F_{Y_{g1}}\left(y\right) = F_{Y_{g2}}\left(y\right) \text{ for all } g1, g2 \in \mathcal{G} \tag{25}$$

will be of interest. This is implied by the sharp null hypothesis of no treatment effect that $Y_{g1}=Y_{g2}$ with probability 1, i.e. no subject's outcome is influenced by the treatment history they choose. Robins (1986, 1997) proves the following.

THEOREM 5.2. *Given (22) for $g\in\mathcal{G}$, (25) holds $\Leftrightarrow$ (23) is the same for all $g \Leftrightarrow \gamma\left(y, \bar{\ell}_m, \bar{a}_m\right)=y \Leftrightarrow$*

$$Y \coprod A\left(k\right) \mid \overline{L}\left(k\right), \overline{A}\left(k-1\right), k=0,\ldots,K\ . \tag{26}$$

5.2. Advantages of SNDMs with a continuous Y. We are now ready to compare the advantages and disadvantages of SNDMs and MSMs for continuous Y. We begin by reviewing the advantages of SNDMs.

1. Although (26) implies $\beta_0=0$ for both a SNDM and a STM, only for a SNDM is (26) equivalent to $\beta_0=0$. What this means causally is the following. For a STM, the null hypothesis $\beta_0=0$ is equivalent to the hypothesis that the distribution of $Y_{\bar{a}}$ is the same for

all non-dynamic regimes $\overline{a}$. This is a weaker hypothesis than the g-null hypothesis that says the distribution of Y_g is the same for all regimes, whether non-dynamic or dynamic. In most cases, it will be the latter null hypothesis (25) that will be of public health interest unless it were not possible to collect data on the covariates L_k which determine the treatment decisions for dynamic regimes.

2. If the $L(k)$ are discrete with only a moderate number of levels, then, even with $f\left[a(k) \mid \overline{\ell}(k-1), \overline{a}(k-1)\right]$ totally unrestricted, an asymptotically distribution-free g-null test of $\beta_0 = 0$ (and thus of (25)) exists for a SNDM but, because of the curse of dimensionality, not for a STM. Specifically, a non-parametric g-null test is equivalent to a test of independence of Y and $A(k)$ within strata defined jointly by $\overline{L}(k), \overline{A}(k-1)$ (Robins, 1997). Thus, even if $A(k)$ is continuous, a test of independence of $A(0)$ and Y within levels of $L(0)$ will be an asymptotic α - level test under (25). In contrast, a test of $\beta_0 = 0$ in a STM (without (25) additionally imposed) requires, by the Remark following Theorem 3.3a, that $\mathcal{W}$ can be consistently non-parametrically estimated which will not be possible due to the curse of dimensionality. (Note that to estimate $\mathcal{W}$, we must be able to consistently estimate the density of $A(k)$ given $\overline{L}(k)$ and $\overline{A}(k-1)$ for all k, which is not possible to do non-parametrically when the $A(m)$ are continuous.) In other words, the stronger hypothesis (25) that $\beta_0 = 0$ for a SNDM is easier to test non-parametrically than the weaker hypothesis that $\beta_0 = 0$ for a STM.

3. Henceforth, assume a correct model for $f\left[a(t) \mid \overline{\ell}(t^-), \overline{a}(t^-)\right]$ is available for all t. (We remind the reader that this would often be a false assumption.) Given a SNDM, with some difficulty the law of Y_g for dynamic g can be estimated using (24). In contrast, the law of Y_g for dynamic g is very hard to estimate given a STM. Specifically, given a SNDM, we estimate the law of Y_g as follows: *(i)* obtain an estimate $\widehat{\beta}$ by g-estimation (Robins, 1997), *(ii)* estimate $F_{\overset{\bullet}{R}(\beta_0)}(u)$ by the empirical law of the $\overset{\bullet}{R}_i(\widehat{\beta})$ for $i = 1, \ldots, n$, *(iii)* specify and estimate a parametric model for $f\Big[L(m) \mid \overline{L}(m-1),$ $\overline{A}(m-1), \overset{\bullet}{R}(\widehat{\beta})\Big]$, *(iv)* and then evaluate the estimated version of the integral (24) by Monte carlo.

   In contrast, given a STM, we must, as discussed in Robins (1997, pg. 114; 1998a, Sec. 11) and Robins et al. (1999), specify a parametric model for $\nu^*\left(y, \overline{\ell}(m), \overline{a}\right)$, where one can choose to define $\nu^*\left(y, \overline{\ell}(m), \overline{a}\right)$ in either of two ways, leading to different parameterizations. Either $\nu^*\left(y, \overline{\ell}(m), \overline{a}\right) \equiv \nu\left(y, \overline{\ell}(m), \overline{a}\right) - \nu\big(y, \{\overline{\ell}(m-1), \ell(m) = 0\}, \overline{a}\big)$ and $\nu\left(y, \overline{\ell}(m), \overline{a}\right)$ maps quantiles of $Y_{\overline{a}}$ given

$\overline{\ell}_m, \overline{a}_{m-1}$ into quantiles of $Y_{\overline{a}}$ given $\overline{\ell}_{m-1}, \overline{a}_{m-1}$, or $\nu^* \left(y, \overline{\ell}(m), \overline{a}\right)$ is defined to be the ratio of the hazard evaluated at y of $Y_{\overline{a}}$ given $\overline{\ell}_m, \overline{a}_{m-1}$ to the hazard at y of $Y_{\overline{a}}$ given $\overline{\ell}_{m-1}, \overline{a}_{m-1}, \ell(m) = 0$. Robins et al. (1999, Sec.8.7a) argue for the second option, since, in contrast to the first option, a parameterization in terms of hazard ratios is variation independent. As discussed in Robins (1997, pp. 114–116; 1998a, Sec. 11) and Robins et al. (1999), estimation of $\nu^* \left(y, \overline{\ell}(m), \overline{a}\right)$ is a computational nightmare; indeed, fully parametric Bayesian or likelihood-based inference for a MSM is computationally extremely burdensome.

4. As discussed in Robins (1997, Sec. 9; 1998bc) and Robins et al. (1999), for SNDMs, it is easy to perform a sensitivity analysis in which the fundamental assumption (22) of ignorable treatment assignment is no longer imposed. For a STM such a sensitivity analysis is somewhat less straightforward and sensitivity analysis methods for MSMs are described in Robins et al. (1999) and Appendix C below.
5. A parameter β_0 of a SNDM, in contrast to that of a STM, can often still be consistently estimated if (22) is false but data are available on an instrumental variable. Specifically, suppose $A(t) = (A_1(t), A_2(t))$ with $A_1(t)$ recording a physician's prescribed treatment and $A_2(t)$ recording treatment actually received. We might suppose (22) is false, but $A_1(t) \coprod Y_g \mid \overline{L}(t^-), \overline{A}(t^-)$ is true if a predictor of Y_g and of $A_2(t)$ was not recorded in $\overline{L}(t^-)$. $A_1(t)$ is often then referred to as an instrumental variable process, particularly when $A_1(t)$ has no direct causal effect, i.e., $Y_{\overline{a}} = Y_{\overline{a}_2}$ w.p.1. In this setting, the parameter of a STM is not identified but the parameter of a SNDM can still in general be consistently estimated by g-estimation (Robins, 1993; 1998b).
4. MSMs, in contrast to SNMs, cannot be used if there exists a value of ℓ_k, say $\ell_k = 0$, such that for all but one $a_k \in \mathcal{A}_k$, $f\left[a_k \mid \overline{\ell}_{k-1}, \ell_k = 0, \overline{a}_{k-1}\right] = 0$, since then the artificial censoring time $C^{\dagger}$ is zero with probability 1. An example would be a study of the effect of an occupational exposure on mortality with $\ell_k = 0$ if a subject is off work at time k, $\ell_k = 1$ otherwise, and subjects off work can only receive exposure level $a_k = 0$.

5.3. Advantages of MSMs with continuous Y or with failure time outcomes.

1. Even in the presence of interaction [i.e., $\gamma\left(y, \overline{\ell}_m, \overline{a}_m\right)$ depends on $\overline{\ell}_m$], given a STM, the distribution of a non-dynamic counterfactual outcome $F_{Y_{\overline{a}}}(y)$ can be estimated by $n^{-1} \sum_i I\{r^{-1}[R_i(\widehat{\beta}), \overline{a}, \widehat{\beta}] > y\}$ without requiring either integration or modelling of the conditional law of $L(m)$. In contrast, as described in point 3 of Sec. 5.2 above, for a SNDM, both integration and modelling are required.

2. Any MSM that can be easily estimated when (8) holds (i.e., $\overline{A}$ is an ancillary process) can be easily estimated when (8) is false. For example, we can use the Cox proportional hazards MSM 2a for a continuous failure time outcome $T_{\overline{a}}$. In contrast, a structural nested Cox model would model the ratio of the conditional hazard given $\overline{\ell}_m, \overline{a}_m$ of $Y_{\overline{a}(m),0}$ to that of $Y_{\overline{a}(m-1),0}$ as a function of an unknown finite-dimensional parameter. Unfortunately, a structural nested Cox model does not admit any simple semiparametric estimators, and even complex estimators will fail due to the curse of dimensionality. Formally, the CODA information bound of Robins and Ritov (1997) for a structural nested Cox model is zero, even when $f\left(a_k \mid \overline{\ell}_k, \overline{a}_{k-1}\right)$ is completely known.

A possible hybrid approach is to impose a MSM model and then specify a model for $\nu^*\left(y, \overline{\ell}\left(m\right), \overline{a}\right)$ is as follows. The g-null hypothesis (26) is true if and only if the distribution of $Y_{\overline{a}}$ given $V^{\dagger}$ is the same for all $\overline{a}$ (i.e., the parameter β_0 of our MSM is zero) and $\nu^*\left(y, \overline{\ell}\left(m\right), \overline{a}\right)$ depends on $\overline{a}$ only through $\overline{a}_{m-1}$ (Robins,1997, Appendix C). Thus, we impose a MSM model depending on a parameter β and an additional model for $\nu^*\left(y, \overline{\ell}\left(m\right), \overline{a}\right)$ that depends on both the parameter β of the MSM model and another parameter $\psi = (\psi_1, \psi_2)$ in such a way that $\beta\psi_1 = 0$ if and only if $\nu^*\left(y, \overline{\ell}\left(m\right), \overline{a}\right)$ depends on $\overline{a}$ only through $\overline{a}_{m-1}$. Specifically, $\nu^*\left(y, \overline{\ell}\left(m\right), \overline{a}\right) / \nu^*\left(y, \overline{\ell}\left(m\right), \left(\overline{a}_{m-1}, a_m = 0, ..., a_K = 0\right)\right)$ depends on (β, ψ) only through the product $\beta\psi_1$ and $\nu^*(y, \overline{\ell}\left(m\right), \left(\overline{a}_{m-1}, a_m = 0, ..., a_K = 0\right))$ depends only on ψ_2. Thus ψ_1 is identified only if $\beta \neq 0$. Such a model can overcome objections 1 and 2 of Sec. 5.2 (but not objections 3–6) while retaining the advantages 1, 2 of Sec. 5.3.

5.4. Structural Nested Mean Models (SNMMs). We now turn to comparing MSMs and SNMs for discrete outcomes. Consider the set up of Sec. 5.1 but with Y discrete. For discrete outcomes, we define structural nested mean models. However, SNMMs are applicable to discrete and continuous outcomes.

Let $\gamma\left(\overline{\ell}\left(m\right), \overline{a}\left(m\right)\right) = E\left[Y_{\overline{a}(m),0} - Y_{\overline{a}(m-1),0} \mid \overline{\ell}\left(m\right), \overline{a}\left(m\right)\right]$. Let $\gamma^{\dagger}$ $\left(\overline{\ell}\left(m\right), \overline{a}\left(m\right)\right) = ln\left\{E\left[Y_{\overline{a}(m),0} \mid \overline{\ell}\left(m\right), \overline{a}\left(m\right)\right] / E\left[Y_{\overline{a}(m-1),0} \mid \overline{\ell}\left(m\right), \overline{a}\left(m\right)\right]\right\}$. An additive structural nested mean model (SNMM) specifies $\gamma(\overline{\ell}\left(m\right), \overline{a}(m))$ $= \gamma\left(\overline{\ell}\left(m\right), \overline{a}\left(m\right), \beta_0\right)$ with $\gamma\left(\overline{\ell}_m, \overline{a}_m, \beta\right)$ a known function satisfying $\gamma(\overline{\ell}_m, \overline{a}_m, \beta) = 0$ if $a_m = 0$ or $\beta = 0$. A multiplicative SNMM specifies $\gamma^{\dagger}(\overline{\ell}(m), \overline{a}(m)) = \gamma\left(\overline{\ell}\left(m\right), \overline{a}\left(m\right), \beta_0\right)$. The g-null mean hypothesis is the hypothesis

$$E\left[Y_{g1}\right] = E\left[Y_{g2}\right], g_1, g_2 \in \mathcal{G}. \tag{27}$$

Robins (1997) proves the following.

THEOREM 5.3. *Given (22), (27) holds if and only if* $\gamma\left(\overline{\ell}\left(m\right), \overline{a}\left(m\right)\right) = 0 \Leftrightarrow \gamma^{\dagger}\left(\overline{\ell}\left(m\right), \overline{a}\left(m\right)\right) = 0 \Leftrightarrow E\left[Y \mid \overline{A}\left(k\right), \overline{L}\left(k\right)\right] = E\left[Y \mid \overline{A}\left(k-1\right), \overline{L}\left(k\right)\right]$, $k = 0, \ldots, K$: *Advantages (1)–(4) and (6) of Sec. 5.2 of a SNM over a*

MSM for continuous Y also will hold (appropriately modified) for discrete Y when considering the g-null mean hypothesis or when estimating $E[Y_g]$.) Advantages (1), (2) in Sec. 5.3 of a MSM over a SNDM for continuous outcome also hold in the discrete case.

An important advantage of MSMs over SNMs with Y dichotomous (or, more generally, when Y has finite support) is that neither an additive SNMM or multiplicative SNMM naturally imposes the fact that, for dichotomous Y, $E[Y_g] \in [0,1]$. In contrast, using the MSM model 1a with $g(\overline{a}, \beta)$ a logistic function, the above restriction is naturally imposed. Analogously, in the setting of MSM model 1d, we can use standard marginal logistic models for the repeated measures outcomes $Y_{\overline{a}}(m)$. There exists logistic SNMMs that do impose that $E[Y_g] \in [0,1]$ (Robins et al., 1999). However, these logistic SNMMs are not very useful for semiparametric inference with high-dimensional data, since the CODA information bound for the parameter ψ of interest is zero even when $f\left(a_k \mid \overline{\ell}_k, \overline{a}_{k-1}\right)$ is known.

5.5. Direct effect models. In this section we show that some of the advantages of MSMs described in Secs. 5.3 and 5.4 are not retained in semiparametric models for the direct effect of a treatment a_1 when a second treatment a_2 is held fixed (set). In such a setting, both MSMs and direct effect SNMs (Robins, 1998a) have important limitations due to the curse of dimensionality if the functional form of the effect of the second treatment a_2 on the outcome is left completely unrestricted. Let $a(u) = (a_1(u), a_2(u))$ and, in a slight abuse of notation, set $\overline{a}(u) = (\overline{a}_1(u), \overline{a}_2(u))$ and $\overline{a} = (\overline{a}_1, \overline{a}_2)$. Continue to assume $V^\dagger = \emptyset$. Consider the following.

Model 3a – direct effect semiparametric regression: Consider the set-up of MSM 1b, with

$$\eta\{E[Y_{\overline{a}}]\} = g[\overline{a}, \beta_0] + g^\dagger(\overline{a}_2)$$

where $g[\overline{a}, \beta_0] = 0$ if $\overline{a}_1 \equiv 0$ and $g^\dagger(\cdot,\cdot)$ is unknown and unrestricted. Since, according to the model, $\eta\{E[Y_{\overline{a}_1,\overline{a}_2}]\} - \eta\{E[Y_{\overline{a}_1\equiv 0,\overline{a}_2}]\} = g(\overline{a}, \beta_0)$, it follows we are modelling the direct effect of treatment $\overline{a}_1$. Furthermore, the main effect of the second treatment $g^\dagger(\overline{a}_2) = \eta\{E[Y_{\overline{a}_1\equiv 0,\overline{a}_2}]\} - \eta\{E[Y_{\overline{a}_1\equiv 0,\overline{a}_2\equiv 0}]\}$ is completely unrestricted. Under sequential randomization assumption (4), the model for the observables O induced by MSM 3a is isomorphic to that induced by MSM 1b with $\overline{A}_2 \equiv \overline{A}_2(K)$ playing the role of $V^\dagger$. In particular, if $\eta(x) = x$ [or $ln(x)$], $\widehat{\beta}(h, \phi)$ will perform well in moderate size samples, provided $f\left[a(t) \mid \overline{L}(t^-), \overline{A}(t^-)\right]$ is known or can be parametrically modelled. However, as discussed in the final remark of Sec. 3.1, if $\eta(x) = ln[x/(1-x)]$, reasonable estimators of β_0 are unavailable because $\overline{A}_2(K)$ will be high-dimensional. Indeed, any choice of $\eta(x)$ that guarantees that $E[Y_{\overline{a}}] \in [0,1]$ will fail to provide reasonable estimators of β_0, negating the advantage of this MSM for dichotomous Y. This reflects the fact that the CODA information bound is zero, even when $f\left(a_k \mid \overline{\ell}_k, \overline{a}_{k-1}\right)$ is known.

Model 3b – direct effect semiparametric Cox proportional hazards model: Consider the set up of MSM 2b, with

$$\lambda_{T_{\overline{a}}}(t) = \lambda_{T_{\overline{a}_1=0,\overline{a}_2}}(t) \exp\left[r\left\{\overline{a}\left(t^-\right), t; \beta_0\right\}\right]$$

with $r\left(\overline{a}\left(t^-\right), t; \beta_0\right) = 0$ if $\overline{a}_1\left(t^-\right) = \mathbf{0}$. This is a model for the direct effect of treatment $\overline{a}_1$ on the hazard of T with the main effect of $\overline{a}_2$ left unrestricted. Given (4), MSM 3b induces a model for the observables isomorphic to that induced by MSM 2b. This implies that, as discussed in the remark in Sec. 3.1, due to the curse of dimensionality, it will not be possible to obtain reasonable estimators of β_0 negating advantage 2 of Sec. 5.3.

Model 3c – direct effect semiparametric time-dependent accelerated failure time model: Strikingly, the accelerated failure time MSM we now develop does not suffer from degradation due to the curse of dimensionality as did model 3b. Consider the model

$$\lambda_{R(\overline{a},\beta_0)}(t) = \lambda_{T_{\overline{a}_1=0,\overline{a}_2}}(t)$$

where $R(\overline{a}, \beta) = r\left(T_{\overline{a}}, \overline{a}, \beta\right)$ satisfies $r(t, \overline{a}, \beta) = t$ if $\overline{a}_1 = \mathbf{0}$ or $\beta = 0$. The model for the observables induced by MSM 3c is isomorphic to that induced by MSM 2c with $\overline{A}_2$ in the role of $V^\dagger$. Hence, the association model 3c can be used to estimate the direct effect of $\overline{a}_1$ on T with the main effect of $\overline{a}_2$ unrestricted. MSM 3c is the natural MSM associated with a structural nested failure time model (SNFTM) (Robins, 1993, App. 1; 1998) since a direct-effect SNFTM without interaction is a MSM 3c. In the presence of interaction, the MSM 3c retains advantage 1 of Sec. 5.3.

APPENDIX

By arguments as in Robins et al. (1994), Theorem 3.1 and 3.3b are easy corollaries of Theorem 3.3a.

A. Sketch of proof of Theorem 3.3a. For convenience, assume the L process and A process jump at times $0^-, 1^-, \ldots$ and $0, 1, \ldots$ respectively. Then by Theorem 3.2 of Robins (1997), Eq. (4) implies the G-computation algorithm formula

$$\begin{aligned} & f_{\overline{Y}_{\overline{a}(k)}}\left[\overline{y}(k) \mid v^\dagger\right] \\ \text{(A.1)} \quad &= \int \prod_{m=0}^{k} f\left[y(m), v(m) \mid \overline{y}(m-1), \overline{v}(m-1), \overline{a}(m-1), v^\dagger\right] \\ &\quad \times \prod_{m=1}^{k} d\mu\left[v(m)\right] d\mu\left(\overset{\bullet}{v}\right), \end{aligned}$$

with $\overset{\bullet}{v} \equiv v(0) \backslash v^\dagger$. Thus, if for some $j < k$, the proposition $f\left[a(j) \mid \overline{a}(j-1), \overline{L}(j), v^\dagger\right] \neq 0$ $w.p.1$ given $V^\dagger$ is false, then (A.1) is not identified. Hence, a MSM model places no (local) restrictions on $f\left[L(m) \mid \overline{L}(m-1), \overline{A}(m-1)\right]$ for $m > C^{\dagger}$. Hence, in semiparametric model *(ii)*, every function of O with mean zero given $O^{\dagger}$ is in the nuisance tangent space for the model. It follows that all members of $\Lambda^{\perp}$ in model *(ii)* depend on the data only through $O^{\dagger}$.

Because of our assumed knowledge of $\Lambda^{\perp,*}$ (the orthogonal complement to the nuisance tangent space under F^{*}), it is sufficient to show that $U \in \Lambda^{\perp} \Leftrightarrow U\mathcal{W} \in \Lambda^{\perp,*}$ when F^{*} is chosen such that $C^{\dagger,*}$ is equal to $C^{\dagger}$. This follows from the fact that $\mathring{\Lambda} = \mathring{\Lambda}^{*}$ where $\mathring{\Lambda} \equiv \Lambda \bigcap \{U_{tp}(\phi)\}^{\perp} \bigcap \{z(O^{\dagger})\}$ and the fact that $E[UB] = E^{*}[U\mathcal{W}B]$ for any $B \in \mathring{\Lambda}$ by Lemma 3.1.

B. Proof. In our model, Eq. (12) states that $E[h(\overline{A}, V^{\dagger})\,\varepsilon\mathcal{W}^{-1}\{h_{eff}(\overline{A}, V^{\dagger})\,\varepsilon\mathcal{W}^{-1} - h_{eff}(\overline{A}, V^{\dagger})\,\mathcal{W}^{-1}E\left[\varepsilon \mid \overline{A}, L(0)\right] + E\left[h_{eff}(\overline{A}, V^{\dagger})\,\mathcal{W}^{-1}E\left[\varepsilon \mid \overline{A}, L(0)\right] \mid L(0)\right]\}] = \kappa(h) \equiv E\Big[h(\overline{A}, V^{\dagger})\,\mathcal{W}^{-1}\,\partial g(\overline{A}, V^{\dagger}, \beta_0)/\partial\beta\Big]$. This can be rewritten as

$$\text{(B.1)}\quad \begin{aligned} &E[h(\overline{A}, V^{\dagger})\,\{h_{eff}(\overline{A}, V^{\dagger})\,\mathcal{W}^{-2}var\left[\varepsilon \mid \overline{A}, L(0)\right] + \mathcal{B}(h_{eff})\}] \\ &\quad = E\left[h(\overline{A}, V^{\dagger})\,\mathcal{W}^{-1}\partial g(\overline{A}, V^{\dagger}, \beta_0)/\partial\beta\right] \end{aligned}$$

where $\mathcal{B}(h_{eff}) = \varepsilon\mathcal{W}^{-1}E\left\{h_{eff}(\overline{A}, V^{\dagger})\,\mathcal{W}^{-1}E\left[\varepsilon \mid \overline{A}, L(0)\right] \mid L(0)\right\}$. Now (B.1) is true for all $h(\overline{A}, V^{\dagger})$ if and only if

$$\text{(B.2)}\quad \begin{aligned} &h_{eff}(\overline{A}, V^{\dagger})\,E\left[\mathcal{W}^{-2}var\left[\varepsilon \mid \overline{A}, L(0)\right] \mid \overline{A}, V^{\dagger}\right] + E\left[\mathcal{B}(h_{eff}) \mid \overline{A}, V^{\dagger}\right] \\ &\quad = E\left[\mathcal{W}^{-1}\partial g(\overline{A}, V^{\dagger}, \beta_0)/\partial\beta \mid \overline{A}, V^{\dagger}\right]. \end{aligned}$$

To simplify (B.2), note for any $q\left[\overline{A}, L(0)\right]$, $E\left[q(\overline{A}, L(0))\,\mathcal{W}^{-1} \mid \overline{A}, V^{\dagger}\right] = f^{*}(\overline{A} \mid V^{\dagger}) \int q(\overline{A}, L(0))\,\{f(\overline{A} \mid L(0))\}^{-1}\{f(\overline{A} \mid L(0), V^{\dagger})\,f[L(0) \mid V^{\dagger}]/f(\overline{A} \mid V^{\dagger})\}\,d\mu(V^{\bullet}) = f^{*}(\overline{A} \mid V^{\dagger})\,\{f(\overline{A} \mid V^{\dagger})\}^{-1} \int q(\overline{A}, L(0))\,f(V^{\bullet} \mid V^{\dagger})\,d\mu(V^{\bullet})$. Thus, we have

$$\text{(*)}\qquad E\left[\mathcal{W}^{-1} \mid \overline{A}, V^{\dagger}\right] = f^{*}(\overline{A} \mid V^{\dagger})/f(\overline{A} \mid V^{\dagger}).$$

$$\text{(**)}\quad \begin{aligned} &E\left[\mathcal{W}^{-2}var\left[\varepsilon \mid \overline{A}, L(0)\right] \mid \overline{A}, V^{\dagger}\right] = \\ &f^{*}(\overline{A} \mid V^{\dagger})\,\{f(\overline{A} \mid V^{\dagger})\}^{-1} \int \mathcal{W}^{-1}var\left[\varepsilon \mid \overline{A}, L(0)\right] f(V^{\bullet} \mid V^{\dagger})\,d\mu(V^{\bullet}) \end{aligned}$$

and

$$E\left[\mathcal{B}\left(h_{eff}\right) \mid \overline{A}, V^{\dagger}\right] =$$

$$(***) \quad \begin{aligned} &f^{*}\left(\overline{A} \mid V^{\dagger}\right)\left\{f\left(\overline{A} \mid V^{\dagger}\right)\right\}^{-1} \int E\left[\varepsilon \mid \overline{A}, L(0)\right] f\left(V^{\bullet} \mid V^{\dagger}\right) d\mu\left(V^{\bullet}\right) \\ &\left\{\int E\left[\varepsilon \mid \overline{a}, L(0)\right] f^{*}\left(\overline{a} \mid V^{\dagger}\right) h_{eff}\left(\overline{a}, V^{\dagger}\right) d\mu\left(\overline{a}\right)\right\} \\ &= \int h_{eff}\left(\overline{a}, V^{\dagger}\right) f^{*}\left(\overline{a} \mid V^{\dagger}\right) d\mu\left(\overline{a}\right) \omega\left(\overline{a}, \overline{A}, V^{\dagger}\right). \end{aligned}$$

Substituting (*), (**), (***) into (B.2) proves the theorem.

C. Sensitivity analysis for continuous and failure-time outcomes. Suppose rather than making the assumption (4) of sequential randomization, we instead assume for a model with a continuous outcome Y measured at end of follow-up at time $K+1^{-}$ (e.g., model 1c of Sec. 2.2) or a continuous failure-time outcome T (models 2a–2c of Sec. 2.2) the existence of a known function $q_m\left(y, \overline{\ell}_m, \overline{a}, a_m^*\right)$ such that for $Y_{\overline{a}}$ the continuous counterfactual variable measured at end of follow-up

$$(\text{C.1}) \quad \begin{aligned} &pr\left[Y_{\overline{a}} < y \mid \overline{\ell}(m), \overline{a}(m-1), a^{*}(m)\right] \\ &= pr\left[q\left(Y_{\overline{a}}, \overline{\ell}(m), \overline{a}, a^{*}(m)\right) < y \mid \overline{\ell}(m), \overline{a}(m)\right] \end{aligned}$$

and, for $T_{\overline{a}}$ the counterfactual failure time variable,

$$(\text{C.2}) \quad \begin{aligned} &pr\left[T_{\overline{a}} < y \mid \overline{\ell}(m), \overline{a}(m-1), a^{*}(m), T \geq m\right] \\ &= pr\left[q\left(T_{\overline{a}}, \overline{\ell}(m), \overline{a}, a^{*}(m)\right) < y \mid \overline{\ell}(m), \overline{a}(m), T \geq m\right]. \end{aligned}$$

The chosen conditional quantile - quantile function $q_m\left(y, \overline{\ell}_m, \overline{a}, a_m^*\right)$ must satisfy

$$(\text{C.3}) \quad q_m\left(y, \overline{\ell}(m), \overline{a}, a^{*}(m)\right) = y \textit{ if } a^{*}(m) = a(m)$$

$$(\text{C.4}) \quad q_m\left(y, \overline{\ell}(m), \overline{a}, a^{*}(m)\right) \textit{ is increasing in } y$$

and, in the failure time case (C.2),

$$(\text{C.5a}) \quad q_m\left(y, \overline{\ell}(m), \overline{a}, a^{*}(m)\right) > m$$

and writing $\mu = q_m\left(y, \overline{\ell}_m, \overline{a}, a_m^*\right)$, then

$$(\text{C.5b}) \quad q_m\left(y, \overline{\ell}_m, \overline{a}, a_m^*\right) \textit{ is a function of } \overline{a} \textit{ only through } \overline{a}\left[\max(y, u)\right].$$

This last restriction follows by consistency assumption (2). Note that the sequential randomization assumption (4) implies that $q_m\left(y, \overline{\ell}_m, \overline{a}, a_m^*\right) \equiv y$.

We now sketch how to construct a regular asymptotically linear (RAL) estimator of the parameter β_0 of a MSM such as model (1c) or model (2a)–(2c). Consider first the continuous outcome Y measured at end of follow-up. We shall replace each subject's observed outcome Y with J pseudo-Y's obtained by use of the following algorithm.

- Step 1: Do for $j = 1, \dots, J$.
- Step 2: Do for $m = 0, \dots, K$.
  - Draw $a_j^*(m)$ from $f\left[a(m) \mid \overline{L}(m), \overline{A}(m-1)\right]$.
- Step 3: Set $Y_{(K+1)j} = Y$.
- Step 4: Do for $m = K, \dots, 0$ $Y_{mj} = q_m\left(Y_{(m+1)j}, \overline{L}(m), \overline{A}, a_j^*(m)\right)$.
- Create a new data set with $n \times J$ observations, $O_{ij} = (\overline{A}_i(K), \overline{L}_i(K), Y_{i0j}), i = 1, \dots, n, j = 1, \dots, J$. Now for each observation O_{ij}, calculate $\widehat{D}_{sm}(\beta, a)$ and $D_{tp}(\phi)$ as described in the paragraph following Lemma 3.1, with Y_{i0j} in place of the actual data Y_i. Then let $\widehat{\beta}(h, \phi)$ solve $0 = \sum_{i=1}^{n} \sum_{j=1}^{J} \widehat{D}_{ij}(\beta, h, \phi)$ where, for each observation O_{ij}, $\widehat{D}(\beta, h, \phi) = \widehat{D}_{sm}(\beta, h)/W + D_{tp}(\phi)$.

Then it can be shown that, subject to regularity conditions, under the model characterized by (C.1), an appropriate MSM, such as model 1c, and (11), $\widehat{\beta}(h, \phi)$ will be a RAL estimator of β_0.

The above algorithm can be modified so as to apply to a study with failure time outcomes under the assumption that the treatment process only jumps at times $0, 1, 2, 3, \dots$ as follows.

To describe our algorithm for failure-time outcomes, we first discuss how to obtain a function $q_m\left(y, \overline{\ell}_m, \overline{a}, a_m^*\right)$ guaranteed to satisfy (C.5a) and (C.5b).

Define, for $m \leq [y-1]$ where $[x]$ is the greatest integer less than or equal to x, the function $q^*\left(x, \overline{\ell}(m), \overline{a}[y], a^*(m)\right)$ by

$$\begin{aligned} & pr\Big[T_{(\overline{a}[y],0)} > u \mid \overline{\ell}(m), \overline{a}(m-1), a^*(m), t \geq m, T_{(\overline{a}[y-1],0)} > [y]\Big] \\ & \quad = pr\Big[q^*\left(T_{(\overline{a}[y-1],0)}, \overline{\ell}(m), \overline{a}[y], a^*(m)\right) \\ & \qquad\qquad > u \mid \overline{\ell}(m), \overline{a}(m-1), a^*(m), T_{(\overline{a}[y-1],0)} > [y]\Big]. \end{aligned} \tag{C.6}$$

Then $q_m\left(y, \overline{\ell}(m), \overline{a}, a^*(m)\right)$ is determined by $q_m^*\left(x, \overline{\ell}(m), \overline{a}[y], a^*(m)\right)$ and $q_m\left(y, \overline{\ell}(m), (\overline{a}[y], 0), a_m^*\right)$ through the following algorithm.

- Step 1: $p \leftarrow q_m\left(y, \overline{\ell}(m), (\overline{a}[y], 0), a_m^*\right)$.
- Step 2: Do for $k = 1, 2, \dots$
  if $p < [y+k]$, stop and declare $q_m\left(y, \overline{\ell}(m), \overline{a}, a^*(m)\right) = p$.
  Otherwise, $p \leftarrow q_m^*\left(p, \overline{\ell}(m), \overline{a}[y+k], a^*(m)\right)$.

In conducting a sensitivity analysis, we choose $q_m(y, \overline{\ell}(m), (\overline{a}[y], 0), a^*(m))$ and $q_m^*\left(x, \overline{\ell}(m), \overline{a}[y], a^*(m)\right)$ restricted only by the fact that the first function q_m is increasing in y, exceeds m and equals y if $a^*(m) = a(m)$ and that the second function q_m^* is increasing in y and exceeds $[y]$. Then we use the above algorithm to compute $q_m\left(y, \overline{\ell}(m), \overline{a}, a_m^*\right)$, which will then be guaranteed to satisfy (C.5a) and (C.5b).

We now describe how to construct a RAL estimator for the parameter of β_0 of a MSM failure time model such as model (2a). We assume we have on each of n subjects the data $\Delta = I(T = C), X = \min(T, C), \overline{A}(X), \overline{L}(X)$ where T is the failure time variable and C is the censoring variable. The algorithm goes as follows.

- Step 1: Do for $j = 1, \ldots, J$
- Step 2: Set $K = [X]$
- Step 3: For $s = K + 1, K + 2, \ldots$
  - Draw $a_j(s)$ from a chosen density $f^*\left[a(s) \mid \overline{A}_K, a_j(K+1), \ldots, a_j(s-1)\right]$
- Step 4: Set $X_{(K+1)j} = X$
- Step 5: Do for $m = K, K-1, \ldots, 0$
  - Draw $a_j^*(m)$ from $f\left[a(m) \mid \overline{L}(m), \overline{A}(m-1), T > m\right]$
  - Define $\overline{A}_j = \left(\overline{A}(K), a_j(K+1), a_j(K+2), \ldots\right)$ and set $X_{mj} = q\left(X_{(m+1)j}, \overline{L}(m), \overline{A}_j, a_j^*(m)\right)$
- Step 6: Create a new data set with $n \times J$ observations

$$O_{ij} = \left(\overline{A}_{ij}(X_{ioj}), X_{ioj}, \Delta_i\right).$$

- We then fit the Cox model (2a) as we described previously in the paper but based on the $n \times j$ observations O_{ij}, with each observation on subject i associated with the same weight $\mathcal{W}_i$, where in calculating the numerator of $\mathcal{W}_i \equiv \mathcal{W}(X_i)$, we must use density f^* that was used in step 3 above. The resulting estimator will be consistent under the assumption that the hazard of censoring at time t given all the data only depends on the observed past.

Robins et al. (1999, Sec. 8.7b) discuss some potential problems with the sensitivity analysis methods discussed in this section due to the lack of a variation independent parameterization.

REFERENCES

CHAMBERLAIN, G., 1987, Asymptotic Efficiency in Estimation with Conditional Moment Restrictions, *Journal of Econometrics*, **34**, 305–324.

CHAMBERLAIN, G., 1988, Efficiency bounds for semiparametric regression, *Technical Report*, Department of Statistics, University of Wisconsin.

GILL, R.D., VAN DER LAAN, M.J., AND ROBINS, J.M., 1997, Coarsening at random: characterizations, conjectures and counterexamples, *Proceedings of the First Seattle Symposium on Survival Analysis*, 255–294.

GILL, R.D. AND ROBINS, J.M., 1999, Causal inference from complex longitudinal data: The continuous case, Unpublished manuscript.

HEITJAN, D.F., AND RUBIN, D.B., 1991, Ignorability and Coarse Data, *The Annals of Statistics*, **19**, 2244–2253.

HOLLAND, P., 1986, Statistics and Causal Inference, *Journal of the American Statistical Association*, **81**, 945–961.

LEWIS, D., 1973, Causation, *Journal of Philosophy*, **70**, 556–567.

LIANG, K-Y., AND ZEGER, S.L., 1986, Longitudinal Data Analysis Using Generalized Linear Model, *Biometrika*, **73**, 13–22.

LIN, D.Y., WEI, L-J., 1989, The robust inference for the Cox proportional hazards model, *Journal of the American Statistical Association*, **84**, 1074–1078.

NEWEY, W.K. AND MCFADDEN, D., 1993, Estimation in large samples, **Handbook of Econometrics, Vol. 4**, Eds. McFadden, D., Engler, R. Amsterdam: North Holland.

PEARL J., 1995, Causal Diagrams for Empirical Research. *Biometrika*, **82**, 669–688.

ROBINS J.M., 1986, A new approach to causal inference in mortality studies with a sustained exposure period - application to control of the healthy worker survivor effect, *Mathematical Modeling*, **7**, 1393–1512.

———, 1987, Addendum to "A new approach to causal inference in mortality studies with sustained exposure periods-Application to control of the healthy worker survivor effect", *Computers and Mathematics with Applications*, **14**, 923–945.

———, 1993, Analytic methods for HIV treatment and cofactor effects, **AIDS Epidemiology – Methodological Issues**, Eds. Ostrow DG; Kessler R. Plenum Publishing, New York, 213–290.

———, 1994, Correcting for non-compliance in randomized trials using structural nested mean models, *Communications in Statistics*, **23**, 2379–2412.

———, 1997, Causal inference from complex longitudinal data, In: **Latent Variable Modeling and Applications to Causality, Lecture Notes in Statistics (120)**, M. Berkane, Editor. NY: Springer Verlag, 69–117.

———, 1998a, Testing and estimation of direct effects by reparameterizing directed acyclic graphs with structural nested models, **Computation, Causation, and Discovery**, Eds. C. Glymour and G. Cooper, Cambridge, MA: The MIT Press, Forthcoming.

———, 1998b, Structural nested failure time models, **Survival Analysis**, P.K. Andersen and N. Keiding, Section Editors, **The Encyclopedia of Biostatistics**, P. Armitage and T. Colton, Editors, Chichester, UK: John Wiley & Sons, 4372–4389.

———, 1998c, Correction for non-compliance in equivalence trials, *Statistics in Medicine*, **17**, 269–302.

———, 1998d, Marginal structural models, *1997 Proceedings of the American Statistical Association, Section on Bayesian Statistical Science*, 1–10.

ROBINS, J.M., AND GREENLAND S., 1989, The probability of causation under a stochastic model for individual risk, *Biometrics*, **45**, 1125–1138.

———, 1994, Adjusting for differential rates of PCP prophylaxis in high- versus low-dose AZT treatment arms in an AIDS randomized trial, *Journal of the American Statistical Association*, **89**, 737–749.

ROBINS, J.M., ROTNITZKY, A., ZHAO LP., 1994, Estimation of regression coefficients when some regressors are not always observed, *Journal of the American Statistical Association*, **89**, 846–866.

ROBINS, J.M. AND RITOV, Y., 1997, A curse of dimensionality appropriate (CODA) asymptotic theory for semiparametric models, *Statistics in Medicine*, **16**, 285–319.

ROBINS, J.M., ROTNITZKY, A., AND SCHARFSTEIN, D.O., 1999, Sensitivity analysis for selection bias and unmeasured confounding in missing data and causal inference models, In: **Statistical Models in Epidemiology**, Halloran E., Editor, Springer-Verlag, Forthcoming.

ROBINS, J.M., ROTNITZKY, A., AND ZHAO LP., 1994, Estimation of regression coefficients when some regressors are not always observed, *Journal of the American Statistical Association*, **89**, 846–866.

ROBINS, J.M., AND TSIATIS A.A., 1992, Semiparametric estimation of an accelerated failure time model with time-dependent covariates, *Biometrika*, **79**, 311–319.

ROBINS, J.M. AND WASSERMAN L., 1997, Estimation of Effects of Sequential Treatments by Reparameterizing Directed Acyclic Graphs, *Proceedings of the Thirteenth Conference on Uncertainty in Artificial Intelligence, Providence Rhode Island, August 1–3, 1997*, Dan Geiger and Prakash Shenoy (Eds.), Morgan Kaufmann, San Francisco, 409–420.

ROSENBAUM, P.R. AND RUBIN, D.B., 1983, The Central Role of the Propensity Score in Observational Studies for Causal Effects, *Biometrika*, **70**, 41–55.

RUBIN, D.B., 1976, Inference and Missing Data, *Biometrika*, **63**, 581–592.

———, 1978, Bayesian Inference for Causal Effects: The Role of Randomization, *The Annals of Statistics*, **6**, 34–58.

SASIENI, P., 1992, Information bounds for the conditional hazard ratio in a nested family of regression models, *Journal of the Royal Statistical Society, Series B*, **54**, 617–635.

P. SPIRTES, C. GLYMOUR, AND R. SCHEINES, 1993, **Causation, Prediction, and Search**, Lecture Notes in Statistics, **81**, New York: Springer-Verlag.

VAN DER VAART, A.W., 1991, On differentiable functionals, *Annals of Statistics*, **19**, 178–204.

NONPARAMETRIC LOCALLY EFFICIENT ESTIMATION OF THE TREATMENT SPECIFIC SURVIVAL DISTRIBUTION WITH RIGHT CENSORED DATA AND COVARIATES IN OBSERVATIONAL STUDIES

ALAN E. HUBBARD*, MARK J. VAN DER LAAN*, AND JAMES M. ROBINS†

Abstract. In many observational studies one is concerned with comparing treatment specific survival distributions in the presence of confounding factors and censoring. In this paper we develop locally efficient point and interval estimators of these survival distributions which adjust for confounding by using an estimate of the propensity score and concurrently allow for dependent censoring. The proposed methodology is an application of a general methodology for construction of locally efficient estimators as presented in Robins (1993) and Robins and Rotnitzky (1992). The practical performance of the methods are tested with a simulation study.

Key words. Right-censored data, asymptotically efficient, asymptotically linear estimator, confounding, Cox proportional hazards model, influence curve.

1. Introduction. In many epidemiological studies, one wishes to estimate the marginal distribution F of a time-variable T. For example, the time-variable of interest could be the time from surgical removal of a malignant tumor to recurrence of cancer. Commonly, this time variable is right-censored due either to drop out or to the end of follow-up. The Kaplan-Meier estimator is the standard method for estimation of the survival distribution when the data are right-censored. The Kaplan-Meier estimator fails to be consistent if the censoring time is informative. As an example, consider a study of the time to a heart attack from onset of a treatment. If those patients who show signs of deterioration have a higher probability of being put on another more aggressive treatment, and thus become censored with regard to the original treatment, then the fact of their censoring can be related to the failure time of interest. In this case, the Kaplan-Meier estimator can be biased.

In simulations not reported here, we investigated the potential bias of the Kaplan-Meier estimator for different levels of informative censoring (about half of the observations were censored). The results show that the bias of the Kaplan-Meier estimator is a monotone function of the correlation between T and C. If T and C are positively correlated, the Kaplan-Meier over-estimates the survival probability. In this paper we will extend the marginal right-censored data structure with the presence of a possibly time-dependent process, $W(t)$, which is observed till end of follow up (we will denote the time-independent covariates with $W(0)$). To salvage estimation in the case of dependent censoring one can appeal to a "coarsening at

*Division of Biostatistics, University of California, Berkeley, CA 94720.
†Harvard School of Public Health, Boston, MA 02115.

random" condition which holds if the dependence between C and T can be explained by the observed covariate process.

In many situations, one wishes to estimate the marginal distribution of failure for different treatments. Of interest in this case is not the marginal distribution of failure within the sub-populations defined by treatment received, but the marginal distribution in the whole population if every subject had received the same treatment. That is, for a treatments s, one is interested in the distribution $F_s(t) \equiv P(T_s \leq t)$ of T_s, where T_s is the time to failure had each subject, possibly contrary to the fact, been treated with treatment s. If one has random assignment of treatments, then $F_s(t) = F_s(t \mid S = s)$. However, when assignment of a treatment or an environmental exposure is not random relative to the failure time (informative assignment), then $F_s(t) \neq F_s(t \mid S = s)$ and thus the effect of treatment is confounded by other factors. As an example of the bias that occurs when estimating F_s by simply applying an existing estimator, such as the Kaplan-Meier, to the sub-groups defined by treatment received, consider the following scenario. Suppose one has two possible treatments for cancer (A and B) that are equivalent (no treatment effect), but treatment A is given more frequently to subjects with poorer prognosis. If one uses the Kaplan-Meier estimate on the subgroups defined by the treatments, then treatment B will appear superior to treatment A.

To salvage estimation in the circumstance of non-random treatment assignment, one can appeal to a missing at random condition (MAR) which assumes that the dependence between the treatment indicator and the failure time can be explained by the time-independent covariates $W(0)$. Specifically, one can assume that assignment and the failure time, T_s, are conditionally independent given a vector of time-independent covariates, $W(0)$. In this paper, following the approach of Robins, et al. (1992) and Robins and Ritov (1997), we will adjust for confounding by $W(0)$ by estimating the distribution of S given $W(0)$.

We will present nonparametric estimators that can use the observed covariates to account for both dependent censoring and for non-random assignment. These estimators can also use the observed covariates to improve efficiency. The specific method (the weighted estimating equation approach) used to construct these estimators was originally proposed by Robins and Rotnitzky (1992) and Robins (1993) and has been applied by these authors to several censored data problems (see appendix 2); in particular, they developed locally efficient estimators based on right-censored data and a surrogate process that is observed till end of follow-up. It has also been applied for the case of delay in reporting of vital status in van der Laan and Hubbard (1998) and to current status data by van der Laan and Robins (1998). The consistency of these estimators rely not on consistently estimating the conditional distribution of failure given the covariates, but on consistently estimating the conditional distribution of censoring given covariates and the conditional probability of treatment assignment given covariates. However, the estimators we propose can use estimates of the conditional distribution of failure in a protected manner to gain efficiency. That is, the consistency and asymptotic normality of our estimators do not rely on consistently estimating the conditional distribution of failure, given the covariate process, but if this is estimated consistently, then our estimators are semiparametrically efficient. In the extreme case that the covariates and the treatment S together perfectly predict T and we estimate this relation consistently, then, provided that, conditional on the failure T, the probability of remaining uncensored until T is always bounded away from zero, our estimator is asymptotically equivalent to the empirical distribution based on the uncensored T's. Thus, in the case of uninformative censoring, we can still improve efficiency relative to the Kaplan-Meier estimator by estimating the conditional distribution of T given the covariates.

1.1. The data structure and model. For simplicity, we will present our estimators in the context of two treatments, A and B; extrapolating to more than two treatments is straightforward. Let T_A be a survival time had the subject been given treatment A, C_A a censoring time had the subject been given treatment A, and $W_A(t) \in \mathbb{R}^k$, $t \in \mathbb{R}_{\geq 0}$ a covariate process had the subject been given treatment A. We define $X_A \equiv (T_A, \bar{W}_A(T_A))$, where for a given t, $\bar{W}(t) = \{W(s) : s \leq t\}$. Then, if the subject is given treatment A, we observe $Z_A \equiv (\tilde{T}_A = T_A \wedge C_A, \Delta_A = I(T_A \leq C_A), \bar{W}_A(\tilde{T}_A))$. Note that $W_A(t)$ is a process that might contain both time-dependent and time-independent covariates. Again, we will denote the time-independent covariates with $W(0)$ (measured at baseline $t = 0$ and so it applies to the subject independent of treatment assignment). If everyone in our population was given treatment A, then we would observe n i.i.d copies of $Z_{A,1}, \ldots, Z_{A,n}$ of Z_A.

Optimally, for each subject one would observe both Z_A and Z_B. More typically subjects may be assigned either treatment A or B, so the data we observe have a missing data structure. Specifically, if S is the random treatment assignment with realizations $s \in \{A, B\}$, we observe $Y = I(S = A)Z_A + I(S = B)Z_B$. The distribution of Y is indexed by the distribution F_{X_s} of X_s, the distributions $G_s(C_s \mid X_s)$ of C_s given X_s and $P(S = s \mid X_A, X_B)$, $s \in \{A, B\}$. In our estimation problem, F_{X_s} will be completely unspecified and we will assume that the joint missingness distribution ($G_s(\cdot \mid X_s)$ and $P(S = s \mid X_A, X_B)$) is such that Y is "coarsening at random" (CAR) for (X_A, X_B). The missingness mechanism satisfies CAR if the joint variable of censoring and treatment assignment are uninformative, given the observed data, as was originally formulated in Heitjan and Rubin (1991) and generalized in Jacobsen, Keiding (1995) and Gill, et al. (1997). It follows that (C_S, S) satisfies CAR, if for $c < T_s$,

$$(1.1)\quad P(S = A \mid X_A, X_B) = P(S = A \mid W(0)) = 1 - P(S = B \mid W(0)).$$
$$\lambda_{C_s}(c \mid X_s) = m_s(c, \bar{X}_s(c)) \text{for some function } m_s \text{ of } (c, \bar{X}_s(c)),$$

where $\lambda_{s,C}(c \mid X)$ is the Lebesgue hazard corresponding to $G_s(dc \mid X_s)$, $s \in \{A, B\}$ (see Robins, 1993), and $P(S = A \mid X_A, X_B)$ is the propensity score of Rosenbaum and Rubin (1983). CAR implies that the likelihood factorizes into a $F_{s,X}$ part, a G_s part and a P_s part (see (5.9) in appendix 3). The appropriateness of the CAR assumption in estimation of F_s in the presence of a time-dependent surrogate process has been argued by Robins and Rotnitzky (1992). They showed that, in many applications, the probability of censoring in $(t, t+\delta)$ may (at least to a good approximation) depend only on the observed covariate history up until time t. For example, a physician decides to change treatment at time t, and this decision is based on the observed surrogate process up until time t.

By the curse of dimensionality (if $W(\cdot)$ is time dependent or if $W(0)$ is high dimensional), asymptotically efficient estimators, like a smoothed nonparametric maximum likelihood estimator, perform poorly in practice. Gill, et al. (1997) have shown that if (1.1) is the only assumption, then the model is saturated so that every regular and asymptotically linear estimator of $F_A(t)$ is asymptotically equivalent and thus efficient. To construct estimators with good finite sample performance, one will typically have to assume a parametric or semiparametric submodel of (1.1) for both $G_s(\cdot \mid X_S)$, $s \in \{A, B\}$, and $P(S = A \mid X_A, X_B)$. Finally, our results for estimation of $F_s(t)$ require that:

$$(1.2) \qquad P(S = s \mid W(0))\bar{G}_s(t \mid X_s) > 0, \;\; F_{X_s} \text{ a.e., } s \in \{A, B\}.$$

The above implies that 1) there must by a positive probability of getting assigned treatment s for all realizable $W(0)$ and 2) there must be a positive probability of observing an uncensored observation beyond t.

1.2. Organization of paper. In section 2, we introduce estimators of $F_A(t)$ for the context that all subjects are given the same treatment A. Here we suppress the subscript A since there is no other treatment. Following the terminology of Robins (1993) and Robins and Rotnitsky (1992), we discuss "inverse probability of censoring weighted" (IPCW) estimators of $F(t)$. Then, we define a locally efficient one-step estimator in terms of our IPCW-estimator plus the empirical mean of an estimate of the efficient influence curve. This efficient influence curve is a function of $F(t \mid \bar{W}(u), \tilde{T} > u) = P(T \leq t \mid \bar{W}(u), \tilde{T} > u)$ and we provide a method for estimating this conditional distribution. We also show that the empirical variance of the estimated efficient influence curve, as needed for the estimator, is an asymptotically conservative estimate of the limit variance of the one-step estimator, and can thus be used to construct conservative confidence intervals.

In section 3, we cover the problem of estimating the distribution of T_s among two treatment groups when these groups have not been assigned randomly. Our solution requires a consistent estimate of the propensity score, $P(S = s \mid W(0))$. In this section, we show how to adjust the efficient influence curve for the one-treatment problem covered in section 2 with the propensity score, which then can be used to construct as in section 2 a locally efficient one-step estimator. Again, the estimate of the efficient influence curve can be used for construction of conservative confidence intervals for $F_s(t)$, $s \in \{A, B\}$. In section 4, we present a simulation study comparing the Kaplan-Meier estimate of the survival distribution to our estimators. We conclude the main body of the paper with a discussion of the simulations and some additional remarks. In the appendix, we present the motivating theory for our estimators, we identify the influence curve of the one-step estimator and we present a method to construct consistent estimates of this influence curve and thus the standard error of our estimator. The proofs of the theorems and lemmas and other technical details are also contained in the appendix.

2. Estimating the marginal distribution when everyone is given the same treatment. In this section, we discuss estimators of the marginal distribution for survival when there is only one existing treatment. Note that the methods described here can be applied to the situation where treatments are assigned completely at random, but, as we will argue in section 3, one can get more efficient estimators by modeling and estimating the probability of treatment assignment ignoring the knowledge that the treatment indicator is independent of the survival time. Because we are talking about the marginal estimation problem with only one relevant treatment, we will drop the treatment (A, B) subscript in this section.

2.1. Inverse probability of censoring weighted estimators. In this section, we discuss an IPCW first proposed by Robins and Rotnitsky (1992). This estimator is referred to as the IPCW estimator because it works by weighting the observed $I(T_i \leq t)$ by the probability of censoring. The motivation for this simple estimator comes from the following identity (given (1.2)), i.e., $\bar{G}(t \mid X) > 0)$),

$$E\left\{\frac{I(T \leq t)\Delta}{\bar{G}(\tilde{T} \mid X)}\right\} = F(t), \tag{2.1}$$

where $\bar{G}$ denotes the conditional survival function of C, given X and $\Delta = I(T \leq C)$. This identity follows directly from

$$E(\Delta \mid X) = P(C \geq T \mid X) = \bar{G}(T \mid X),$$

which shows that the conditional expectation given X of the left-hand side of (2.1) equals $I(T \leq t)$. This suggest the following ad hoc estimator of $F(t)$:

$$F_n^0(t) = \frac{1}{n}\sum_{i=1}^{n} \frac{I(T_i \leq t)\Delta_i}{\bar{G}_n(\tilde{T}_i \mid X_i)}. \tag{2.2}$$

where $\bar{G}_n$ is an estimator of $\bar{G}$ assuming a given model for G. Note that by the coarsening at random assumption (1.1), $\bar{G}(\tilde{T} \mid X)$ is only a function of $Y = (\tilde{T} = C \wedge T, \Delta = I(T \leq C), \bar{W}(\tilde{T}))$ so that $F_n^0(t)$ indeed only depends on $Y_1, \ldots, Y_n$. If one assumes a Cox proportional hazard model

$$\lambda_C(t \mid X) = \lambda_0(t) \exp(\alpha^T L(t)),$$

where $L(t) = f(\bar{W}(t))$ is a set of covariates extracted from the process $\bar{W}(t)$ for some given $\mathbb{R}^k$-valued function f, then one can use standard software to obtain the maximum (partial) likelihood estimator of the baseline hazard and the regression coefficients α. If one assumes that C is completely independent of X, then one can consistently estimate $\bar{G}$ with the Kaplan-Meier estimator based on the n observations of $(\tilde{T} = C \wedge T, 1 - \Delta)$, where T now plays the role of the censoring variable for C. In the latter case $F_n^0(t)$ in fact equals the Kaplan-Meier estimator.

However, as shown in Robins and Rotnitsky (1992) and in simulations later in this paper, to increase efficiency one should preferably use a estimate of $G(\cdot \mid X)$, even when C is independent of T (see lemma 5.1 in appendix 1). Heuristically, one is adjusting for the possibility of a chance empirical association between C and T through $W(\cdot)$ due to random sampling. This is equivalent to adjusting for a covariate that is empirically related to the outcome in the given sample even when one knows a priori that the covariate is independent of the outcome in the population. A concrete example is adjusting for smoking in a study of the effect of a risk factor on the development of lung cancer. In this case, we might know that the risk factor is statistically independent of smoking status so that consistent estimators of the regression effect of the risk factor on lung cancer can be obtained without adjusting for smoking status. By chance, however a particular sample might show that for each subsample of subjects defined by levels of the risk factor we have very different proportions of smokers and non-smokers. As a consequence, the estimator that does not adjust for smoking status is less efficient than the adjusted estimator. The gain in performance for a particular sample relative to the unadjusted estimator, even when C is independent of T, is greater the stronger the empirical association between T and C. Thus, the gain in efficiency from modeling $G(\cdot \mid X)$, even when C is independent of $W(\cdot)$, is greater the stronger the dependence between T and $W(\cdot)$.

If censoring depends on T through the observed covariates, i.e. the independent censoring assumption of the Kaplan-Meier estimator fails to hold, then the Kaplan-Meier estimator will be inconsistent. However, by using an estimate of G under a correct model (as non-parametric as sample size permits), the IPCW estimator will remain consistent.

2.2. The locally efficient one-step estimator. In this section, we construct a locally efficient one-step estimator by adding to the estimator $F_n^0(t)$ (2.2) an estimate of the empirical mean of the estimated efficient influence function. Although in this paper we restrict attention to locally efficient one-step estimators, other types of locally efficient estimators exist for this problem. For instance, Robins and Rotnitzky (1992) and Robins (1993) have proposed alternative locally efficient estimators. Our first task is to provide a representation of the efficient influence function at a given data generating distribution (F_X, G), which will then be estimated by simple substitution of estimators of the unknown components of F_X and G. This representation has two pieces. The first is given by the influence function of $F_n^0(t)$ when using the known G:

$$IC_0^F(Y \mid G, F(t)) \equiv \frac{I(T \leq t)\Delta}{\bar{G}(\tilde{T} \mid X)} - F(t),$$

where the superscript F indicates that this is a influence curve for the full data model in which all individuals receive the treatment of interest. This notation will become useful in section 3 where one either receives treatment A or treatment B and where the efficient influence curve is a function of IC_0^F. The second piece is a projection in $L_0^2(P_{F_X,G})$ of IC_0^F on the nuisance tangent space of G only assuming CAR (for a detailed discussion of the relevant Hilbert space projections, see appendices 1 and 2). We will denote this function of Y by IC_{nu}^{*F}, and it is defined by:

$$\text{(2.3)} \qquad IC_{nu}^{*F}(Y \mid F_X, G) = -\int_0^t F(t \mid \bar{W}(u), \tilde{T} > u)\frac{dM(u)}{\bar{G}(u \mid X)},$$

where

$$dM(u) \equiv I(C \in du, \Delta = 0) - \Lambda_C(du \mid X)I(\tilde{T} > u)$$

and $F(t \mid \bar{X}(u), \tilde{T} > u)$ is the conditional probability that $T \leq t$, given $\bar{W}(u)$ and $\tilde{T} > u$. It is important to emphasize that, for any function $H(u, \bar{L}(u))$, the stochastic integral

$$\int_0^t H(u, \bar{W}(u))dM(u) = H(C, \bar{X}(C))(1 - \Delta)I(C \leq t) - \int_0^{\tilde{T} \wedge t} H(u, \bar{W}(u))\Lambda_C(du \mid X)$$

is a function of the observed data Y because $\lambda_C(u \mid X)$ depends on X only through $\bar{W}(u)$. Also note that $IC_{nu}^*(\cdot \mid F_X, G)$ only depends on F_X through $F(t \mid \bar{W}(u), \tilde{T} > u)$ for various u.

In appendices 1 and 2 it is shown that the efficient influence curve IC^{*F} at (F_X, G) for estimation of $F(t)$ is given by:

$$\text{(2.4)} \qquad IC^{*F}(Y \mid G, F_X, F(t)) = IC_0^F(Y \mid G, F(t)) - IC_{nu}^{*F}(Y \mid F_X, G).$$

For our one-step estimator we will slightly modify this representation of the efficient influence curve and this modification will typically result in a more efficient one-step estimator when the model for F_X is misspecified. For the following, we use the notation $IC^*_{nu}(Y \mid F^1_X, G)$ for the expression (2.3) with the true conditional distribution $F(t \mid \bar{W}(u), \tilde{T} > u)$ replaced by a wrong $F^1(t \mid \bar{W}(u), \tilde{T} > u)$. We define for a given F^1_X, $G, F(t)$:

$$IC^{*F}(Y \mid F^1_X, G, F(t)) \equiv IC^F_0(Y \mid G, F(t)) - c(F^1_X, G, F(t)) IC^{*F}_{nu}(Y \mid F^1_X, G), \tag{2.5}$$

where

$$c(F^1_X, G, F(t)) \equiv \frac{E\left\{IC^F_0(Y \mid G, F(t)) IC^{*F}_{nu}(Y \mid F^1_X, G)\right\}}{E\left\{(IC^{*F}_{nu}(Y \mid F^1_X, G))^2\right\}}.$$

Here the expectation is always taken w.r.t. the true distribution $P_{F_X,G}$ of Y. Since $IC^*_{nu}(Y \mid F_X, G)$ equals the projection $IC_0(Y \mid G, F(t))$ it follows that $c(F_X, G, F(t)) = 1$, whereas $c(F^1_X, G, F(t)) \neq 1$ for $F^1_X \neq F_X$. In other words, the adjustment only has an effect if the estimating model for F_X is misspecified. Since

$$\begin{aligned} &var\left\{IC^F_0(Y \mid G, F(t)) - U(Y)\right\} \geq \\ &var\left\{IC^F_0(Y \mid G, F(t) - \frac{E(IC_0(Y)U(Y))}{EU^2(Y))} U(Y)\right\} \end{aligned}$$

with equality if and only if the projection of IC_0 on U equals U, where U plays the role of $IC^{*F}_{nu}(\cdot \mid F^1_X, G)$ (the limit of our estimator $IC^{*F}_{nu}(\cdot \mid F_{X,n}, G_n)$), the adjusted efficient influence curve at $(F^1_X, G, F(t))$ has a smaller (or equal, if $F^1_X = F_X$) variance than the unadjusted influence curve at $(F^1_X, G, F(t))$.

To estimate IC^{*F}, one must substitute the estimators of $F(t \mid \bar{W}(u), \tilde{T} > u)$ and G into the representation (2.5). In the next subsection, we propose an estimator of $F(t \mid \bar{W}(u), \tilde{T} > u)$. $c(F_X, G, F(t))$ can be estimated as

$$c_n = \frac{\sum_{i=1}^n IC^F_0(Y_i \mid G_n, F^0_n(t)) IC^{*F}_{nu}(Y_i \mid F_{X,n}, G_n)}{\sum_{i=1}^n \{IC^{*F}_{nu}(Y_i \mid F_{X,n}, G_n)\}^2}, \tag{2.6}$$

where $F_{X,n}$ denotes the estimator of $F(t \mid \bar{W}(u), \tilde{T} > u)$. Now, we estimate the efficient influence curve IC^{*F} by substituting these estimators in the representation (2.5):

$$\begin{aligned} &IC^{*F}(Y \mid F_{X,n}, G_n, F^0_n(t)) = \\ &IC^F_0(Y \mid G_n, F^0_n(t)) - c_n IC^{*F}_{nu}(Y \mid F_{X,n}, G_n), \end{aligned} \tag{2.7}$$

where F^0_n is the IPCW-estimator defined in (2.2).

Now one can estimate $F(t)$ with the one step estimator:

$$F^1_n(t) = F^0_n(t) + \frac{1}{n} \sum_{i=1}^n IC^{*F}(Y_i \mid F_{X,n}, G_n, F^0_n(t)) \tag{2.8}$$

$$= F_n^0(t) + \frac{1}{n}\sum_{i=1}^{n}\left\{IC_0^F(Y_i \mid G_n, F_n^0(t)) - c_n IC_{nu}^{*F}(Y_i \mid F_{X,n}, G_n)\right\}.$$

Note that $c_n IC_{nu}^{*F}(\cdot \mid F_{X,n}, G_n)$ is just the least squares projection of $IC_0(\cdot \mid G_n, F_n^0(t))$ onto $IC_{nu}^{*F}(\cdot \mid F_{X,n}, G_n)$. One could also just set $c_n = 1$ and still obtain a locally efficient estimator. However, if $F(t \mid \bar{W}(u), \tilde{T} > u)$ is estimated inconsistently, then the estimator using the empirical c_n is typically more efficient than the estimator using $c_n = 1$, whereas if $F(t \mid \bar{W}(u), \tilde{T} > u)$ is estimated consistently, then $c_n \to 1$.

Let $Pf \equiv \int f dP$ for a probability measure P and measurable function f. Let P_n be the empirical cumulative density function (CDF), so that $P_n f = 1/n \sum_{i=1}^n f(Y_i)$. Note $P_n IC_0^F(\cdot \mid G_n, F_n^0(t)) = 0$, and therefore one can delete the IC_0^F-term in (2.8). We chose to retain the IC_0^F-term to show that $F_n^1(t)$ is just the classical one-step estimator as defined in Bickel, et al. (1993).

If $W(u)$ only contains time independent variables, i.e., $W(u) = W(0)$, then

$$F(t \mid \bar{W}(u), \tilde{T} > u) = I(t > u)\frac{F(t \mid W(0)) - F(u \mid W(0))\}}{1 - F(u \mid W(0))}.$$

In this case, the one-step estimator reduces to

$$(2.9) \quad F_n^1(t) = \frac{1}{n}\sum_{i=1}^{n}\frac{\Delta_i I(T_i \le t)}{\bar{G}_n(T_i \mid X_i)} + c_n \int \frac{I(t > u)}{\bar{G}_n(u \mid X_i)} \frac{(F_n(t \mid W_i(0)) - F_n(u \mid W_i(0)))}{1 - F_n(u \mid W_i(0))} dM_{i,G_n}(u).$$

Theorem 5.1 in appendix 1 can be used as a template to prove the local efficiency result for the one-step estimator $F_n^1(t)$. Generally speaking, theorem 5.1 shows that if G is estimated consistently, then the estimator $F_n^1(t)$ is asymptotically linear and if IC_{nu}^{*F}, i.e. $F(t \mid \bar{W}(u), \tilde{T} > u)$, is also estimated consistently, then $F_n^1(t)$ is even asymptotically efficient. The protection against inconsistent estimation of this conditional probability comes from the fact that $M(u)$ is a Martingale. This implies that $E(dM(u) \mid X, C > u) = 0$ (Anderson, et al., 1993) and thus $\int H(u, \bar{W}(u) dM(u)$ has conditional mean zero, given X, for any function H.

2.3. Estimation of the conditional distribution of failure. Consider the case that $W(u) = W(0)$ only contains time independent covariates. In this case, one can assume for $F(\cdot \mid W(0))$ a classical parametric or semi-parametric model and estimate it with standard methods. In particular, one could assume the Cox-proportional hazards model.

If one has time-dependent covariates, or $F(t \mid \bar{W}(u), \tilde{T} > u)$ is difficult to estimate by traditional methods, one can estimate this conditional probability by using a general regression approach. Note that

$$(2.10)\quad F(t \mid \bar{W}(u), \tilde{T} > u) = E\left[\frac{I(T \leq t)\Delta\bar{G}(u \mid X)}{\bar{G}(\tilde{T} \mid X)} \mid \bar{W}(u), \tilde{T} > u\right].$$

Robins (1993) and Robins and Rotnitzky (1992) originally suggested representing the conditional probability as a regression of a random variable $O_G(Y)$ on observed covariates. If one has an estimate of $G(\cdot \mid X)$, and thus of $dM(u)$, then it remains to estimate the conditional expectation of the random variable:

$$O_G \equiv \frac{I(\tilde{T} \leq t)\Delta\bar{G}(u \mid X)}{\bar{G}(\tilde{T} \mid X)},$$

given $\bar{W}(u)$, $\tilde{T} > u$ at u's corresponding with the observed censoring times. This is because if the censoring distribution is estimated with either Cox regression or the Kaplan-Meier estimator, then $d\hat{M}(u)$ only has mass at the observed censoring times. Given an estimate G_n of G and for a given t, O_{G_n} is an observed random variable. Consequently, for every u corresponding with an observed C_i, one can carry out a parametric or nonparametric regression estimation of O_{G_n} on one or a number of relevant (for T) summary measures $W_1, \ldots, W_k$ of $\bar{W}(u)$, only using the observations with $\tilde{T}_i > u$. For example, one could use the SPLUS function gam (Hastie and Tibshirani, 1990) to fit an additive logistic regression of O_{G_n} on $W_1, \ldots, W_k$:

$$E(O_{G_n} \mid W_1, \ldots, W_k) = \frac{\exp(f_1(W_1) + \ldots + f_k(W_k))}{1 + \exp(f_1(W_1) + \ldots + f_k(W_k))},$$

where gam allows the user to specify the number of degrees of freedom used to fit f_i, $i = 1, \ldots, k$. In the simulations presented in section 4 we will report the results for both the estimate using this general regression approach and that using an explicit formulation where $F(t \mid \bar{W}(u))$ is estimated directly with Cox regression.

2.4. The one-step estimator when one guesses an extreme model for the conditional failure time distribution. It is straightforward to prove the following lemma.

LEMMA 2.1. *If $F(t \mid W(0)) = I(T \leq t)$, then*

$$IC^{*F}(Y \mid F_X, G, F(t)) = I(T \leq t) - F(t).$$

In fact the finite sample analogue of this lemma is also true, namely the one step estimator $F_n^1(t)$ using $c_n = 1$ and setting $F(t \mid \bar{W}(u), \tilde{T} > u) = I(T \leq t)$ reduces to the empirical distribution of the T's. This lemma provides us with the following interesting application of our one-step estimator. Suppose one can predict T at baseline using the time-independent covariates, $W(0)$; we will call this predicted failure time T^*.

Note that to get an estimate of IC^{*F}_{nu} we need an estimate of $F(t \mid T^*, T > u)$. If one acts as if $T = T^*$ then one "estimates" $F(t \mid W(0) = T^*, T > u)$ with $I(T^* \leq t)$. In this case, the one-step estimator (2.9) reduces to,

$$F^1_n(t) = \frac{1}{n}\sum_{i=1}^{n} \frac{\Delta_i I(T_i \leq t)}{\bar{G}_n(T_i)} + c_n I(T^*_i \leq t) \int \frac{dM_{G_n}(u)}{\bar{G}_n(u)}, \tag{2.11}$$

where we used the fact that the $P_n IC^F_0(Y_i \mid G_n, F^0_n(t)) = 0$. This estimator is always consistent, asymptotically normal and it is even asymptotically equivalent to the empirical distribution of the T_i's if $T^* = T$.

Though the consistency of $F_n(t)$ is not affected by the discrepancy between T^*_i and T_i, the efficiency of $F_n(t)$ will be. In fact, this estimator is not guaranteed to be more efficient than the Kaplan-Meier estimator if T^* deviates substantially from T. Even when T^* is a poor estimate of T, one can modify the one step estimator (2.11) to guarantee it will be asymptotically more efficient than the Kaplan-Meier estimator. This can be arranged using precisely the same methodology as presented above, the only difference being one must use a different initial influence curve, IC^F_0. Theorem 5.1 shows that the one-step estimator $F^1_n(t)$ is asymptotically linear with an influence curve $IC^F(Y)$ which is guaranteed to have smaller variance than $IC^F_0(Y)$. In this paper we chose (for the sake of simplicity) $IC^F_0(Y) = I(T \leq t)\Delta/\bar{G}(T \mid X) - F(t)$. However, one can also select IC^F_0 to be the influence curve of a good initial estimator. In that case, the one-step estimator is guaranteed to be more efficient than the initial estimator, at any level of misspecification of $F(t \mid \bar{W}(u), \tilde{T} > u)$. In particular, if censoring and failure are independent, one can substitute the influence curve of the Kaplan-Meier estimator, $IC^F_{0,KM}$, for IC^F_0. First, the influence curve of the Kaplan-Meier estimator is,

$$\begin{aligned} &IC^F_{0,KM}(Y \mid F, G, F(t)) = \\ &\frac{I(T \leq t)\Delta}{\bar{G}(T \mid X)} - F(t) - \int \frac{F(t) - F(u)}{1 - F(u)} I(u < t) \frac{dM(u)}{\bar{G}(u)}. \end{aligned}$$

Let $IC^{*F}_{nu,KM}$ be the projection of $IC^F_{0,KM}$ on the orthogonal complement of the tangent space so that $IC^F_{0,KM} - IC^{*F}_{nu}$ equals the efficient influence curve (proposition 5.1 in the appendix 1):

$$\begin{aligned} IC^{*F}_{nu,KM}(Y \mid F_X, G) = &- \int_0^t F(t \mid W(0) = T^*, \tilde{T} > u) \frac{dM(u)}{\bar{G}(u)} \\ &- \int_0^t \frac{F(t) - F(u)}{1 - F(u)} \frac{dM(u)}{\bar{G}(u)}. \end{aligned}$$

To get an estimate of $IC^{*F}_{nu,KM}$ we need an estimate of $F(t \mid T^*, T > u)$ and the marginal distributions F and G. If one acts as if $T = T^*$ then one estimates $F(t \mid W(0) = T^*, T > u)$ with $I(T^* \leq t)$. Let F_{KM} be the Kaplan-Meier estimator of F and recall that G_n is the Kaplan-Meier estimator of G as above. Substitution of these estimators in $IC^{*F}_{nu,KM}$ results in an estimator $\widehat{IC}^{*F}_{nu,KM}$. Let $\widehat{IC}^{F}_{0,KM} = IC_0^F(\cdot \mid F_{KM}, G_n, F_{KM}(t))$. Finally, as in (2.6) we let $c_n = \sum_i \widehat{IC}^{F}_{0,KM}(Y_i)\widehat{IC}^{*F}_{nu,KM}(Y_i)/\sum_i\{\widehat{IC}^{*F}_{nu,KM}(Y_i)\}^2$. Now, we define the one-step estimator as in (2.9):

$$F_n^1(t) = F_{KM}(t) + \frac{1}{n}\sum_{i=1}^{n} IC_{0,KM}^F(Y_i \mid G_n, F_{KM}, F_{KM}(t))$$
$$-c_n\left\{\int_0^t I(T_i^* \leq t)\frac{dM_{G_n}(u)}{\bar{G}_n(u)} + \int_0^t \frac{F_{KM}(t) - F_{KM}(u)}{1 - F_{KM}(u)}\frac{dM_{G_n}(u)}{\bar{G}_n(u)}\right\}$$

Even if this estimate $I(T^* \leq t)$ of $F(t \mid W(0) = T^*, T > u)$ demonstrates unfounded optimism in the accuracy of the prediction of failure, this estimator still remains at least as asymptotically efficient as the Kaplan-Meier estimator. If a clinician at baseline interview is quite good at predicting survival for a patient, then this could be a practical way to incorporate the prediction to increase efficiency relative to the Kaplan-Meier estimator. The appeal of this estimator is that it naturally incorporates the clinician's subjective judgements of a patient's prognosis. More importantly, even if the judgement of the clinician is poor, the estimator still remains asymptotically more efficient than the initial Kaplan-Meier estimator.

2.5. Construction of conservative confidence intervals. Consider the one-step estimator (2.9) which is given by $F_n^0(t) + 1/n\sum_{i=1}^n \widehat{IC}^F(Y_i)$, where $\widehat{IC}^F(Y) \equiv IC^{*F}(Y \mid F_{X,n}, G_n, F_n^0(t))$ defined by (2.7). Under the conditions of theorem 5.1, $F_n^1(t)$ is asymptotically linear with influence curve having variance smaller than or equal to the variance of $IC^{*F}(Y \mid F_X^1, G, F(t))$ ($IC^{*F}(Y \mid F_X^1, G, F(t))$ represents the limit for $n \to \infty$ of $\widehat{IC}^F(Y)$).

Therefore a conservative estimate of the asymptotic variance of $F_n^1(t)$ is given by

$$\widehat{\sigma}^2 = \frac{1}{n}\sum_{i=1}^{n}\{\widehat{IC}^F(Y_i)\}^2.$$

This can be used to construct a conservative 95% confidence interval for $F(t)$:

$$F_n^1(t) \pm 1.96\frac{\widehat{\sigma}}{\sqrt{n}}. \tag{2.12}$$

This confidence interval is asymptotically correct if one consistently estimates $F(t \mid \bar{W}(u), \tilde{T} > u)$ and it is asymptotically conservative otherwise. This confidence interval is very practical since one gets if for free after having computed the estimator $F_n^1(t)$. In appendix 3, we provide an asymptotically correct confidence interval. However, simulations in section 4 suggest that the confidence interval (2.12) can be very close to the correct confidence interval, even at a high degree of misspecification.

3. Non-random assignment. Suppose that in addition to the covariate process, $W(\tilde{T})$, we also have k levels of a treatment or environmental exposure, $S = (S_1, S_2, \ldots, S_k)$. Examples of S are treatment doses or levels of cigarette consumption. Suppose one wishes to estimate the survival distribution of the population if everyone belonged to the risk group of interest, that is, one wishes to estimate the distribution $F_s(\cdot)$ of T_s. If the data come from an observational study, then the data might be generated from two possible situations. First, and least likely, the "assignment" or group membership in a risk group (S) is random w.r.t. the failure time. In this lucky scenario, we have effective randomization of group membership and one can simply estimate the marginal distribution on the subsamples defined by group membership to get an estimate of $F_s(\cdot)$, because in this case $F_s(t \mid S = s) = F_s(t)$. More generally, there is some assignment bias w.r.t. group membership, that is assignment of group membership is not random w.r.t. the failure time, and thus $F_s(t \mid S = s) \neq F_s(t)$. In this case, an estimate of the marginal distribution in the subsample defined by group membership will give an estimate of $F_s(t \mid S = s)$. In this section, we will propose a locally efficient method for estimating $F_s(\cdot)$ that applies to both scenarios.

Rosenbaum and Rubin (1983, 1984, 1985) and Rosenbaum (1984, 1987, 1988) considered estimating the causal effect of a dichotomous treatment S on an outcome Y by modeling $P(S = A \mid W(0))$, which they referred to as the propensity score. They proposed an ad hoc method which requires subclassification or matching on the propensity score. Robins, et al. (1992) used a locally efficient estimating equation approach to estimate β in the model $Y = \beta S + h(W) + e$, $h(W)$ unspecified, by modeling the expectation of exposure conditional on the confounders (the W). Robins and Ritov (1997) describe locally efficient estimators that utilized the weighted estimating equation approach of Robins (1993) and Robins and Rotnitzky (1992). None of these previous locally efficient estimators allowed for concurrent dependent censoring as we shall do here.

3.1. The efficient influence curve. Let (Z_A, Z_B) play the role of the full data and let S be the censoring variable. The observed data is $Y = I(S = A)Z_A + I(S = B)Z_B$. Note that the missingness process is now $P(S = s \mid Z_A, Z_B)$, which equals by assumption (1.1) the propensity score, $P(S = A \mid W(0))$. Let $D(Z_A)$ be the efficient influence curve (i.e. the optimal estimating equation) for $F_A(t)$ in this full data model, where we actually observe Z_A, Z_B for every subject. Since this nonparametric full data model is saturated (Gill, et al., 1997), the optimal estimating equation is $D(Z_A) = IC^{*F}(Z_A)$, where IC^{*F} is the efficient influence curve defined in (2.4). The weighted estimating equations theory in Robins and

Rotnitzky (1992) outlined in appendix 2 provides a method to optimally adjust this efficient influence curve $D(Z_A)$ with the propensity score to obtain the efficient influence curve (i.e. the optimal estimating equation) for the observed data Y.

A natural ad hoc way of adjusting $D(Z_A)$ is the following:

$$U_{P(S=A|W(0))}(D(Z_A)) = \frac{I(S=A)}{P(S=A \mid W(0))} D(Z_A). \tag{3.1}$$

Secondly, we subtract the projection, in the Hilbert space of functions of Y with inner product being the covariance, of $U_{P(S|W(0))}(D(Z_A))$ on the space of missingness scores corresponding with the nonparametric MAR-model for S (see appendix 1 for more detail). It is straightforward to show that this space consists of all functions $\Phi(S, W(0))$ for which $E(\Phi(S, W(0)) \mid W(0)) = 0$. The projection of a function (3.1) on this space is:

$$\frac{I(S=A) - P(S=A \mid W(0))}{P(S=A \mid W(0))} E(D(Z_A) \mid W(0), S=A).$$

This results in the following adjustment of $D(Z_A)$ for estimation of $F_A(t)$:

$$\frac{I(S=A)}{P(S=A \mid W(0))} D(Z_A) \\ - \frac{I(S=A) - P(S=A \mid W(0))}{P(S=A \mid W(0))} E(D(Z_A) \mid W(0), S=A).$$

In fact, it can be shown that for any given full data model for (Z_A, Z_B) any influence curve for $F_A(t)$ can be obtained by an appropriate choice of $D(Z_A)$. In our nonparametric model assuming only (1.1), the optimal (and only) choice of D is $D(Z_A) = IC^{*F}(Z_A)$ defined in (2.4). This results in the efficient influence curve for estimation of $F_A(t)$ based on observing Y:

$$\begin{aligned} IC^*(Y) = & \frac{I(S=A)}{P(S=A \mid W(0))} IC^{*F'} \\ & - \frac{I(S=A) - P(S=A \mid W(0))}{P(S=A \mid W(0))} E(IC^{*F'} \mid W(0), S=A) - F_A(t), \end{aligned}$$

where $IC^{*F'}(Z_A) = IC^{*F}(Z_A) + F_A(t)$. We note that

$$\begin{aligned} E(IC^{*F'} \mid W(0), S=A) &= E\left(\frac{I(T_A \leq t)\Delta_A}{\bar{G}_A(T_A \mid X_A)} \mid W(0), S=A\right) \\ &= F(t \mid W(0), S=A). \end{aligned}$$

Substituting (2.4) for $IC^{*,F}$ results in the following representation of IC^* $(Y \mid F_{X_A}, P(S=A \mid W(0)), G_A, F_A(t))$:

$$IC^*(Y) = \frac{I(S=A)}{P(S=A \mid W(0))}$$

$$\left\{\frac{I(T_A \le t)\Delta_A}{\bar{G}_A(T_A \mid X_A)} + \int F_A(t \mid \bar{W}_A(u), \tilde{T}_A > u)\frac{dM_A(u)}{\bar{G}_A(u \mid X_A)}\right\}$$

$$-\frac{I(S = A) - P(S = A \mid W(0))}{P(S = A \mid W(0))} F_A(t \mid W(0), S = A) - F_A(t). \tag{3.2}$$

3.2. The IPCW estimator. In this section we develop a version of the IPCW estimator (2.2) that accounts for non-random assignment using the above ad hoc recipe (3.1). Similar to the IPCW estimator developed above, this estimator utilizes the following equality:

$$E\left[\frac{I(T_A \le t)\Delta_A I(S = A)}{\bar{G}_A(T_A \mid X_A)P(S = A \mid W(0))}\right] = F_A(t). \tag{3.3}$$

This identity follows from first conditioning on the full data (Z_A, Z_B) and by applying (1.1),

$$E(I(S = A) \mid Z_A, Z_B) = P(S = A \mid W(0)).$$

Finally, by arguments given in section 2.1 the conditional expectation given X_A of the left hand side of (3.3) equals $I(T_A \le t)$. This suggests the following ad hoc estimator of $F_A(t)$:

$$F^0_{A,n}(t) = \frac{1}{n}\sum_{i=1}^{n} \frac{I(S_i = A)I(T_{A,i} \le t)\Delta_i}{\bar{G}_{A,n}(T_{A,i} \mid X_{A,i})P_n(S_i = A \mid W_i(0))}. \tag{3.4}$$

To calculate this estimate, one needs an estimate of the propensity score $P(S = A \mid W(0))$. One obvious choice for two to K treatment groups is polychotomous regression. For $K = 2$ this reduces to the standard logistic regression model:

$$P(S = A \mid W(0)) = \frac{\exp(f(W(0)))}{1 + \exp(f(W(0)))},$$

where $f(W(0)) = f_1(W_1) + \ldots + f_k(W_k)$ is assumed to be additive in the components of $W(0)$. Smooth estimation of f_j, $j = 1, \ldots, k$ has been implemented in the SPLUS function *gam* (Hastie and Tibshirani, 1990) and standard generalized linear regression is implemented in the SPLUS function *glm*.

Since one must model the propensity score consistently to get consistent estimates of $F_A(t)$ and the asymptotic efficiency only increases when one increases the dimension of the model by the arguments given in section 2.1, it makes sense to estimate the score as non-parametrically as sample size permits. However, one should also realize that the second order asymptotics will depend heavily on how efficient one estimates the propensity score. Thus, to expect a good finite sample behavior of the estimator $P(S = A \mid W(0))$ one will need to choose the appropriate dimension of the model for $P(S = A \mid W(0))$.

3.3. The locally efficient estimator. To implement the locally efficient estimator for $F_A(t)$, one must estimate the following components of the efficient influence curve IC^* (3.2): $P(S = A \mid W(0))$, $F_A(t \mid W(0), S = A)$, $F_A(t \mid \bar{W}_A(u), \tilde{T}_A > u)$ and $G_A(u \mid X_A)$. Since S is independent of the Z_A, given $W(0)$, we have:

$$P(T_A \leq t \mid \bar{W}_A(u), \tilde{T}_A > u) = P(T_A \leq t \mid \bar{W}_A(u), \tilde{T}_A > u, S = A)$$
$$P(C_A > t \mid X_A) = P(C_A > t \mid X_A, S = A).$$

Thus, one possible method of deriving estimates of $G_A(\cdot \mid X_A)$ and $F_A(t \mid \bar{W}_A(u), \tilde{T}_A)$ is to estimate them as discussed in section 2, using the subsample with $S = A$. Another possibility is by using the traditional approach that includes a treatment dummy variable in a regression model.

We have already discussed in the previous section possible estimates of the propensity score. Thus, it remains to estimate $F_A(t \mid W(0), S = A)$. If C_A is independent of T_A, given $W(0)$, then one could assume, for example, a Cox-proportional hazards model with time-independent covariates $W(0)$ and estimate $F_A(t \mid W(0), S = A)$ with the partial likelihood estimator based on the sub-sample defined by $S = A$. However, since we are not assuming such conditional independence, we recommend use of the relation

$$F_A(t \mid W(0)) = E\left(\frac{I(T_A \leq t)\Delta_A}{\bar{G}_A(T_A \mid X_A)} \mid W(0), S = A\right).$$

As discussed in section 2.3, this can be estimated as a regression of $I(T_A \leq t)\Delta_A / \bar{G}_{A,n}(T_A \mid X_A)$ on $W(0)$ using a flexible regression routine, such as the gam-function in Splus on the sub-sample defined by $S = A$.

When all the components have been estimated, then we can represent our estimator, just as we did in section 2.2 (see 2.8), as a one-step estimator:

$$(3.5)\quad F^1_{A,n}(t) = F^0_{A,n}(t) + \frac{1}{n}\sum_{i=1}^{n} IC^*(Y_i \mid G_{A,n}, P_n(S = A \mid W(0)), F_{X_A,n}, F^0_{A,n}(t)),$$

where $F^0_{A,n}(t)$ is (3.4). Theorem 5.1 demonstrates that, under regularity conditions, if G_A and $P(S = A \mid W(0))$ are estimated consistently, then the estimator $F^1_{A,n}(t)$ is asymptotically linear. In addition, if $F_A(t \mid \bar{W}_A(u), \tilde{T}_A > u)$ and $F_A(t \mid W(0), S = A)$ are also consistently estimated, then $F^1_{A,n}(t)$ is asymptotically efficient.

3.4. Construction of a conservative confidence interval. Under the conditions of theorem 5.1, $F^1_{A,n}(t)$ is asymptotically linear having an influence curve with variance smaller than or equal to the variance of $IC^*(Y \mid F^1_{X_A}, P(S = A \mid W(0)), G_A, F_A(t))$, where $IC^*(Y \mid F^1_{X_A}, P(S = A \mid W(0)), G_A, F_A(t))$ represents the limit of $\widehat{IC}(Y) \equiv IC^*(Y \mid F_{X_A,n}, P_n(S = A \mid W(0)), G_{A,n}, F^0_{A,n}(t))$.

Therefore a conservative estimate of the asymptotic variance of $F^1_{A,n}(t)$ is given by

$$\widehat{\sigma}^2 = \frac{1}{n}\sum_{i=1}^{n}\{\widehat{IC}(Y_i)\}^2.$$

This can be used to construct a conservative 95% confidence interval for $F_A(t)$:

$$F^1_{A,n}(t) \pm 1.96\frac{\widehat{\sigma}}{\sqrt{n}}. \tag{3.6}$$

4. Simulation results. A simulation study was performed to examine the relative performance of the locally efficient one-step, the IPCW and the Kaplan-Meier estimators. The simulation section is split into two subsections. The first subsection contains the results of simulations corresponding to the single treatment context. We examine the performance of our estimators under both dependent and independent censoring and include simulations when there exists a relevant time-dependent covariate process. In the second subsection, we present simulations where two relevant treatments are assigned according to a MAR model and one is interested in the estimate of the corresponding survival functions. We include simulations for both conditionally independent assignment and assignment completely at random. Our potential gain over traditional estimators should be a reduction in bias for the former and a reduction in variance for the latter. We discuss the results of these simulations in the Discussion and conclusions section.

4.1. One relevant treatment. Three different types of simulations are reported in this section. First, we report the results of simulations investigating the relative performance of our estimators when the censoring time is marginally independent of the failure time, but mean failure time is a function of a time-independent covariate ($W = W(0)$). Although the Kaplan-Meier estimator remains consistent in this context, our estimators should have superior efficiency. Next, results from a simulation in which a time-independent covariate is relevant to both censoring and failure are reported. In this simulation, because C and T are no longer independent, the Kaplan-Meier estimator is inconsistent, but our estimators can incorporate the relevant covariate information to reduce the bias. Finally, we examine the relative performance of our locally efficient estimator when there exists a time-dependent surrogate process.

Simulation 1. For this set of simulations and for simulation 2, both the censoring and failure times are generated from a logistic distribution:

$$F(t \mid W) = \frac{1}{1+exp(-(\beta_0^T+\beta_1^T t+\beta_2^T w))}$$

$$G(c \mid W) = \frac{1}{1+exp(-(\beta_0^C+\beta_1^C c+\beta_2^C w))}.$$

Like the normal distribution, the logistic distribution is symmetric and we chose it as the model for $F(t \mid W)$ because one can conveniently vary the variance of this conditional distribution by modifying the β_1 parameter; the variance of $T \mid W$ is proportional to $1/\beta_1^3$. The information about T contained in W is a function of the variance of $T \mid W$. As the variance goes to 0, then $W \to T$ and thus the covariates becomes perfectly informative about T. We use the ratio of the standard deviations of the the distribution of $T \mid W$ over that of T, $\tau \equiv \frac{\sigma_{T|W=w}}{\sigma_T}$, as a measure of the relative information about T contained in W. For the conditional failure distribution, we use two sets of coefficients. The first results in a relatively large variance of $T \mid W$ and so one should not expect the locally efficient estimator to gain much over the Kaplan-Meier (see table 1). The second set of coefficients results in a conditional distribution with relatively small variance (see table 2). In this simulation, W is highly predictive of the location of T and so the locally efficient estimator should gain over the Kaplan-Meier estimator by incorporating W, as discussed in section 2. In this set of simulations (tables 1 and 2), the coefficients β_i^C are fixed at -9, 1, and 0, respectively, which results in independent censoring and an average of just over 50 percent censored observations per sample. Because the censoring times are marginally independent of the failure times, the Kaplan-Meier estimator is consistent for these data-generating distributions and thus the gain in efficiency from using our estimators will come solely from a reduction in variance. For all the simulations in this section $W \sim U(-1,1)$, the sample size is 100, we perform 625 replicates, and we determine the estimates at 3 quantiles (25th, 50th and 75th).

To calculate the IPCW estimator (2.2) we need an estimate of $\bar{G}(\cdot \mid W)$ and for these simulations we use Cox regression to get this estimate. Note that we ignore the fact that C is independent of W, but as discussed in section 2.1 this should improve the performance of this estimator. We report the results of three asymptotically equivalent locally efficient one-step estimates: 1) the locally efficient estimator using an explicit representation of IC^*_{nu} (2.9) with all components known (called "all known"), 2) the locally efficient estimator using an explicit representation of IC^*_{nu} with the distributions estimated (called "explicit"), and 3) the locally efficient estimator using a regression approach (2.10) to estimate IC^*_{nu} (called "expectation"). For all these locally efficient estimators, we are assuming the constant, $c(F_X^1, G, F(t)) = 1$ in (2.5). However in practice, one can expect greater efficiency by estimating this constant.

The three methods for estimating the efficient influence curve were done to contrast approaches for estimating the relevant distributions. Because the "all known" estimator uses the efficient influence curve with the known F_X and G, this estimator represents the optimal scenario for our locally efficient estimator and corresponds to the efficiency one would expect when estimating $F(\cdot \mid W)$ with a correctly specified parametric model. Generally, our one-step estimator will require an estimate of both

TABLE 1
Independent censoring with weak covariate. $MSE \times 10^2(RMSE)$ *for estimation of* $F(t)$ *at three quantiles:* $\tau = 0.85$, $(\beta_0^T, \beta_1^T, \beta_2^T) = (-10, 1, 2)$.

Estimator	25th	50th	75th
Kaplan-Meier	0.27(1.0)	0.55(1.0)	1.27(1.0)
Simple	0.27(1.0)	0.53(1.0)	1.32(1.0)
L.E.(all known)	0.26(1.0)	0.51(1.1)	1.22(1.0)
L.E.(expectation)	0.26(1.0)	0.52(1.1)	1.28(1.0)
L.E.(explicit)	0.26(1.0)	0.52(1.1)	1.28(1.0)

TABLE 2
Independent censoring with strong covariate. $MSE \times 10^2(RMSE)$ *for estimation of* $F(t)$ *at three quantiles:* $\tau = 0.20$, $(\beta_0^T, \beta_1^T, \beta_2^T) = (-30, 3, 17)$.

Estimator	25th	50th	75th
Kaplan-Meier	0.19(1.0)	0.45(1.0)	2.52(1.0)
Simple	0.19(1.0)	0.36(1.2)	2.41(1.0)
L.E.(all known)	0.18(1.0)	0.29(1.5)	1.14(2.2)
L.E.(expectation)	0.18(1.0)	0.34(1.3)	2.25(1.1)
L.E.(explicit)	0.18(1.0)	0.32(1.4)	2.33(1.1)

F_X and G and for the "explicit" estimator we used Cox regression and the Kaplan-Meier estimator, respectively. Note that because sample sizes are small and $F(\cdot \mid W)$ is estimated semi-parametrically, the resulting finite sample efficiency will be less than if a correct parametric estimating model were used. For the expectation estimator, to get an estimate of $E\left(\frac{I(\tilde{T} \le t)\Delta}{\bar{G}(\tilde{T}|X)} \mid \bar{X}(u), \tilde{T} > u\right)$, we chose a large set of u's and performed smooth regression at each u of the random variable $\frac{I(T \le t)\Delta}{\bar{G}(\tilde{T}|X)}$ against W for only those observations where $\tilde{T} > u$ (see section 2.3). The smooth regression was done using the super-smoother (Friedman, 1984). The expectation approach provides a general method for estimating F_X and can be particularly useful when traditional methods, such as Cox regression, are either invalid or more difficult to use, as with time-dependent covariates. We still need an estimate of G for this estimator and again we use the Kaplan-Meier estimator. We use the ratio of the mean-squared error (MSE) of the Kaplan-Meier estimator over that of the competing estimator, based on the 625 iterations of each simulation, as a measure of the performance of our estimators (see tables 1 and 2). Because all estimators are consistent for this set of simulations $MSE \approx Variance$.

The results demonstrate the potential advantage of using the locally efficient estimators. For the simulation reported in table 1, the distribution of $T \mid W$ has relatively large variance ($\tau = 0.85$) and so W contains only weak information about T. Thus, the locally efficient estimators will have little potential to improve over the Kaplan-Meier estimator and this is precisely what these simulations show. However, the locally efficient estimators do not lose in efficiency relative to the Kaplan-Meier estimator and so in this case, one is not hurt by trying to utilize the covariate information. For the simulation reported in table 2, the distribution of $T \mid W$ has a relatively tight distribution around the mean ($\tau = 0.20$) and so W contains precise information about the location of T. Thus, the locally efficient estimator should be able to utilize this information to improve efficiency and this simulation demonstrates this potential. Note in particular the "all known" estimator which reduces the MSE relative to the Kaplan-Meier estimator by a factor of 2 for estimation of $S(t)$ at the 75th quantile. The other locally efficient estimators gain little over the Kaplan-Meier at the 75th quantile because, due to censoring, the semi-parametric estimates of $F(t \mid W)$ and $G(\cdot \mid W)$ are highly variable in the upper tail of the distribution. However, at the 50th quantile (the median), both these estimators have significantly lower mean-squared errors relative to the Kaplan Meier ($RMSE = 1.3$). Note that all estimators are essentially equivalent at the 25th quantile. This is because, on average, few observations have been censored by $t = F^{-1}(0.25)$ in this simulation and so the variance of the Kaplan-Meier estimator is nearly the same as the empirical distribution. Given that the locally efficient estimator can be no more efficient than the empirical distribution, there is little room to gain in efficiency over the Kaplan-Meier estimator for t's where there has yet to be much censoring.

To examine the performance of confidence intervals when the model for $F(t \mid \bar{W}(u), T > u)$ is misspecified, we examine both the coverage rate of the conservative confidence interval (2.12), that is a confidence interval based on an estimate of the variance making the naive assumption that we have estimated $F(t \mid \bar{W}(u), T > u)$ consistently (call "naive"), and that based on the projection shown in lemma 5.3 (call "robust"). Our data generating models are:

$$F(t \mid w) = \frac{1}{1 + \exp(-(-20 + 2t + 5w + 5w^2))}$$

$$G(c \mid w) = \frac{1}{1 + \exp(-(-8 + c))}.$$

In this case, we inconsistently estimate F_X using Cox regression entering only a linear term for W. Table 3 gives the results of confidence intervals that use both the "naive" and the "robust" estimates of the asymptotic variance. As one can see, both the naive and robust estimators of the asymptotic variance perform equivalently in this simulation suggesting that misspecification can be ignored for at least these data-generating distributions.

Simulation 2. The only difference between this simulation and simulation 1 is that T and C are dependent through W ($\beta_2^C = 2$) and the sample

TABLE 3
Percent of the confidence intervals containing the true $F(t)$ for both naive and robust estimates at three quantiles, $(\beta_0^T, \beta_1^T, \beta_2^T) = (-30, 3, 17)$..

CI	25th	50th	75th
Naive	94	93	93
Robust	94	96	96

TABLE 4
Dependent censoring. $MSE \times 10^2(RMSE)$ for estimation of $F(t)$ at three quantiles: $(\beta_0^T, \beta_1^T, \beta_2^T) = (-30, 3, 8)$, $(\beta_0^C, \beta_1^C, \beta_2^C) = (-10, 1, 2)$.

Estimator	25th	50th	75th
Kaplan-Meier	0.33(1.0)	1.16(1.0)	1.24(1.0)
Simple	0.048(6.9)	0.073(15.9)	0.13(9.6)
L.E.(explicit)	0.044(7.5)	0.070(16.6)	0.059(21.1)

size is 500. In this simulation, the Kaplan-Meier is biased and so the potential gain in efficiency from using our estimators comes not only from reducing the variance, but by eliminating the bias. Here we only report the explicit locally efficient estimator where both $G(\cdot \mid W)$ and $F(\cdot \mid W)$ are estimated with Cox regression (see table 4). Because the Kaplan-Meier estimator is badly biased in this simulation (for the 625 simulations the average Kaplan-Meier estimates are 0.26, 0.60, 0.85 for the 25th, 50th and 75th quantile, respectively), both the IPCW and the locally efficient estimators have substantially lower MSE's. The reduction in MSE from using the IPCW estimator is mainly by eliminating bias whereas not only is the locally efficient estimator consistent, it also has lower variance than the IPCW estimator by optimally using the information contained in the covariate. This simulation confirms that our estimators can still salvage estimation when censoring and failure are dependent through observed covariates.

Simulation 3. In this set of simulations, C is marginally independent of T and at at evenly spaced times c_j's (every 0.15 units) less than $\tilde{T}$ and at $\tilde{T}$, the analyst observes a surrogate process $W(c_j)$. This simulation is motivated by a clinical setting where patients come in for regular visits. During those visits, the clinician records some measure of the health of the patient that is related to the failure time of interest (e.g., CD4 counts for HIV+ patients). Thus, as more measurements are taken, more information is available about the prognosis of the patient and our estimators can optimally use this information.

The data generating distributions are as follows:

$$T \sim U(0.5, 1.5)$$
$$C \sim U(0, 1.25)$$

TABLE 5
$MSE \times 10^2 (RMSE)$ for estimation of $F(t)$ at three quantiles where one observes a time-dependent surrogate process, $W(u) = T + \sigma e$. γ is the ratio of σ over the standard deviation of T.

Estimator	γ	25th	50th	75th
Kaplan-Meier	.	0.14(1.0)	0.23(1.0)	0.25(1.0)
L.E.	0.001	0.079(1.9)	0.11(2.1)	0.071(3.5)
L.E.	0.032	0.066(2.12)	0.10(2.2)	0.070(3.6)
L.E.	0.100	0.080(1.7)	0.10(2.2)	0.085(3.0)
L.E.	0.316	0.12(1.2)	0.14(1.6)	0.12(1.9)
L.E.	0.707	0.18(0.69)	0.23(0.86)	0.30(0.85)

$$W(c_j) = T + \sigma e,$$

where $e \sim N(0, 1)$. At each monitoring time one observes another observation of T plus an error, where the variance of the error is σ^2. Thus, as the number of observations of $W(c_j)$ on a person increases, the more accurately one can estimate the person's failure time. In this case, we estimate G consistently using the Kaplan-Meier estimator. As discussed as a possibility in section 2.4, we use an extreme model for estimating $F(t \mid \bar{W}(u), T > u)$: $\hat{F}(t \mid \bar{W}(u), T > u) = I(\widehat{T}(u) < t)$, where $\widehat{T}(u)$ is the predicted failure time based the surrogate process as:

$$\widehat{T}(u) = \frac{1}{n_j} \sum_{c_j \leq u} W(c_j),$$

where n_j is the number of monitoring times less than or equal to u. We report the results of five simulations, each with a different value of σ. As a measure of the information about T contained in $W(c_j)$, we define γ as the ratio of σ over the standard deviation of the marginal distribution of T. If γ is small, then $W(c_j)$ will be very informative about the location of T, if it is large, then the process will contain relatively little information about T. When σ is very large (and thus γ is large) then $\widehat{T}(u)$ is a very poor estimate of T and thus $I(\widehat{T}(u) < t)$ is a very bad estimate of $F(t \mid W(u))$. In the case that one does not use the constant, c_n (see section 2.4), then our locally efficient estimator is not guaranteed to be better than the Kaplan-Meier estimator (for this simulation, we do not modify our influence curve with the constant). For simulations where σ is relatively small, then the surrogate process is a very good predictor of T and our estimator should do relatively well. In the extreme case where $\sigma = 0$, then $F(t \mid \bar{W}, T > u) = I(\widehat{T}(u) < t)$ and as shown above our one-step estimator is equivalent to the estimator based on the empirical distribution of the T's.

The results of this set of simulations are in table 5. As one can see, when γ is small (and so $W(c_j)$ is very close to T) then our locally efficient estimator has much lower MSE than the Kaplan-Meier estimator; because the Kaplan-Meier estimator is consistent for these simulations, the gain in efficiency (reduction in MSE) comes soley from a reduction in the variance of estimation. However, if γ is very large (0.707 in table 5) then the locally efficient estimator, while still consistent, now has greater variance than the Kaplan-Meier estimator. This is because the model for $F(t \mid W(u))$ is badly misspecified and if one does not modify the influence curve by using the constant, c_n (section 2.4), then the locally efficient estimator can suffer relative to the Kaplan-Meier estimator. It is interesting to note that even when γ is relatively large (0.316 in table 5) and so $I(\hat{T}(u) < t)$ is a poor estimator of $F(t \mid W(u))$, the locally efficient one-step estimator still significantly out-performs the Kaplan-Meier estimator.

4.2. Two relevant treatments. In this subsection, we present two simulations that examine the performance of our one-step estimator (3.5) when one is interested in the marginal treatment survival curve and two or more treatments exist. The first simulation examines the performance when treatment assignment and the failure time are marginally dependent, but these random variables are conditionally independent given the covariate. In this case, the simple Kaplan-Meier estimator performed on each treatment group is inconsistent, so the advantage of our estimator is a reduction in bias. In the second simulation, treatment assignment is done completely at random, but there exists a binary covariate (W) that strongly predicts failure. In this case, the performance of our estimator should be superior to that of the Kaplan-Meier by reducing the variance of estimation. As discussed above, the reduction in variance occurs by accounting for the non-uniform distribution of W within each sub-sample defined by the treatment group. In this way, the one-step estimator reduces the bias within a realized random sample. Although the Kaplan-Meier estimator is consistent for repeated experiments under this scenario, it can be significantly biased in any realized sample if by bad luck W is unevenly distributed among the treatment groups.

For both simulations, we use the same families of data-generating models:

$$\begin{aligned} F(t \mid W, S) &= \frac{1}{1+\exp(-(\beta_0^T + \beta_1^T t + \beta_2^T W + \beta_3^T S))} \\ G(c \mid W, S) &= \frac{1}{1+\exp(-(-10+c))}, \end{aligned} \tag{4.1}$$

where $W = (0, 1)$ with equal probability, $S = (0, 1)$. The β's and $P(S = 1 \mid W = w)$ vary with the simulation. In the first simulation, we simply use the known values of G, $F(t \mid W, S)$ and $P(S = 1 \mid W)$ when calculating our estimators. In the second simulation, we again use the known values of G and $F(t \mid W, S)$, but we estimate $P(S \mid W)$ even though treatment assignment and W are independent. As discussed above and shown formally in appendix 1, our one-step estimator should improve over the estimator that uses the known values of the propensity score.

Simulation 4. For this simulation:

$$(\beta_0^T, \beta_1^T, \beta_2^T, \beta_3^T) = (-10, 1, 5, -5)$$
$$P(S = 1 \mid W = 1) = 0.90$$
$$P(S = 1 \mid W = 0) = 0.10.$$

Thus, those subjects with $W = 1$ have a shorter mean survival time than those with $W = 0$. If a subject has $W = 1$, however, then they have a much higher probability of receiving treatment ($S = 1$) relative to those subjects with $W = 0$. Furthermore, those with treatment have a higher mean survival than controls ($S = 0$). Thus, W confounds the relationship of treatment and survival because the treatment group will contain differentially more subjects with shorter survival times. This will result in an over-estimation of $F_{S=1}(t)$ and under-estimation of $F_{S=0}(t)$ by the stratified Kaplan-Meier estimator. However, our one-step estimator should successfully adjust for the confounding of assignment and treatment effect that occurs through W.

Instead of reporting the results of repeated iterations, we present the graphical results of a single iteration (figure 1). As one can see, the Kaplan-Meier estimator performed on the two subsamples ($S = 0$ and $S = 1$) provides a biased estimate of the marginal treatment distribution. As anticipated, the Kaplan-Meier estimator underestimates the treatment survival distribution and overestimates the control distribution. However, the locally efficient one-step estimator consistently estimates both distributions.

Simulation 5. For this simulation:

$$(\beta_0^T, \beta_1^T, \beta_2^T, \beta_3^T) = (-30, 3, 15, -15)$$
$$P(S = 1 \mid W = 1) = 0.50$$
$$P(S = 1 \mid W = 0) = 0.50.$$

In this case, assignment is done completely at random, however W has such a strong effect on survival that non-uniform distribution of W among the subjects in the two treatment groups can have a strong confounding effect for any one sample. Thus, we should gain over the Kaplan-Meier by modeling $P(S \mid W)$.

The graphical results of four iterations of this simulation are shown in figure 2. Because for this simulation, the Kaplan-Meier estimates of the treatment distributions are consistent (treatment assignment was done completely at random), these estimates do not depart from the true distributions as dramatically as in simulation 4. However, by estimating the propensity score, the one-step estimator (3.5) provides an estimate of the treatment survival distribution that is closer, on average, to the true distribution than the Kaplan-Meier estimator. Note that the improvement

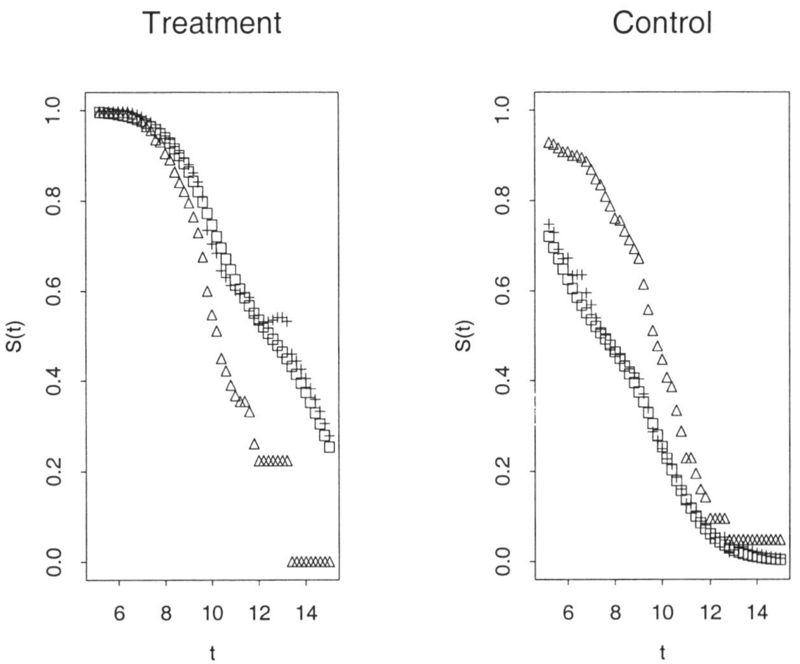

FIG. 1. *Estimates of the distribution function under non-random assignment, simulation 4.* $\square$ *= truth,* $+$ *= one-step, and* $\triangle$ *= Kaplan-Meier.*

over the Kaplan-Meier estimator in this circumstance will be a function of how strongly W affects survival. In this case, W significantly affects the mean survival and so small discrepancies in the distribution of W between subsamples defined by treatment group ($S = 0$ and $S = 1$) will result in confounding by W within any *realized* sample. Thus, one can substantially improve efficiency relative to the Kaplan-Meier estimator by modeling the propensity score.

5. Discussion and conclusions. The simulations have supported the potential gain in efficiency (relative to the Kaplan-Meier estimator) offered by our one-step estimator. Simulation 1 (tables 1 and 2) shows that when censoring is independent of failure, the one-step estimator can have significantly lower variance that the Kaplan-Meier estimator, particularly if W, the covariate, is highly predictive of T. These simulations also suggest that one might want to guess a parametric model for $F(t \mid \bar{W}(u), T > u)$ if sample sizes are relatively small. When we use a semi-parametric model for $F(t \mid \bar{W}(u), T > u)$ at small sample sizes, we gain little over the Kaplan-Meier estimator. However, a parametric model can yield significant gains (see "all known" in table 2). In fact, in simulations not reported here we show how a misspecified parametric model for $F(t \mid \bar{W}(u), T > u)$ can still

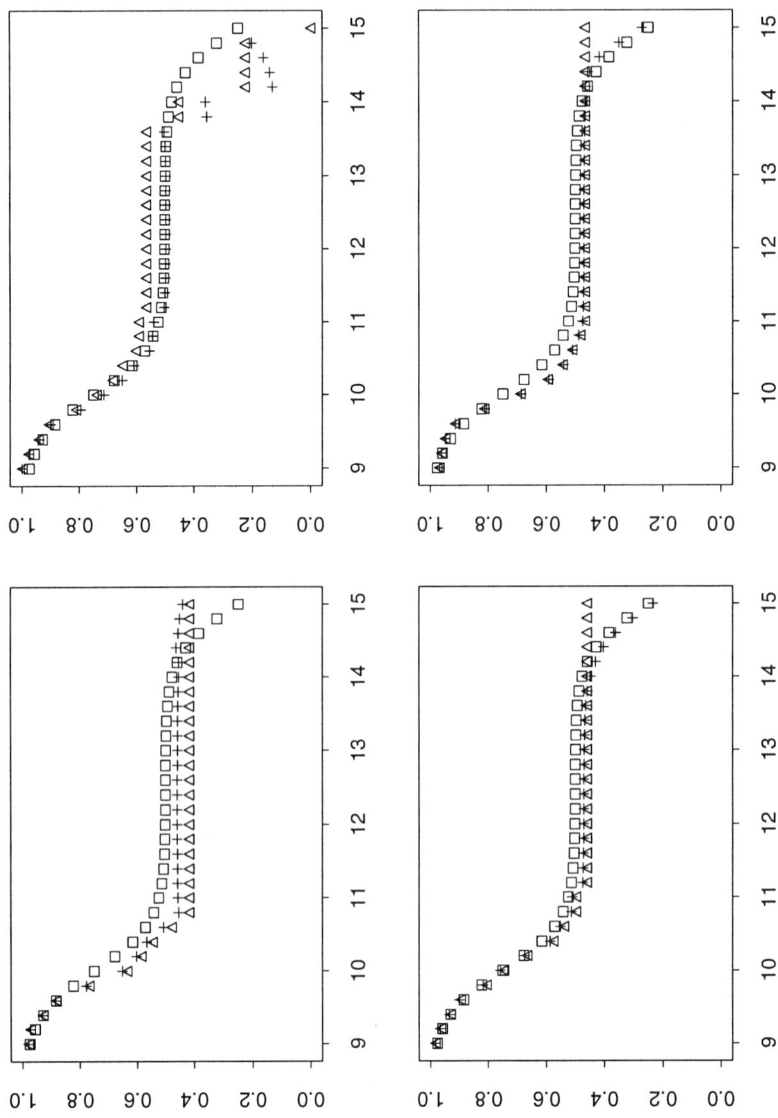

FIG. 2. *Estimates of the distribution function under random assignment, simulation 5.* □ *= truth,* + *= one-step, and* △ *= Kaplan-Meier.*

gain significant efficiency relative to the Kaplan-Meier estimator.

Simulation 2 (table 4) demonstrates that when T is not independent of C, the one-step and IPCW estimators offer a consistent method of estimation of $F(t)$ if covariates that explain the dependence between them have been collected. Simulation 3 (table 5) shows that a surrogate process that is highly predictive of T can be utilized in a simplified way to get consistent, and possibly efficient estimates of the distribution function. In this case, as the surrogate nearly perfectly predicts T, our ad hoc estimator (using $I(\widehat{T}(u) < t)$ to estimate $F(t \mid \bar{W}(u), T > u)$) is nearly as efficient as the empirical distribution based on the unobserved T's. Thus, if a physician can make accurate judgments about the prognosis of a patient based on measurements made up to that time, this approach can yield significant improvements over the Kaplan-Meier estimator. Note also that only when the surrogate process is very noisy (γ is large) does the one-step estimator lose against the Kaplan-Meier estimator. However, if we would have implemented the one-step estimator with IC_0 being the influence curve of the Kaplan-Meier estimator (see section 2.4), then the one-step estimator would never lose (asymptotically) against the Kaplan-Meier estimator.

Simulations 4 (figure 1) demonstrate that if treatment assignment is not marginally independent of failure time, but conditionally independent given the baseline covariates, the one-step estimator can provide consistent estimates of the treatment distributions, whereas the Kaplan-Meier is typically biased. In simulation 5 (figure 2), where treatment assignment is independent of T, we show that the one-step estimator gains efficiency by using an estimated propensity score. Specifically, by modeling $P(S = A \mid W)$ even when assignment is known to be independent of failure, one accounts for random associations of T with S through the observed covariates.

Our method for estimating the marginal treatment distribution relies on consistently estimating the censoring distributions, that is, $P(S = A \mid W(0))$ and $G_A(c \mid X)$. However, one might also estimate the marginal treatment distribution by assuming a model for the conditional failure distribution given treatment and the confounders, such as the Cox regression model. If the model is correct, then integrating over the empirical distribution of covariate values for a fixed treatment effect will provide a consistent estimate of the treatment distribution. In addition, one can estimate the conditional distribution of failure given the treatment and covariates as nonparametrically as sample size permits, the same approach we use to estimate $P(S = A \mid W(0))$ and $G_A(c \mid X)$. Of course, if one estimates the conditional failure distribution nonparametrically, then the information bound of the estimator of the marginal treatment distribution based on this nonparametric estimate will be the same as our locally efficient estimator. This leads to the question of which approach should be preferred; the one that relies on consistent estimates of the censoring distributions or one that relies on consistent estimate of the conditional failure distribution. The answer to this question will be data specific. If one feels that they understand the censoring process better, then our approach should be preferred and the other approach should be used if one feels that the failure process is better understood. In biomedical applications, one often has a reasonably good understanding of why patients are lost to follow-up or how treatments are assigned. In some circumstances one will have good reason to believe that the censoring process is independent of failure (e.g., fixed follow-up time, random assignment of treatments). In these circumstances, provided that the estimating models for the censoring distributions include independence of censoring and failure, our estimators should be preferred.

We have presented a semi-parametric, locally efficient estimator of the survival distribution when the data are right-censored. In addition, we have extended our estimators to estimation of "treatment" distributions when two or more possible treatments (or environmental exposures) exist. Besides a recipe for calculating these estimates we have showed that the estimate of the efficient influence curve yields a confidence interval which is either conservative or correct depending on the level of misspecification of the model for $F(t \mid \bar{W}(u), \tilde{T} > u)$. In the most general sense, our estimators can improve over existing estimators by incorporating covariate information. We have shown that when the covariates are perfectly predictive of T, then these estimators can attain the efficiency of the empirical distribution. These estimators are and their standard errors have explicit formulas and they can be calculated with existing statistical software, such as Splus and STATA. These locally efficient estimators not only have the potential to improve estimation after data have been collected, but can be utilized in sample size planning in clinical trials so that the relevant covariates are collected and the number of requisite subjects is reduced. In many circumstances, it may be far more cost-effective to collect more informative covariates on each subject than to enroll more subjects. Thus, the locally efficient estimator provides a compelling alternative to the Kaplan-Meier estimator in both observational studies and clinical trials.

Acknowledgement. This research was supported by a FIRST award from the National Institute of General Medical Sciences, National Institute of Health (GM53722).

THE APPENDIX. The appendix is split into three major sections, appendices 1, 2 and 3. In appendix 1, we present the locally efficient theorem and the sketch of a proof. We also present a lemma that demonstrates how optimal estimation of an orthogonal nuisance parameter (in this case the censoring distribution) leads to an asymptotic improvement of the estimator. In appendix 2, we give a summary of the weighted estimating equation approach presented in Robins (1993) and Robins and Rotnitsky (1992). In addition, we provide an alternative method to find the efficient influence curve presented in Bickel, et. al. (1993). An estimate of this influence curve is then used to construct a one-step, locally efficient estimator. Finally, in appendix 3, we provide explicit formulas and methods to estimate the components of the influence curve under misspecification of F_X. This influence curve can then be used to estimate the variance of the one-step estimator. Note, we presented a method of estimating a simple and conservative variance (if model for F_X is misspecified) in the main body of the paper and we believe this estimate will usually suffice. However, appendix 3 provides an estimate of the variance that is consistent even under misspecification.

Appendix 1 - The locally efficient theorem.

An alternative representation of the data. In order to simplify the theoretical development, we provide an alternative way of representing the one-step estimator $F^1_{A,n}(t)$ that allows a unified treatment of the one-step estimators $F^1_{A,n}(t)$ and $F^1_n(t)$ as defined in (3.5) and (2.8), respectively. In sections 2 and 3, we chose to develop our estimators in a two step fashion by developing the locally efficient estimator in the single treatment context and then adding treatment assignment as a second form of censoring. Presenting these estimators in this two step process provides an intuitive understanding and a recipe for how estimators such as these can be constructed. First, find the efficient influence curve (i.e. the efficient estimator) for the censored problem where the entire population gets the identical treatment, then modify the efficient influence curve with the propensity score of treatment assignment to account for missing data on the counterfactual. However, one could develop the data model in an equivalent fashion that finds the locally efficient estimator in just one step, similar to the development in section 2.2. For estimation of $F_A(t)$, one is only interested in the distribution of $X_A = (T_A, \bar{W}(T_A))$. Because we model the effect of treatment nonparametrically, we assume no relation between X_A and X_B, and thus we can define X_A as the full data. Now, define C^*_A to be the censoring variable, such that $C^*_A = C_A$ if $S = A$, and $C^*_A = 0$ if $S \neq A$. Then, one observes:

$$Y = (\tilde{T}^*_A \equiv \min(C^*_A, T_A), \Delta^*_A \equiv I(T_A < C^*_A) \\ = I(T_A < C_A)I(S = A), \bar{W}_A(\tilde{T}^*_A)). \tag{5.1}$$

Note that $\bar{W}_A(0) = W(0)$ is the time-independent component of W_A and W_B and so is observed regardless of treatment assignment. The efficient influence curve for $F_A(t)$ based on observing the data (5.1) equals the efficient influence curve based on observing $I(S = A)Z_A + I(S = B)Z_B$.

Since the data structure (5.1) is equivalent to the data structure studied in section 2 the same methodology can be applied. We just replace, in section 2.2, C by C^*_A and G by G^*_A, where

$$G^*_A(c \mid X_A) = P(S = A \mid X_A)G_A(c \mid X_A). \tag{5.2}$$

So define as in section 2.2

$$IC_0(Y \mid G^*_A, F_A(t)) = \frac{I(T_A \leq t)\Delta^*_A}{\bar{G}^*(T_A \mid X_A)} - F_A(t)$$

$$IC^*_{nu}(Y \mid F_{X_A}, G^*_A) = -\int F_A(t \mid \bar{W}_A(u), \tilde{T}^*_A > u)\frac{dM^*_A(u)}{\bar{G}(u \mid X_A)}, \tag{5.3}$$

where

$$dM_A^*(u) = I(C_A^* \in du, \Delta_A^* = 0) - \Lambda_{C_A^*}(du \mid X_A) I(\tilde{T}_A^* > u).$$

Then the efficient influence curve for $F_A(t)$ at (F_{X_A}, G_A^*) is given by:

$$IC^*(Y \mid F_{X_A}, G_A^*, F_A(t)) = IC_0(Y \mid G_A^*, F_A(t)) - IC_{nu}^*(Y \mid F_{X_A}, G_A^*). \tag{5.4}$$

Note that

$$\begin{aligned} F_A(t \mid \bar{W}_A(u), \tilde{T}_A^* > u) &= F_A(t \mid \bar{W}_A(u), \tilde{T}_A > u, S = A) \text{ for } u > 0 \\ F_A(t \mid \bar{W}_A(0), \tilde{T}_A^* > 0) &= F_A(t \mid W(0), S = A). \end{aligned} \tag{5.5}$$

Suppose one parameterizes G_A^* as a product of G_A with $P(S = A \mid W(0))$ as in (5.2) and one-estimates $F_A(t \mid \bar{W}_A(u), \tilde{T}_A^* > u)$ using the representation (5.5) in terms of $F_A(t \mid W(0), S = A)$ and $F_A(t \mid \bar{W}_A(u), \tilde{T}_A > u, S = A)$. Then an estimate of IC^* based on the new representation (5.4) involves estimation of the same components as needed using the representation (3.2), namely $P(S = A \mid W(0))$, $G_A(u \mid X_A)$, $F_A(t \mid \bar{W}_A(u), \tilde{T}_A > u, S = A)$ and $F_A(t \mid W(0), S = A)$. It is straightforward to verify that both representations (3.2) and (5.4) are indeed the same functions of these components. In other words, the representations (3.2) and (5.4) in terms of the four components of the efficient influence curve are equivalent.

Thus using the representation (5.4) yields exactly the same one-step estimator as $F_{A,n}^1(t)$ (3.5):

$$F_{A,n}^1(t) = F_{A,n}^0(t) + \frac{1}{n}\sum_{i=1}^{n} IC^*(Y_i \mid F_{X_A}^n, G_{A,n}^*, F_{A,n}^0(t)). \tag{5.6}$$

As in section 2, we can adjust the representation (5.4) of the efficient influence curve with the constant c. Namely, we define for a given $F_{X_A}^1, G_A, F_A(t)$:

$$\begin{aligned} IC^*(Y \mid F_{X_A}^1, G_A^*, F_A(t)) &\equiv IC_0(Y \mid G_A^*, F_A(t)) \\ &\quad - c(F_{X_A}^1, G_A^*, F_A(t)) IC_{nu}^*(Y \mid F_{X_A}^1, G_A^*), \end{aligned} \tag{5.7}$$

where

$$c(F_{X_A}^1, G_A^*, F_A(t)) \equiv \frac{E\left\{IC_0(Y \mid G_A^*, F_A(t)) IC_{nu}^*(Y \mid F_{X_A}^1, G_A^*)\right\}}{E\left\{(IC_{nu}^{*F}(Y \mid F_{X_A}^1, G_A^*))^2\right\}}.$$

Here the expectation is always taken w.r.t. the true distribution $P_{F_{X_A}, G_A^*}$ of Y. If we use this representation of the efficient influence curve in (5.6), then we obtain the equivalent of the one-step estimator (2.9) as defined in section 2, using the empirical c_n:

$$F^1_{A,n}(t) = F^0_{A,n}(t) + \frac{1}{n}\sum_{i=1}^{n} IC_0(Y_i \mid G^*_{A,n}, F^0_{A,n}(t))$$
$$-c_n IC^*_{nu}(Y_i \mid F_{X_A,n}, G^*_{A,n}).$$

The above representation of the data model and representation of the one-step estimator unifies section 2 and 3 and is therefore convenient for proving the asymptotic results of the one-step estimator.

Asymptotic linearity and efficiency. Suppose we observe n i.i.d. copies of Y defined in (5.1). In other words, we throw away the data on a subject with $S = B$, but we still know for that observation that $S = B$. An estimator $F_{A,n}(t)$ of $F_A(t)$ is asymptotically linear with influence curve $IC(Y \mid F_{X_A}, G^*_A)$ at (F_{X_A}, G^*_A) if

$$\sqrt{n}(F_{A,n}(t) - F_A(t)) = \frac{1}{\sqrt{n}}\sum_{i=1}^{n} IC(Y_i \mid F_A, G^*_A) + o_P(1).$$

A regular estimator is asymptotically efficient at (F_{X_A}, G^*_A) if and only if it is asymptotically linear with influence curve equal to the efficient influence curve $IC^*(Y \mid F_{X_A}, G^*_A)$ as defined in (3.2). The efficient influence curve is formally defined as the canonical gradient of the pathwise derivative of the parameter $F_A(t)$ (see Bickel, et al., 1993).

Definition of tangent spaces. To characterize the efficient influence curve and the limit distribution of our one-step estimator we will need the notion of a tangent space. Denote the Hilbert space of functions of Y with finite variance and mean zero, endowed with the covariance norm $\|v\|_{P_{F_{X_A},G^*_A}} = \sqrt{\int v^2 dP_{F_{X_A},G^*_A}}$, by $L^2_0(P_{F_{X_A},G^*_A})$. The tangent space $T^A_1(P_{F_{X_A},G^*_A})$ for the parameter F_{X_A} is, by definition, the closure of the linear extension in $L^2_0(P_{F_{X_A},G^*_A})$ of the scores corresponding to all parametric submodels through F_{X_A}. The tangent space $T^A_2(P_{F_{X_A},G^*_A})$ for the parameter G^*_A is the closure of the linear extension in $L^2_0(P_{F_{X_A},G^*_A})$ of the scores corresponding with all parametric submodels (of the given model $G^*_{A,\alpha}$) through G^*_A. For convenience, we will sometimes denote these tangent spaces by T_1 and T_2 suppressing the dependence on $P_{F_{X_A},G^*_A}$ and dropping the A index. The CAR assumption (1.1) implies that the likelihood of the data factorizes is in a G^*_A part and an F_{X_A} part and thus the spaces T_1 and T_2 are orthogonal.

The theorem. The following theorem provides the asymptotic distribution of the one-step estimator $F^1_{A,n}(t)$ and proves that when the models for $F_A(t \mid \bar{X}_A(u), \tilde{T}^*_A > u)$ and $F_A(t \mid W(0), S = A)$ happen to be correctly specified, then $F^1_{A,n}(t)$ is asymptotically efficient. Further, the theorem shows that $F^1_{A,n}(t)$ remains consistent and asymptotically normal if the specified model for $\bar{G}^*_A(u \mid X_A)$ is correct, even if the models for $F_A(t \mid \bar{X}_A(u), \tilde{T}^*_A > u)$ and $F_A(t \mid W(0), S = A)$ are misspecified. In the latter case, the asymptotic variance of $F^1_{A,n}(t)$ will depend on the model for the nuisance parameter $G^*_A(\cdot \mid X_A)$.

THEOREM 5.1. *Recall the notation* $Pf = \int f(x)dP(x)$. *Let* t *be given and consider the one-step estimator*

$$F^1_{A,n}(t) = F^0_{A,n}(t) + \frac{1}{n}\sum_{i=1}^{n} IC^*(Y_i \mid F_{X_A,n}, G^*_{A,n}, F^0_{A,n}(t))$$

using the representation (5.7) or (5.4).

We assume

(i) $\bar{G}^*_A(t \mid X_A) > \delta$, F_{X_A}*-a.e. for some* $\delta > 0$.

(ii) $IC^*(\cdot \mid F_{X_A,n}, G^*_{A,n}, F^0_{A,n}(t))$ *falls in a* $P_{F_{X_A},G^*_A}$*-Donsker class with probability tending to 1.*

(iii) For some $F^1_{X_A}$ *we have*

$$\|IC^*(\cdot \mid F_{X_A,n}, G^*_{A,n}, F^0_{A,n}(t)) - IC^*(\cdot \mid F^1_{X_A}, G^*_A, F_A(t))\|_{P_{F_{X_A},G^*_A}} \to 0$$

in probability.

(iv) Define for a G_1

$$\Phi(G_1) = P_{F_{X_A},G^*_A}\{IC^*(\cdot \mid F^1_{X_A}, G_1, F_A(t))\}.$$

Assume that

$$P_{F_{X_A},G^*_A}\{IC^*(\cdot \mid F_{X_A,n}, G^*_{A,n}, F^0_{A,n}(t)) - IC^*(\cdot \mid F_{X_A,n}, G^*_A, F^0_{A,n}(t))\}$$
$$= \Phi(G^*_{A,n}) - \Phi(G^*_A) + o_P(1/\sqrt{n})$$

(v) $\Phi(G^*_{A,n})$ *is an asymptotically efficient estimator of* $\Phi(G^*_A)$ *for a model containing the true* G^*_A *with tangent space* $T_2(P_{F_{X_A},G^*_A})$.

Then $F^1_{A,n}(t)$ *is asymptotically linear with influence curve given by*

$$IC \equiv \Pi(IC^*(\cdot \mid F^1_{X_A}, G^*_A, F_A(t)) \mid T_2^{\perp}(P_{F_{X_A},G^*_A})).$$

In particular, if $IC^*_{nu}(\cdot \mid F^1_{X_A}, G^*_A) = IC^*_{nu}(\cdot \mid F_{X_A}, G^*_A)$ *(i.e.* $F_A(t \mid \bar{W}_A(u), \tilde{T}_A > u, S = A)$ *and* $F_A(t \mid W(0), S = A)$ *are both estimated consistently), then* $F^1_{A,n}(t)$ *is asymptotically efficient.*

In appendix 3 we provide the projection on T_2 for the Cox-proportional hazards model in closed form and use this result to construct an asymptotic confidence interval.

Proof of Theorem 5.1

We have

$$F_{A,n}^1(t) = F_{A,n}^0(t) + (P_n - P_{F_{X_A},G_A^*})\{IC^*(\cdot \mid F_{X_A,n}, G_{A,n}^*, F_{A,n}^0(t))\}$$
$$+P_{F_{X_A},G_A^*}\{IC^*(\cdot \mid\mid F_{X_A,n}, G_{A,n}^*, F_{A,n}^0(t))\}.$$

For empirical process theory we refer to van der Vaart and Wellner (1996). Condition (ii) and (iii) in the theorem imply that the empirical process term on the right-hand side is asymptotically equivalent with $(P_n - P_{F_{X_A},G_A^*})$ $\{IC^*(\cdot \mid F_{X_A}^1, G_A^*, F_A(t))\}$ plus a $o_P(1/\sqrt{n})$. The last term we can write as:

$$P_{F_{X_A},G_A^*}\{IC^*(\cdot \mid F_{X_A,n}, G_{A,n}^*, F_{A,n}^0(t)) - IC^*(\cdot \mid F_{X_A,n}, G_A^*, F_{A,n}^0(t)\}$$
$$+P_{F_{X_A},G_A^*}\{IC_{nu}^*(\cdot \mid F_{X_A,n}, G_A^*, F_{A,n}^0(t))\}.$$

Because $P_{F_{X_A},G_A^*} IC_0(\cdot \mid G_A^*, F_{A,n}^0(t)) = F_A(t) - F_{A,n}^0(t)$ and $P_{F_{X_A},G_A^*} IC_{nu}^*$ $(\cdot \mid F_{X_A,n}, G_A^*) = 0$ the second term equals $F_A(t) - F_{A,n}^0(t)$. By assumption (iv) we have that the first term equals

$$\Phi(G_{A,n}^*) - \Phi(G_A^*) + o_P(1/\sqrt{n}).$$

We conclude that $F_n^1(t)$ is asymptotically linear with influence curve $IC^*(\cdot \mid F_{X_A}^1, G_A^*, F_A(t)) + IC_{nu}(\cdot \mid F_{X_A}, G_A^*)$, where $IC_{nu}(\cdot \mid F_{X_A}, G_A^*)$ is the influence curve of $\Phi(G_{A,n}^*)$. Now, the same argument as given in the proof of lemma 5.1 below proves that this is given by:

$$\Pi(IC^*(\cdot \mid F_{X_A}^1, G_A^*, F_A(t)) \mid T_2^{\perp}).$$

Finally, the efficiency statement for the case that $IC_{nu}^*(\cdot \mid F_{X_A}^1, G_A^*) = IC_{nu}^*(\cdot \mid F_{X_A}, G_A^*)$ follows from the fact that $IC_0(\cdot \mid G_A^*, F_A(t)) - IC_{nu}^*(\cdot \mid F_{X_A}, G_A^*)$ equals the efficient influence curve which has no component in $T_1^{\perp} \supset T_2$ (proposition 5.1). □

Discussion of theorem. The theorem above can be used as a template to prove the local efficiency result for a one-step estimator $F_{A,n}^1(t)$. Condition (ii) in the theorem is an empirical process condition. For empirical process theory we refer to van der Vaart and Wellner (1996). This condition is technical and depends on the chosen models for the unknown parameters. After having assumed that $\bar{G}_A^*(t \mid X_A) > \delta > 0$ this condition can typically be considered as a regularity condition. Condition (iii) basically says that $G_{A,n}^*$ needs to be consistent and $F_{A,n}(t \mid \bar{W}_A(u), \tilde{T}_A^* > u)$ needs to converge to some function $F_A^1(t \mid \bar{X}_A(u), \tilde{T}_A^* > u)$, which does not necessarily equals the true $F_A(t \mid \bar{X}_A(u), \tilde{T}_A^* > u)$. It can be shown that a sufficient condition for condition (iv), assuming condition (i) so that denominators are bounded away from zero, is that for some function $F_A^1(t \mid \bar{X}_A(u), \tilde{T}_A^* > u)$ (not necessarily equal to the true $F_A(t \mid \bar{X}_A(u), \tilde{T}_A^* > u)$) the product $\|G_{A,n}^*(u \mid \bar{X}_A) - G_A^*(u \mid \bar{X}_A)\|_{\infty} \|F_{A,n}(t \mid \bar{X}_A(u), \tilde{T}_A^* > u) - F_A^1(t \mid \bar{X}_A(u), \tilde{T}_A^* > u)\|_{\infty}$ is $o_P(1/\sqrt{n})$, where $\|\cdot\|_{\infty}$ is the supremum norm over u and the support of $\bar{X}_A(u)$. Since smooth functionals of nonparametric or parametric maximum likelihood estimators for a given model are efficient under regularity conditions, condition (v) will hold under regularity conditions if $G^*_{A,n}$ is a (non)parametric maximum likelihood estimator of G^*_A under a given model. Condition (v) is not a condition on the choice of model for G^*_A; it just states that whatever correct model one chooses for G^*_A, one should use an estimation procedure which is efficient for that model.

The fact that $F^1_{A,n}(t)$ remains a consistent and asymptotically normal estimator even when our model for $F_A(t \mid \bar{W}_A(u), \tilde{T}^*_A > u)$ is misspecified is due to the fact that (5.3) represents IC^*_{nu} as $IC^*_{nu} = \int H(u, \bar{W}_A(u))\, dM^*_A(u)$ for some given function H depending on $F_A(t \mid \bar{W}_A(u), \tilde{T}^*_A > u)$ and G^*_A, where M^*_A is a Martingale w.r.t. the increasing sigma-field $\mathcal{F}_u$ generated by X_A and $\{C^*_A > u\}$. Thus $\int H_n(u, \bar{X}_A(u))dM^*_A(u)$ has conditional mean zero, given X_A, for any $\mathcal{F}_u$-adapted function H_n. This explains why $F^1_{A,n}$ will still be consistent even if H, i.e. $F_A(t \mid \bar{W}_A(u), \tilde{T}^*_A > u)$, is estimated inconsistently.

It is interesting to consider what the distribution of $F^1_{A,n}(t)$ would be when $G^*_A(\cdot \mid x)$ is known and its known value is used in the one-step estimator. In that case, T_2 is empty. Thus, by theorem 5.1 the influence curve of $F^1_{A,n}(t)$ is given by $IC^*(\cdot \mid F^1_{X_A}, G^*_A, F_A(t))$, which has variance greater than or equal to that of the influence curve IC based on $G^*_A(\cdot \mid X)$ estimated by $G^*_{A,n}$. Lemma 5.1 below, which is used in the proof of the theorem, provides a general understanding of the fact that efficient estimation of a known orthogonal nuisance parameter often leads to improvements in efficiency.

LEMMA 5.1. *Let $Y \sim P_{F_{X_A}, G^*_A}$, G^*_A satisfying the coarsening at random condition (1.1). Denote the tangent space for the parameter F_{X_A} with $T_1(P_{F_{X_A}, G^*_A})$. Consider the parameter $F_A(t)$ which is a real valued functional of F_{X_A}. Let $F_{A,n}(t, G^*_A)$ be an asymptotically linear estimator of $F_A(t)$ with influence curve $IC_0(\cdot \mid F_{X_A}, G^*_A)$ which uses the true $G^*_A(\cdot \mid x)$. Assume now that for an estimator $G^*_{A,n}$*

$$F_{A,n}(t, G^*_{A,n}) - F_A(t) = F_{A,n}(t, G^*_A) - F_A(t) + \Phi(G^*_{A,n}) - \Phi(G^*_A) + o_P(1/\sqrt{n})$$

for some functional Φ of $G^*_{A,n}$. Assume that $\Phi(G^*_{A,n})$ is an asymptotically efficient estimator of $\Phi(G^*_A)$ for the model $\{G^*_{A,\eta} : \eta \in \Gamma\}$ with tangent space $T_2(P_{F_{X_A}, G^*_A})$. Then $F_{A,n}(t, G^*_{A,n})$ is asymptotically linear with influence curve

$$IC_1(\cdot \mid F_{X_A}, G^*_A) = \Pi(IC_0(\cdot \mid F_{X_A}, G^*_A) \mid T_2(P_{F_{X_A}, G^*_A})^{\perp}).$$

Proof. We decompose $L^2_0(P_{F_{X_A}, G^*_A})$ orthogonally in $T_1(P_{F_{X_A}, G^*_A}) + T_2(P_{F_{X_A}, G^*_A}) + T_{\perp}(P_{F_{X_A}, G^*_A})$, where $T_{\perp}(P_{F_{X_A}, G^*_A})$ is the orthogonal complement of $T_1 + T_2$. The assumptions in the lemma imply that $F_{A,n}(t, G^*_{A,n})$

is asymptotically linear with influence curve $IC = IC_0 + IC_{nu}$, where IC_{nu} is an influence curve corresponding with an estimator of the nuisance parameter $\Phi(G_A^*)$ estimated under the model with nuisance tangent space T_2. Let $IC_0 = a_0 + b_0 + c_0$ and $IC_{nu} = a_{nu} + b_{nu} + c_{nu}$ according to the orthogonal decomposition of $L_0^2(P_{F_{X_A}, G_A^*})$ above. From now on the proof uses the following two general facts about influence curves of regular asymptotically linear estimators; 1) an influence curve is orthogonal to the nuisance tangent space and 2) the efficient influence curve lies in the tangent space. Since IC_{nu} is an influence curve of $\Phi(G_A^*)$ in the model where nothing is assumed on F_{X_A} it is orthogonal to T_1; i.e. $a_{nu} = 0$. Since $\Phi(G_{A,n}^*)$ is efficient IC_{nu} lies in the tangent space T_2 and hence $c_{nu} = 0$ as well. We also have that $IC_0 + IC_{nu}$ is an influence curve for an estimator of μ and hence it is orthogonal to T_2: so $b_0 + b_{nu} = 0$. Consequently, we have that

$$IC_1 = IC_0 + IC_{nu} = a_0 + c_0 = \Pi(IC_0 \mid T_2^{\perp}).$$

This completes the proof. □

Appendix 2 - Computation of the efficient influence curve. In this section, we provide two methods for constructing the efficient influence curve for the right-censored data model with competing treatments. The first method (method 1) is an application of the weighted estimating equation approach presented in Robins (1993) and Robins and Rotnitsky (1992). The second method (method 2) applies the theory for finding the efficient influence curve presented in Bickel, et al. (1993). These methods result, of course, in the same efficient influence curve, which can then be used to construct a locally efficient one-step estimator.

Method 1. LEMMA 5.2. *(Robins and Rotnitzky) Suppose that the distribution F_X of the full data is unspecified and that we only assume that the conditional distribution G of C, given X, satisfies coarsening at random. Suppose that the parameter of interest is given by μ which is some real valued functional of F_X. Let $L_0^2(P)$ be the Hilbert space of functions of $Y \sim P$ with finite variance and mean zero endowed with the inner product $\langle f, g\rangle_P = E_P(f(Y)g(Y))$. Let $D(Y) \equiv IC^{*F}(Y \mid F_X, G, \mu)$ be the efficient influence curve of μ in the full-data model. Let $U_G(D)(Y) \in L_0^2(P)$ be a function of Y only depending on D and G which satifies $E(U_G(D)(Y) \mid X) = D(X)$. Consider the Hilbert space $T_{CAR}(G) = \{h \in L_0^2(P) : E_G(h(Y) \mid X) = 0\}$, which is the tangent space of G when only assuming CAR. Then the efficient influence curve of μ for the observed data Y is given by:*

$$IC^*(Y) \equiv U_G(D)(Y) - \Pi(U_G(D)(Y) \mid T_{CAR}(G)),$$

where $\Pi(\cdot \mid T_{CAR}(G))$ is the projection operator in $L_0^2(P)$ onto $T_{CAR}(G)$. We can find the efficient influence curve for μ for the data Y applying this lemma twice in a row. Firstly, let the full data be $X^1 = (X_A, X_B)$, let the censoring variable be $C^1 = (C_A, C_B)$ and the observed data is (Z_A, Z_B). Here we make no assumptions on the distribution of X^1, but assume CAR on the conditional distribution of C^1, given X^1, which corresponds with the assumptions (1.1). The parameter of interest is $\mu = F_A(t)$. One can reduce the data to Z_A without loss of information for estimation of μ. In other words, we are just interested in finding the efficient influence curve for μ when observing Z_A for every subject, where X_A is the full data. We apply the lemma to find the efficient influence curve for estimation of μ when observing Z_A. For the right-censored data structure, explicit forms of both the projection operator on $T_{CAR}(G)$ and $U_G(D)$ are established in Robins (1993) and Robins and Rotnitzky (1992). Therefore we actually obtain the efficient influence curve IC^{*F} from their results. The efficient influence curve and the corresponding locally efficient estimator for this problem are presented in section 2.

Secondly, we let $X^2 = (Z_A, Z_B)$ be the full data, S the censoring variable while the observed data is $Y = I(S = A)Z_A + I(S = B)Z_B$. Since we only assumed CAR on G_A, G_B for the data structure Z_A, Z_B, respectively, and we assumed no relation between X_A, X_B, we can use a result in Gill, et al., (1997) to conclude that the model of the full data X^2 is saturated . In addition, our assumption on $P(S = s \mid Z_A, Z_B)$ corresponds with assuming CAR on Y with X^2 being the full data. Thus we can apply the lemma to find the efficient influence curve IC^* as a function of IC^{*F}. This requires finding a $U_{P(S=A|(W(0))}(IC^{*F})(Y)$ and the projection on the tangent space of $P(S = s \mid W(0))$. The efficient influence curve IC^* and its relation to IC^{*F} are presented in section 3.

Method 2. To apply the method in Bickel, et al. (1993), define, as we did in appendix 1, the full data to be X_A and C^*_A as the censoring variable. Let

$$IC_0(Y \mid G^*_A, F_A(t)) = \frac{I(T_A \leq t)\Delta^*_A}{\bar{G}^*_A(T_A \mid X_A)} - F_A(t)$$

be the influence curve of $F^0_{A,n}(t)$ in the model with $G^*_{A,n} = G^*_A$ known. Bickel, et al. (1993) show that the projection of any initial influence curve on the scores for a model gives the efficient influence function for that model. In the model with G^*_A known, T_1 represents all the scores of the model. Therefore by projecting the initial influence curve IC_0 on T_1 we obtain the efficient influence curve IC^* for estimating $F_A(t)$ in the model with G^*_A known (since IC_0 is an influence curve of an estimator in the model with G^*_A). However, IC^* is also the efficient influence curve for estimating $F_A(t)$ in any CAR model for G^*_A. This reflects the fact that $F_A(t)$ is a functional of F_{X_A} and T_1 and T_2 are mutually orthogonal, so that the efficient influence function IC^* in the model with G^*_A known has no projection on the tangent spaces T_2 for G^*_A in a model where G_A is unknown. Hence, we can represent the efficient influence curve as in (5.4), where $IC^*_{nu} = \Pi(IC_0 \mid T_1^{\perp})$ and $T_1^{\perp}$ is the orthogonal complement of T_1. Note that Gill, et al. (1997) show that if CAR is the only assumption, $T_1^{\perp} = T_{CAR}(G)$. Here $\Pi(\cdot \mid T_{CAR}(G))$: $L^2(P_{F_{X_A},G^*_A}) \rightarrow L^2(P_{F_{X_A},G^*_A})$ is the projection operator on $T_{CAR}(G)$. The explicit form of IC^*_{nu} has been given in (5.3) and this is proved in proposition 5.1 below.

PROPOSITION 5.1. *If* $IC_0(\cdot \mid G^*_A, F_A(t)) \in L^2_0(P_{F_{X_A},G_A})$, *where* IC_0 *is defined in (5.3), then*

$$IC^*_{nu}(\cdot \mid F_{X_A}, G^*_A) \equiv \Pi(IC_0 \mid T_{CAR}(G)) = -\int E\left(\frac{I(\tilde{T}^*_A \le t)\Delta^*_A}{\bar{G}_A(\tilde{T}^*_A \mid X_A)} \mid \bar{W}_A(u), \tilde{T}^*_A > u\right) dM^*_A(u),$$

where

$$dM^*_A(u) \equiv I(C^*_A \in du, \Delta^*_A = 0) - \Lambda_{C^*_A}(du \mid X_A) I(\tilde{T}^*_A > u).$$

Proof. In Robins and Rotnitzky (1992, appendix) it is shown that

$$T_{CAR}(G) = \{\int H(u, \bar{W}_A(u)) dM^*_A(u) : H\}.$$

Moreover, it is shown that for any function $D(X_A)$

$$\Pi(D(X_A)\Delta^*_A \mid T_1^{\perp}) = -\int E(D(X_A)\Delta^*_A \mid \bar{W}_A(u), \tilde{T}^*_A > u) dM^*_A(u). \tag{5.8}$$

Now, note that $IC_0(Y \mid G^*_A, F_A(t))$ can be represented as

$$IC_0(Y \mid G^*_A, F_A(t)) = D(X_A)\Delta^*_A - F_A(t)$$

where $D(X_A) = I(T_A \le t)/\bar{G}_A(T_A \mid X_A)$. Apply (5.8) to this $D(X_A)\Delta_A$ and note that the projection of a function of X_A (like $F_A(t)$) on all functions of Y with conditional mean zero, given X_A, equals zero. This proves proposition 5.1. □

Appendix 3 - Projections.

Finding the influence curve under misspecification. Theorem 5.1 states that to estimate IC (since we cannot assume that the guessed models for both $F_A(t \mid \bar{W}_A(u), \tilde{T}_A > u, S = A)$ and $F(t \mid W(0), S = A)$ are correctly specified) one must define and estimate the projection on $T_2^{\perp}$. First, note that

$$\Pi(IC^*(\cdot \mid F^1_{X_A}, G^*_A, F_A(t)) \mid T_2^{\perp}(P_{F_{X_A},G^*_A})) = IC^*(\cdot \mid F^1_{X_A}, G^*_A, F_A(t)) - \Pi(IC^*(\cdot \mid F^1_{X_A}, G^*_A, F_A(t)) \mid T_2(P_{F_{X_A},G^*_A})).$$

To find this projection, we will utilize the fact that T_2 can be divided into two orthogonal components, T_2^a and T_2^b, which correspond to the model of C_A given X_A and that of the model of treatment assignment ($P(S = A \mid X_A) = P(S = A \mid W(0))$), respectively. Note that given (1.1), $G_A^*(c \mid X_A) = G_A(c|X_A)P(S = A \mid W(0))$, we estimate G_A^* by estimating parametric or semi-parametric submodels $G_{A,\alpha}$ and $P_\beta(S = A \mid W(0))$. Because we assume no common parameters for these models, the likelihood of C_A^* factorizes into G_A part and a $P(S = A \mid W(0))$ part (see appendix 1), and thus T_2 can be represented as a sum of two orthogonal tangent spaces:

$$T_2 = T_2^a \oplus T_2^b$$

Thus, one can represent the projection of IC^* (3.2)onto T_2 as $\Pi(IC^* \mid T_2) = \Pi(IC^* \mid T_2^a + T_2^b) = \Pi(IC^* \mid T_2^a) + \Pi(IC^* \mid T_2^b)$, and the influence curve of the one-step estimator is:

$$IC = \Pi(IC^* \mid T_2^\perp) = IC^* - \Pi(IC^* \mid T_2^a) - \Pi(IC^* \mid T_2^b).$$

Next we will present the influence curves of our one-step estimator (3.5) for the case that $G_A(\cdot \mid X_A)$ is modeled with Cox regression and that the propensity score, $P(S = A \mid W(0))$ is modeled with logistic regression. If it is known that C_A is independent of X_A, then one could either estimate G_A marginally (using Kaplan-Meier) or one could model $G_A(\cdot \mid X_A)$ using a regression model that contains the marginal Kaplan-Meier estimator as a sub-model; Cox regression is such a procedure. Note that modeling C_A in this fashion should increase the efficiency of the one-step estimator if F_{X_A} is misspecified, even if C_A is independent of X_A (lemma 5.1). We will prove the following lemma.

LEMMA 5.3. *Let $T_2^a(P_{F_{X_A},G_A^*})$ be the tangent space of the Cox-proportional hazards model for the distribution G_A given X_A:*

$$\lambda_{C_A}(t \mid X_A) = \lambda_0(t)\exp(\alpha^\top L(t)),$$

where $L(t) = f(\bar{W}_A(t))$ is a k-vector of covariates extracted from $\bar{W}_A(t)$, α is the vector of unknown coefficients and λ_0 is the unspecified baseline hazard. Let $T_2^b(P_{F_{X_A},G_A^*})$ be the tangent space of the following logistic regression model for $P(S = A \mid W(0))$:

$$log\left[\frac{P(S = A \mid W(0))}{1 - P(S = A \mid W(0)}\right] = \beta_0 + \beta_1 V_1 + \cdots + \beta_p V_p,$$

where $\vec{V} = h(W(0))$ is a p-dimensional vector of covariates extracted from $W(0)$ and β is the vector of unknown regression coefficients. In this lemma we use the following shorthand notation: $IC^* = IC^*(\cdot \mid F_{X_A}^1, G_A^*, F_A(t))$ (5.7) and $IC^{*F} = IC^{*F}(\cdot \mid F_{X_A}^1, G_A, F_A(t))$ (2.5). Then $\Pi(IC^* \mid T_2^a + T_2^b) = I(S = A)\left[\int I(t > u)\, E\left\{F_A(t \mid \bar{W}_A(u), \tilde{T}_A > u, S = A) - \right.\right.$ $\left. F_A^1(t \mid \bar{W}_A(u), \tilde{T}_A > u, S = A) \mid \tilde{T}_A = u, \Delta_A = 0, S = A\right\} \frac{dM_A(u)}{\bar{G}_A(u|X_A)} +$

$E(IC^{*F}\phi^{\top}(Z_A))\left\{E(\phi(Z_A)\phi(Z_A)^{\top})\right\}\phi(Z_A)] + E(IC^*(Y)U_\beta(Y)^{\top})I_\beta^{-1}U_\beta$ $(S, W(0))$, *where* $U_\beta(S, W(0))$ *is the p-dimensional vector of scores of the logistic regression coefficients,* I_β *is the corresponding Fisher's Information matrix and* $\phi(Z_A) = I(S = A)\int\left[\vec{L}(u) - E(\vec{L}(u) \mid \tilde{T}_A = u, \Delta_A = 0, S = A)\right]$ $dM_A(u)$.

Proof of lemma 5.3.

Note that given (1.1)

$$\begin{array}{ll} G_A^*(c \mid X_A) = G_A(c|X_A)P(S = A \mid W(0)) & c \geq 0 \\ G_A^*(c \mid X_A) = 1 - P(S = A \mid W(0)) & c = 0. \end{array}$$

This leads to the following likelihood of the nuisance parameters:

$$\begin{aligned} \mathcal{L}_{nu} &= P(S = A \mid W(0))^{I(S=A)}(1 - P(S = B \mid W(0)))^{(1-I(S=A))} * \\ &\quad G_A(\tilde{T}_A \mid X_A)^{I(S=A)\Delta_A} g_A(\tilde{T}_A \mid X_A)^{I(S=A)(1-\Delta_A)} \end{aligned} \tag{5.9}$$

Because we assume no common parameters for G_A and $P(S = A \mid W(0))$, the likelihood factorizes into a G_A part that depends only on those observations with $S = A$ and a $P(S = A \mid W(0))$ part that depends on all the data. Now T_2 can be represented as:

$$T_2 = T_2^a \oplus T_2^b$$

Thus, one can represent the projection of IC^* (3.2)onto T_2 as $\Pi(IC^* \mid T_2) = \Pi(IC^* \mid T_2^a + T_2^b) = \Pi(IC^* \mid T_2^a) + \Pi(IC^* \mid T_2^b)$, and the influence curve of the one-step estimator is:

$$IC = \Pi(IC^* \mid T_2^{\perp}) = IC^* - \Pi(IC^* \mid T_2^a) - \Pi(IC^* \mid T_2^b).$$

Therefore, one needs the explicit form of these projections, under the estimating model, to estimate the influence curve and its asymptotic variance.

The proof of lemma 5.3 is essentially given in Robins (1996), but will presented here for the sake of completeness. The tangent space for Cox regression is (Ritov and Wellner, 1988)

$$T_2^a(P_{F_{X_A}, G_A^*}) = I(S = A)\left(\int \vec{L}_A(u)dM_A(u) + \left\{\int g(u)dM_A(u) : g\right\}\right).$$

If we define H_0 as $\left\{\int g(u)dM_A(u) : g\right\}$, then (Robins, 1996)

$$\begin{aligned} \Pi\left(\int H(u, X_A)dM_A(u) \mid H_0\right) \\ = \int E(H(u, X_A) \mid \tilde{T}_A = u, \Delta_A = 0)dM_A(u). \end{aligned} \tag{5.10}$$

Now, by defining $U(Z_A) \equiv \int \vec{L}_A(u)dM_A(u)$ we can split T_2^a into two orthogonal components as:

$$T_2^a = [U(Z_A) - \Pi(U(Z_A) \mid H_0)] + H_0,$$

where $U(Z_A) = I(S = A) \int \vec{L}_A(u) dM_A(u)$. By (5.10) we can formulate the tangent space for Cox regression as:

$$T_2^a(P_{F_{X_A}, G_A^*}) = I(S = A)$$
$$\left\{ \int \vec{L}_A(u) dM_A(u) - \int E\left[\vec{L}_A(u) \mid \tilde{T}_A = u, \Delta_A = 0\right] dM_A(u) \right\}$$
$$+ \left\{ I(S = A) \int g(u) dM_A(u) : g \right\}. \tag{5.11}$$

The projection can be done separately on the to orthogonal components of T_2^a. However, first we can simplify matters by projecting on a larger space first $T_2^l \supset T_2^a$ where T_2^l consists of all functions of Z_A. It is straightforward to show that $\Pi(V(Y) \mid T_2^l) = E(V(Y) \mid Z_A)$. Now $\Pi(IC^* \mid T_2^l) = E(IC^* \mid Z_A) = IC^{*F}(Z_A)$, because the only random variable remaining is $I(S = A)$ and $E[I(S = A) \mid Z_A] = P(S = A \mid W(0))$. So, now we must project IC^{*F} onto T_2^a as defined in (5.11). Recall that $IC^{*F}(Z_A \mid G_A, F_{X_A,1}) = IC_0^F(Z_A \mid G_A, F_A(t)) - IC_{nu}^{*F}(Z_A \mid G_A, F_{X_A,1})$ where

$$IC_0^F(Z_A \mid G_A) = \frac{I(T_A \leq t)\Delta_A}{\bar{G}_A(T_A \mid X_A)}$$
$$IC_{nu}^{*F}(Z_A \mid G_A, F_{X_A,1}) = -\int \frac{F_A^1(t \mid \bar{W}_A(u), \tilde{T}_A > u)}{\bar{G}_A(u \mid X_A)} dM_A(u).$$

Recall that F_A^1 represents the limit of the estimator used in our one-step estimator. Since $H_0 \subset T_1^\perp$ we can represent the projection of IC^{*F} on H_0 as:

$$\Pi(IC^{*F} \mid H_0) = \Pi(\Pi(IC^{*F} \mid T_1^\perp) \mid H_0).$$

Proposition 5.1 implies that $\Pi(IC_0(\cdot \mid G_A) \mid T_1^\perp) = IC_{nu}^{*F}(\cdot \mid G_A, F_{X_A})$ and that $IC_{nu}^{*F}(\cdot \mid G_A, F_{X_A}^1) \in T_1^\perp$. Thus

$$\Pi(IC^{*F} \mid T_1^\perp) = \int \left\{ F_A(t \mid \bar{W}_A(u), \tilde{T}_A > u) - F_A^1(t \mid \bar{W}_A(u), \tilde{T}_A > u) \right\} \frac{dM_A(u)}{\bar{G}_A(u)}.$$

Now, we can apply the projection formula (5.10) on H_0 with

$$H(u, X) = \frac{1}{\bar{G}_A(u)} \left\{ F_A(t \mid \bar{X}_A(u), \tilde{T} > u) - F_A^1(t \mid \bar{X}_A(u), \tilde{T}_A > u) \right\}.$$

The projection on the other component of the Cox scores is just a finite-dimensional projection of IC^{*F} on the functions $\phi(Z_A) \equiv I(S = A) \int \vec{L}_A(u) dM_A(u) - I(S = A) \int E\left[\vec{L}_A(u) \mid \tilde{T}_A = u, \Delta_A = 0\right] dM_A(u)$, as done in lemma 5.3.

That completes the proof of the projection on T_2^a. The projection of IC^* onto T_2^b is a straightforward finite-dimensional projection as given in lemma 5.3.

Construction of confidence interval. This section provides a method for estimating the above projection and thus for a confidence interval for our estimator, assuming that one uses Cox regression to estimate $G_A(\cdot \mid X_A)$ and logistic regression to estimate $P(S = A \mid W(0))$. In this case, the projections in lemma 5.3 apply. In addition to the scores (U_β) and Fisher information matrix (I_β), in order to estimate this projection, one needs estimates of:

$$E\left[F_A(t \mid \bar{W}_A(u), \tilde{T}_A > u, S = A) \mid C_A = u, \Delta_A = 0, S = A\right]$$
$$E\left[F_A^1(t \mid \bar{W}_A(u), \tilde{T}_A > u, S = A) \mid C_A = u, \Delta_A = 0, S = A\right]$$
$$E\left[\bar{L}_A(u) \mid C_A = u, \Delta_A = 0\right]$$
$$E(\phi(Z_A)IC^{*F})$$
$$E(\phi^2(Z_A))$$
$$E(IC^*(Y), U_\beta(S, W(0))).$$

When $C_A \perp T_A$, then (we can always delete $S = A$ by our CAR-assumption) $E\left[F_A(t \mid \bar{W}_A(u), \tilde{T}_A > u) \mid C_A = u, \Delta_A = 0\right] = F_A(t \mid T_A > u)$ reduces to just a function of the marginal distribution of T_A, and thus it can be estimated using the IPCW estimator (3.4).

One can estimate both

$$E\left[F_A^1(t \mid \bar{W}_A(u), \tilde{T}_A > u, S = A) \mid C_A = u, \Delta_A = 0, S = A\right]$$

and $E\left[\bar{L}_A(u) \mid C_A = u, \Delta_A = 0, S = A\right]$ as a non-parametric (smooth) regression of $F_{A,n}(t \mid \bar{W}_A(u), \tilde{T}_A > u, S = A)$ and $\bar{L}_A(u)$, respectively, against the censoring times, C_A's, limited to observations where $S = A$. The last three quantities can be estimated with method of moments as follows:

$$\widehat{E}_j(\phi(Z_A)IC^{*F}(Z_A)) = \frac{1}{n}\sum_{i=1}^{n} I(S_i = A)\widehat{\phi}_j(Z_{A,i})IC^{*F}(Z_{A,i} \mid G_{A,n}, F_{X_A,n})$$

$$\widehat{E}_j(\phi(Z_A))^2 = \frac{1}{n}\sum_{i=1}^{n} I(S_i = A)\widehat{\phi}_j^2(Z_{A,i})$$

$$\widehat{E}_j(U_\beta(S, W(0))IC^*(Y))$$
$$= \frac{1}{n}\sum_{i=1}^{n} IC^*(Y_i \mid G_{A,n}^*, F_{X_A,n}, F_{A,n})U_{\beta_{j,n}}(S_i, W_i(0)).$$

Now let $\widehat{IC} = \widehat{IC}^* - \widehat{\Pi}(\widehat{IC}^* \mid T_2)$ be the estimator of the influence curve of $F_{A,n}^1(t)$ obtained by substitution of the above estimators into the projection formula in lemma 5.3. Its asymptotic variance, and a 95% confidence interval for $F_A(t)$ can be estimated, respectively, as:

$$\widehat{\sigma}^2 = \frac{1}{n}\sum_{i=1}^{n}\widehat{IC}^2$$

$$F^1_{A,n}(t) \pm 1.96\frac{\widehat{\sigma}}{\sqrt{n}}.$$

For the case that C_A and T_A are dependent through a covariate process we refer to Robins (1996) for a method of estimation of the projection formulas.

REFERENCES

[1] ANDERSEN, P.K., BORGAN, O., GILL, R.D. AND KEIDING, N, (1993), *Statistical models based on counting processes*, Springer, New York.

[2] BICKEL, P.J., KLAASSEN, A.J., RITOV, Y. AND WELLNER, J.A., (1993), *Efficient and adaptive inference in semi-parametric models*, Johns Hopkins University Press, Baltimore.

[3] FRIEDMAN, J, (1984), *A variable span smoother*, Department of Statistics, Technical report LCS, Stanford University, Stanford, CA.

[4] GILL, R.D., VAN DER LAAN, M.J. AND ROBINS, J.M, (1997), *Coarsening at Random: Characterizations, Conjectures and Counter-Examples*, Proceedings of the First Seattle Symposium in Biostatistics, (1995), D.Y. Lin and T.R. Fleming (editors), Springer Lecture Notes in Statistics, 255–294.

[5] HASTIE, T.J. AND TIBSHIRANI, R.J, (1990), *Generalized Additive Models*, Chapman and Hall, London.

[6] HEITJAN, D.F. AND RUBIN, D.B, (1991), *Ignorability and coarse data*, Annals of Statistics, **19**, 2244–2253.

[7] JACOBSEN, M. AND KEIDING, N, (1995), *Coarsening at random in general sample spaces and random censoring in continuous time*, Ann. Statist, **23**, 774–786.

[8] ROBINS, J.M, (1993), *Information recovery and bias adjustment in proportional hazards regression analysis of randomized trials using surrogate markers*, Proceedings of the Biopharmaceutical section, American Statistical Association, 24–33.

[9] ROBINS, J.M, (1996), *Locally efficient median regression with random censoring and surrogate markers*, Lifetime Data: Models in Reliability and Survival Analysis, Ed. N.P. Jewell et al., Kluwer Academic Publishers, 263–274.

[10] ROBINS, J.M., MARK, S.D. AND NEWEY, W.K, (1992), *Estimating exposure effects by modeling the expectation of exposure conditional on confounders*, Biometrics, **48**, 479–495.

[11] ROBINS, J.M. AND RITOV, Y, (1997), *Toward a curse of dimensionality appropriate (CODA) asymptotic theory for semiparametric models*, Statistics in Medicine, **16**, 285–319.

[12] *Robins, J.M. and Rotnitzky, A*, (1992), *Recovery of information and adjustment for dependent censoring using surrogate markers*, Aids Epidemiology, Methodological issues, Birkhäuser, 297–331, Rosenbaum, P.R., (1984), Conditional permutation tests and the propensity score in observational studies, JASA, **79**, 565–574.

[13] ROSENBAUM, P.R, (1987), *Model-based direct adjustment*, JASA, **82**, 387–394.

[14] ROSENBAUM, P.R, (1988), *Permutation tests for matched pairs with adjustments for covariates*, Applied Statistics, **37**, 401–411.

[15] ROSENBAUM, P.R. AND RUBIN, D.B, (1983), *The central role of the propensity score in observational studies for causal effects*, Biometrika, **70**, 41–55.

[16] ROSENBAUM, P.R. AND RUBIN, D.B, (1984), *Reducing bias in observational studies using subclassification on the propensity score*, JASA, **79**, 516–524.

[17] ROSENBAUM, P.R. AND RUBIN, D.B, (1985), *Constructing a control group using multivariate matched sampling methods that incorporate the propensity score*, JASA, **39**, 33–38.

[18] VAN DER LAAN, M.J. AND HUBBARD, A.E, (1998), *Locally Efficient Estimation of the Survival Distribution with Right Censored Data and Covariates when Collection of Data is Delayed*, to appear in, Biometrika.

[19] VAN DER LAAN, M.J. AND ROBINS, J.M, (1998), *Locally efficient estimation with current status data and high-dimensional covariates*, to appear in Journal of the American Statistical Association.

[20] VAN DER VAART, A.W. AND WELLNER, J.A, (1996), *Weak convergence and empirical processes*, Springer Verlag.

ESTIMATION OF DISEASE RATES IN SMALL AREAS: A NEW MIXED MODEL FOR SPATIAL DEPENDENCE*

BRIAN G. LEROUX †, XINGYE LEI† , AND NORMAN BRESLOW†

Abstract. In this paper, a new model is proposed for spatial dependence that includes separate parameters for overdispersion and the strength of spatial dependence. The new dependence structure is incorporated into a generalized linear mixed model useful for the estimation of disease incidence rates in small geographic regions. The mixed model allows for log-linear covariate adjustment and local smoothing of rates through estimation of the spatially correlated random effects. Computer simulation studies compare the new model with the following sub-models: intrinsic autoregression, an independence model, and a model with no random effects. The major finding was that regression coefficient estimates based on fitting intrinsic autoregression to independent data can have very low precision compared with estimates based on the full model. Additional simulation studies demonstrate that penalized quasi-likelihood (PQL) estimation generally performs very well although the estimates are slightly biased for very small counts.

Key words. Random effect, log-linear model, penalized quasi-likelihood, Gaussian intrinsic auto-regression, generalized linear mixed model, Monte Carlo simulation.

AMS(MOS) subject classifications. Primary 62M40, 62F11, 62J12, 62M30, 92D30.

1. Introduction. Epidemiologists often use maps to illustrate geographic variation in disease incidence or mortality rates in small regions such as U.S. counties. Producing such maps is complicated by the fact that raw incidence rates are typically unstable because of small incidence counts, and also by the presence of spatial correlation in the rates. Note that spatial dependence may exist in rates of non-infectious diseases such as cancer, possibly because of the presence of environmental risk factors which are themselves spatially correlated.

Statistical models for use in producing stable estimates of rates must be able to accommodate all of the features of the data, including non-normal distributions of count data, the effects of explanatory variables, and spatial correlation. One approach involves the use of generalized linear mixed models (GLMMs) in which a generalized linear model (GLM) is augmented by unobserved normally distributed random effects that explain spatial correlation as well as overdispersion (Clayton and Kaldor, 1987). Conditional on a random effects vector b, the observed incidence counts y_i follow a log-linear GLM with conditional means μ_i given by

$$\log \mu_i = \log E_i + x_i'\alpha + b_i, \tag{1.1}$$

*This research was supported in part by United States Public Health Service Grants CA40644 and CA09168.

†Department of Biostatistics, University of Washington, Seattle WA 98195, USA, E-mail: leroux@biostat.washington.edu

where x_i is a vector of explanatory variables for the ith region, α is the vector of regression coefficients, and E_i is the expected count, which may be based on the age distribution in the region and a set of standard rates. Possible models for the random effects have been discussed by Besag, York, and Mollié (1991).

In this article, we propose a new spatial dependence model that includes separate parameters for overdispersion and the strength of the spatial dependence. We study the performance of this model as a basis for estimation of parameters and prediction of SMRs in individual regions through computer simulation and compare it to intrinsic autoregression, as well as to an independence model and a model with no random effects. An additional purpose of the article is to examine the performance of the penalized quasi-likelihood (PQL) method of parameter estimation (Breslow and Clayton, 1993).

2. A new model for spatial dependence. Under Gaussian intrinsic autoregression (Besag et al., 1991), b has a (singular) multivariate normal distribution with mean 0 and a covariance matrix D with Moore-Penrose generalized inverse $D^- = R/\sigma^2$, where R is determined by the neighbourhood structure of the regions. The typical element of R is

$$R_{ij} = \begin{cases} n_i, & i = j \\ -I\{i \sim j\}, & i \neq j \end{cases},$$

where n_i is the number of neighbours of region i, $i \sim j$ indicates that regions i and j are neighbours, and I is the indicator function. Typically, neighbours are those regions which share a border, although other ways of defining neighbours may be used instead. Under intrinsic autoregression, the conditional mean of the random effect for any region given all the other random effects is equal to the mean of the random effects for the neighbouring regions, and the conditional variance is inversely proportional to the number of such neighbours (Besag, 1974).

A limitation of intrinsic autoregression is that the parameter σ^2 serves both to represent overdispersion and spatial dependence. A few ways of separating overdispersion and spatial dependence have been suggested. In one approach, a proportionality constant is introduced into the conditional mean, but the form of the conditional variance is unchanged (Cressie, 1991). Besag et al. (1991) note that this model can have unappealing properties when the proportionality constant is close to 0; note that in this model the conditional variance is inversely proportional to the number of neighbours even in the independence case. In Clayton and Kaldor's (1987) model, this problem is avoided by using a constant conditional variance, but the conditional mean then becomes proportional to the sum (rather than the mean) of the neighbours. An alternative approach uses two additive random effect components, one an intrinsic autoregression and the other an independence (white noise) process (Besag et al., 1991).

We propose a different model based on specification of the generalized inverse of the covariance matrix D as follows:

$$\sigma^2 D^- = (1-\lambda)I + \lambda R, \tag{2.1}$$

where I is the identity matrix, R is the intrinsic autoregresion matrix given above, and λ is a spatial dependence parameter lying in the interval $[0,1]$. This specification yields the independence case ($D = \sigma^2 I$) if $\lambda = 0$, and intrinsic autoregression ($D = \sigma^2 R^-$) if $\lambda = 1$. A test of the null hypothesis $H_0 : \lambda = 0$ is available in Singh and Shukla's (1983) test for autoregression, but this test does not extend to other values of λ because the model used by these authors coincides with (2.1) only for $\lambda = 0$.

The local conditional moments corresponding to (2.1) take the form

$$E(b_i|b_{-i}) = \frac{\lambda}{1-\lambda+\lambda n_i}\sum_{j\sim i} b_j$$

and

$$\mathrm{var}(b_i|b_{-i}) = \frac{\sigma^2}{1-\lambda+\lambda n_i},$$

where b_{-i} denotes the random effect vector with the ith component deleted. The conditional mean can be written as a weighted average of the local mean $\sum_{j\sim i} b_j/n_i$ based on the intrinsic autoregression (with weight λn_i), and the mean value 0 based on the independence model (with weight $1-\lambda$):

$$E(b_i|b_{-i}) = \frac{1-\lambda}{1-\lambda+\lambda n_i} \times 0 + \frac{\lambda n_i}{1-\lambda+\lambda n_i} \times \frac{1}{n_i}\sum_{j\sim i} b_j.$$

Note that the weight assigned to the local mean depends on the number of neighbors (as well as the dependence parameter λ), which is intuitively reasonable because the number of neighbors affects the precision of the local mean. The conditional variance can similarly be written as a weighted average of the local variance from the intrinsic autoregression and the variance from the independence model:

$$\mathrm{var}(b_i|b_{-i}) = \frac{1-\lambda}{1-\lambda+\lambda n_i} \times \sigma^2 + \frac{\lambda n_i}{1-\lambda+\lambda n_i} \times \frac{\sigma^2}{n_i}.$$

3. Penalized quasi-likelihood estimation. Here we will briefly describe the implementation of the PQL estimation procedure (Breslow and Clayton, 1993) for the proposed model. The main advantage of this method over others such as maximum-likelihood and Bayesian techniques is that PQL estimates can be computed more quickly and easily with fewer convergence problems. The method produces biased estimates, but it can be expected to perform very well for nearly normal responses such as large counts or binomial proportions with large denominators. The performance of PQL estimates is unknown in many situations, including that of small counts with spatial correlation.

Consider a general model corresponding to (1.1), in which the conditional mean vector μ is modeled via a given link function g as $\eta = g(\mu) = \text{Offset} + X\alpha + b$, for a known offset vector, a fixed effect $X\alpha$, and random effect vector b. The conditional variance is specified as $\sigma^2 V(\mu)$, for a known variance function V. In the application described in the previous section, the offset is given by the term $\log E_i$ in (1.1), and the Poisson link function ($g(\mu) = \log \mu$) and variance function ($V(\mu) = \mu$) are used.

The PQL fitting algorithm combines features of the standard algorithms for fitting GLMs and linear mixed models. At each step, the usual GLM adjusted dependent variate (McCullagh and Nelder, 1989) is calculated as

$$Y = \hat{\eta} + (y - \hat{\mu})\frac{d\hat{\eta}}{d\hat{\mu}}, \tag{3.1}$$

where $\hat{\mu}$ and $\hat{\eta}$ denote the current vector of fitted values and estimate of the linear predictor, respectively. The covariance matrix of Y is approximated by

$$\hat{V} = \hat{W}^{-1} + \hat{D}, \tag{3.2}$$

where $\hat{D}$ is the random effects covariance matrix evaluated at the current estimates for the variance parameters, and $\hat{W}$ is the diagonal matrix of GLM weights given by $\hat{w}^{-1} = V(\hat{\mu})(\frac{d\hat{\eta}}{d\hat{\mu}})^2$. Updated estimates of the fixed effect vector α and random effect vector b are obtained through solution of the so-called mixed model equations as follows:

$$\hat{\alpha} = (X'\hat{V}^{-1}X)^{-1}X'\hat{V}^{-1}(Y - \text{Offset}), \tag{3.3}$$

and

$$\hat{b} = \hat{D}\hat{V}^{-1}(Y - \text{Offset} - X\hat{\alpha}). \tag{3.4}$$

Then updated estimates of the variance parameters σ and λ are obtained by a Newton-Raphson or Fisher scoring step as follows:

$$\begin{pmatrix} \hat{\sigma} \\ \hat{\lambda} \end{pmatrix}^{\text{new}} = \begin{pmatrix} \hat{\sigma} \\ \hat{\lambda} \end{pmatrix}^{\text{old}} + I^{-1}s, \tag{3.5}$$

where s is the score vector and I is either the observed (Newton-Raphson) or expected (Fisher scoring) information based on the REML likelihood for Y (see Appendix). The variance parameters are restricted to their natural ranges ($\sigma \geq 0, 0 \leq \lambda \leq 1$); estimates outside of these ranges are set at the appropriate boundary values.

Convenient starting values for the fitting algorithm are $\sigma = 0.5$, $\lambda = 0.5$, and 0 for the regression coefficients. Iteration is terminated when changes in parameter estimates are less than a specified tolerance level (0.001 in the simulation studies reported below). Achieving convergence can be difficult, particularly with regard to the variance parameters. A single iteration of equations (3.1)–(3.5) is usually most efficient, but in a small number of cases iteration to convergence of equations (3.1)–(3.4) at each step improves convergence of the algorithm. The Marquardt technique of inflating the diagonal terms of the information matrix is generally useful to control the step size in the early iterations. Expected information tends to be more stable than observed information; however, a switch to observed information sometimes avoids alternating between distinct solutions. Note that the PQL method does not provide an objective function that could be used to evaluate multiple solutions. Approximate standard errors for $\hat{\sigma}$ and $\hat{\lambda}$ are obtained from the information matrix in the usual way, and, for $\hat{\lambda}$, from the matrix $X'\hat{V}^{-1}X$, which represents the information matrix for λ with the variance parameters fixed.

4. Application to the Scottish lip cancer data. Here we apply the model to a set of data on lip cancer in Scotland (Clayton and Kaldor, 1987). The response variable is the number of incident male cases of lip cancer in each of the 56 Scottish counties over a six-year period. The expected counts (E_i) were estimated by Clayton and Kaldor using the county age distributions, but are assumed to be known constants for illustrative purposes; they range from 1.1 to 88.7, with median equal to 6.3. The observed counts range from 0 to 39 with median 8.

Clayton and Kaldor examined the effect of the percentage of the work force employed in agriculture, fishing, or forestry divided by 10 (AFF). Based on an observation by Kemp et al. (1985) and results of Yasui and Lele (1997) that suggested northern counties had higher rates, we decided to explore the effect of latitude. By overlaying a map of the counties onto a population density map (Kemp et al., 1985), approximate centers of mass of the county populations were located and approximate latitudes of these were recorded to the nearest 0.2° using a rectangular grid. These values ranged from $54.8°N$ to $60.2°N$. We fit the following log-linear GLMM to these data:

$$\log \mu_i = \log E_i + \alpha_0 + \alpha_1 \mathrm{AFF}_i + \alpha_2 \mathrm{LAT}_i + b_i, \tag{4.1}$$

where LAT = latitude − $56°N$ ($56°N$ being the approximate mean latitude). Both intrinsic autoregression and our new spatial dependence model were used. The estimated regression coefficients (and standard errors) are given in table 1.

Note that $\hat{\lambda}$ based on the full model was less than one, indicating weaker spatial dependence than assumed by the intrinsic model, although the uncertainty in $\hat{\lambda}$ is large. The estimated coefficients for the two models

TABLE 1

Results for fitting model (4.1) to the Scottish lip cancer data (estimated regression coefficients with standard errors in parentheses) using the full spatial dependence structure given in (2.1) and the intrinsic model (i.e., with λ set to 1).

Dependence Model	α_0	α_1	α_2	σ	λ
Intrinsic	−.32(.15)	.39(.12)	.30(.22)	.70(.13)	1(NA)
Full Model	−.35(.28)	.40(.12)	.36(.17)	.69(.13)	.86(.38)

are quite similar although they are uniformly larger in magnitude for the full model. A major difference between the models concerns the latitude variable; in particular, there is greater evidence for the existence of a latitude effect under the full model, partly because of a smaller standard error. Simulation studies described below show that intrinsic autoregression produces less precise estimates of the latitude effect than the full model if the spatial dependence is weaker than assumed by the intrinsic model.

Another difference between the models is the larger standard error for the intercept under the full model. The larger standard error is not due to additional uncertainty introduced by the estimation of λ because the standard error for the fixed effects estimated using $X'\hat{V}^{-1}X$ does not account for this uncertainty. Rather, the larger standard error results simply from $\hat{\lambda}$ being less than one. Based on simulation studies reported below, such inflation of the standard error is an unusual occurrence.

We also fit the model excluding the latitude variable, and in this case the full spatial model estimated λ to be 1 and the other parameters to be $\hat{\alpha}_0 = -.18(.12), \hat{\alpha}_1 = .36(.12)$ and $\hat{\sigma} = .73(.13)$, as reported by Breslow and Clayton (1993). Comparing these results with table 1 indicates that the inclusion of the latitude covariate explained a small portion of the spatial random variation and had a small influence on the estimated effect of AFF.

Figure 1 illustrates the predicted values of the standardized morbidity ratio, SMR $= 100 \times \hat{\mu}_i/E_i$ where $\hat{\mu}_i$ are the fitted values from the full spatial model, plotted against the raw SMR based on the observed count $(100 \times y_i/E_i)$. Note that the model predictions are closer to the mean than the raw values, particularly for the extreme cases, which tend to correspond to small expected counts.

A simulation study was conducted to compare parameter estimates and SMR predictions from the full spatial model with those from 1) the intrinsic model, 2) the independence model and 3) a GLM with no random effects which does not allow for overdispersion. The simulations were based on the model in (4.1) with expected counts taken from the Scottish lip cancer data. The random effects covariance matrix of (2.1) was used with the neighbourhood structure of the Scottish counties. The parameter values were set approximately equal to the values obtained for the lip cancer data ($\alpha_0 = -.4$, $\alpha_1 = .4$, $\alpha_2 = .4$, and $\sigma = 1$), except that λ was set to 0

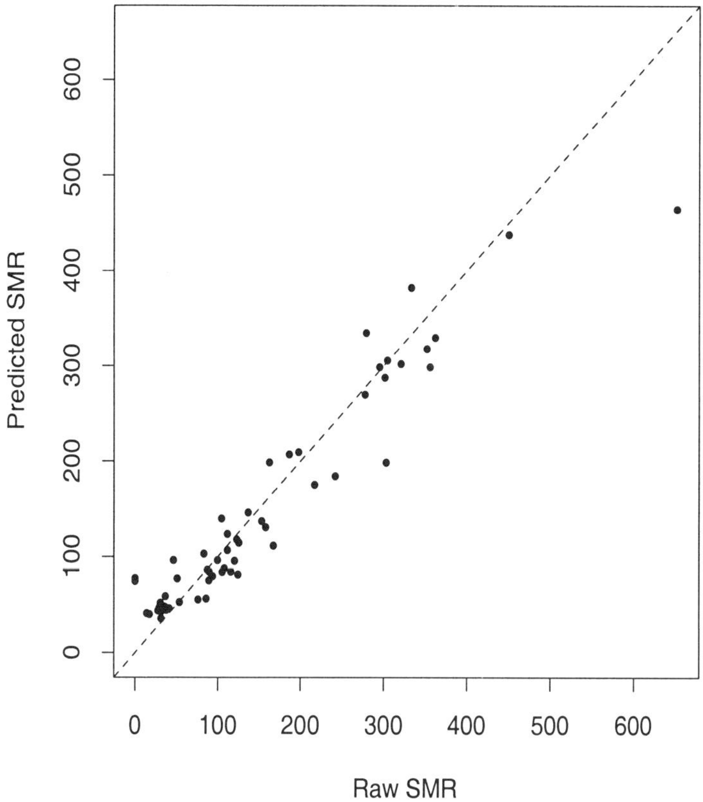

FIG. 1. *Scatterplot of predicted SMR versus raw SMR for the Scottish lip cancer data based on fitting the model (4.1) with dependence structure given by (2.1).*

(Independent Model), 0.5, or 1 (Intrinsic Model), in order to determine the effect of the true dependence structure. For each model, 400 data sets were simulated.

Table 2 gives the mean and standard deviation of the parameter estimates obtained from the four models for data simulated under the independence and intrinsic models. For each simulated data set we also calculated the bias of the predicted log SMRs (denoted BIAS) as the average across counties of the prediction errors (predicted log SMR minus actual value), the standard deviation of the prediction errors (denoted SD), and the root mean square error across counties as RMSE $= \sqrt{(\text{BIAS})^2 + (\text{SD})^2}$.

When data were simulated under the independence model, coefficient estimates obtained using intrinsic autoregression were more variable than those obtained using the independence and full models. The difference was very large for LAT, with the standard deviation for intrinsic autoregres-

TABLE 2

Mean values of parameter estimates, prediction bias of the log SMRs (BIAS), and root mean square error (RMSE) of the prediction error from models with various assumptions on the dependence structure: $\sigma = 0$ (GLM), $D = \sigma^2 I$ (Independent), $\sigma^2 D^- = R$ (Intrinsic), and $\sigma^2 D^- = \lambda I + (1-\lambda) R$ (Full Model). Standard deviations are given in parentheses. Results are based on 400 simulated data sets from the model (4.1) with the spatial dependence structure given in (2.1), $\alpha_0 = -.4, \alpha_1 = .4, \alpha_2 = .4, \sigma = 1$ and λ = 0 (Independent Case) or 1 (Spatial Case).

Model	α_0	α_1	α_2	σ	λ	BIAS	RMSE
			Independent Case ($\lambda = 0$):				
GLM	.05	.41	.38	0	–	.45	1.11
	(.36)	(.33)	(.17)	–	–	(.16)	(.14)
Independent	−.32	.39	.39	.95	0	.08	.43
	(.23)	(.21)	(.14)	(.12)	–	(.06)	(.06)
Intrinsic	−.31	.39	.37	1.99	1	.08	.45
	(.33)	(.27)	(.36)	(.28)	–	(.06)	(.06)
Full Model	−.32	.39	.39	1.01	.05	.08	.43
	(.23)	(.21)	(.14)	(.15)	(.09)	(.06)	(.06)
			Intrinsic Case ($\lambda = 1$):				
GLM	−.31	.46	.50	0	–	.18	.73
	(.37)	(.28)	(.41)	–	–	(.19)	(.19)
Independent	−.40	.43	.44	.65	0	.04	.36
	(.26)	(.21)	(.36)	(.14)	–	(.06)	(.06)
Intrinsic	−.38	.41	.40	.97	1	.03	.32
	(.19)	(.15)	(.30)	(.15)	–	(.06)	(.04)
Full Model	−.38	.41	.41	.92	.81	.03	.32
	(.20)	(.15)	(.30)	(.17)	(.25)	(.06)	(.04)

sion approximately 2.5 times as large as for the other two methods. The intrinsic model estimates tended to be further away from the true value of 0.4 than the estimates from the full model (figure 2). However, the estimates from the intrinsic model did not exhibit appreciable bias, so that the phenomenon cannot be attributed to ordinary confounding by the spatial random effect. Interestingly, the large variation in the LAT coefficient estimate from the intrinsic model had essentially no impact on SMR prediction (table 2).

There was very little bias in the estimates of the covariate effects for any method. The intercept estimates were all biased, and the log SMRs were also biased as a consequence; however, this bias contributed little to the RMSE of the log SMR predictions. The naive GLM which assumes no random effects gave unbiased estimates for the two regression coefficients although the variability was somewhat higher than for the independence and full models. The intercept and SMRs were estimated poorly using the GLM.

When data were simulated under intrinsic autoregression, the estimates obtained from the independence model were somewhat more variable

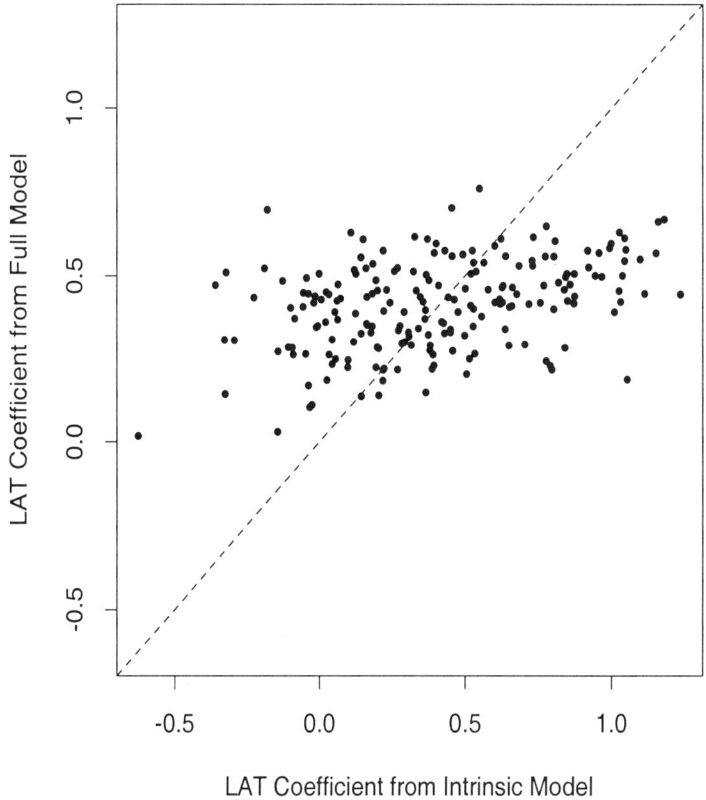

FIG. 2. *Scatterplot of estimates of the LAT coefficient using the full model (2.1) versus intrinsic autoregression for 400 data sets simulated from the model (4.1) with independent random effects.*

than those from the intrinsic and full models. Unlike the results obtained in the independence case, the estimates of the intercept as well as the covariate coefficients were approximately unbiased for the three random effects models. The GLM produced biased estimates of the fixed effects and, as in the independence case, poor SMR predictions.

It is noteworthy that in both situations considered, fitting the full model gave results which were essentially the same as those obtained by fitting the correct model (either independence or intrinsic autoregression). Results for the case $\lambda = 0.5$ (not shown) were intermediate between the independence and intrinsic cases, and the differences between the three random effects models were smaller. The simulations were repeated with $\sigma = 2$ and the results were qualitatively the same.

Additional simulations were conducted to determine how well the PQL

TABLE 3

Mean values of PQL parameter estimates, prediction bias of the log SMRs (BIAS), and root mean square error (RMSE) of the prediction error, based on 400 simulated data sets from the model (4.1) with the spatial dependence structure given in (2.1). True parameter values are given in parentheses.

$\bar{E}$	α_0 (−.4)	α_1 (.4)	α_2 (.4)	σ (1)	λ (.5)	BIAS	RMSE
.2	−.26	.35	.40	.70	.44	.08	.77
.5	−.29	.39	.40	.79	.45	.11	.65
1	−.26	.37	.38	.86	.51	.09	.57
2	−.36	.42	.41	.90	.49	.07	.48
5	−.34	.40	.40	.89	.43	.05	.38
10	−.38	.41	.39	.91	.47	.03	.30
20	−.36	.41	.37	.95	.50	.02	.23

estimation method performs with small to moderately large counts. Data were simulated as before, except that the expected counts were scaled so that the median value (denoted $\bar{E}$) was equal to .2, .5, 1, 2, 5, 10, or 20. Note that the means (μ_i) vary substantially between counties around the typical value of $\bar{E}$ because of the covariate effects and the random effects. For each model, 400 data sets were simulated. In non-convergent cases (three for $\bar{E} = .2$ and one each for $\bar{E} = 0.5, 1$) the final parameter estimates obtained after 50 iterations were used.

Mean values of the PQL parameter estimates, as well as the BIAS and RMSE of the prediction errors, are given in table 3. The estimate of the intercept was biased for small expected counts. The intercept tended to be underestimated in magnitude (estimates closer to 0 than true value), in agreement with Zeger, Liang, and Albert (1988). However, the PQL estimate of the regression coefficients had negligible bias even for very small counts. The estimate of the random effects standard deviation had a large negative bias for smaller counts, but only a small bias for $\bar{E} \geq 2$. There was little bias in the estimate of λ. For small expected counts a small positive bias was present in the PQL predictions, corresponding to overestimation of the SMRs by approximately 10%. This bias was reduced as the expected count increased, and in all cases the bias was small enough that the RMSE was determined primarily by the SD.

The simulation standard deviations and the mean values of the estimated standard errors are given in table 4. Standard errors for the regression coefficients were estimated very accurately. In particular, no evidence was found that the coefficient standard errors were underestimated because of the failure to account for uncertainty in the variance parameter estimates. Estimated standard errors for σ and λ performed well for large counts, but for the smaller counts the estimated standard errors tended to be too large. Improved methods are needed for assessing uncertainty of PQL estimates, and for performing inference on variance parameters, in particular.

TABLE 4
Mean values of the estimated standard errors for PQL estimates and simulation standard deviations in parentheses, based on 400 simulated data sets from the model (4.1) with the spatial dependence structure given in (2.1) and parameter values $\alpha_0 = -.4, \alpha_1 = .4, \alpha_2 = .4, \sigma = 1, \lambda = 0.5$.

$\bar{E}$	α_0	α_1	α_2	σ	λ
.2	.44 (.44)	.40 (.41)	.32 (.32)	.75 (.44)	.61 (.44)
.5	.33 (.32)	.28 (.30)	.24 (.25)	.43 (.34)	.54 (.41)
1	.33 (.29)	.23 (.25)	.22 (.22)	.30 (.26)	.45 (.37)
2	.29 (.29)	.20 (.21)	.20 (.21)	.24 (.23)	.38 (.32)
5	.25 (.24)	.17 (.17)	.17 (.17)	.20 (.20)	.31 (.28)
10	.26 (.25)	.15 (.16)	.17 (.19)	.18 (.19)	.29 (.28)
20	.27 (.25)	.15 (.15)	.17 (.19)	.18 (.18)	.28 (.18)

5. Discussion. The new spatial dependence structure proposed here provides a flexible way of describing spatial data, including separate parameters describing overdispersion and spatial dependence. The model provides a useful framework for obtaining stable estimates of incidence rates or SMRs based on small counts. A computer simulation study showed that regression coefficient estimates assuming intrinsic autoregression can have very low precision when there is no spatial correlation. Fitting the full model, including estimation of the spatial dependence parameter, produced good results under both independence and intrinsic autoregression models.

Further research is necessary to compare our proposed model with the additive model of Besag et al. (1991). Our model allows interpretation in terms of the local conditional moments and is particularly convenient for maximum-likelihood estimation using Markov Chain Monte Carlo techniques, for which direct use of the inverse variance matrix avoids repeated matrix inversion and allows efficient computation (results to be presented elsewhere).

Computer simulation showed that PQL parameter estimates provide nearly unbiased assessment of the effect of explanatory variables, even for very small expected counts. This property may be related to the fact that the log-linear form of the regression relationship is the same for the marginal mean as for the conditional mean; i.e., $\log E(y_i) = \log E_i + x_i'\alpha + D_{ii}/2$, as compared with equation (1.1). Zeger, Liang, and Albert (1988) gave a similar formula for models with independent random effects. The magnitudes of the intercept and the random effects standard deviation were somewhat underestimated by PQL for small expected counts, and this was associated with a small positive bias in estimates of the SMRs. However, this bias was not too serious and relatively small compared with the prediction standard deviation.

Our results show that PQL is a useful approximate method for analysing spatial incidence data. Improved methods, perhaps using maximum-likelihood or Bayesian techniques, are needed for analysing very small counts, which arise in subgroup analyses or the study of very rare diseases. The spatial dependence structure proposed here in terms of the inverse variance matrix is particularly amenable to these methods of estimation.

APPENDIX

The REML likelihood for the variance parameters σ and λ is (Breslow and Clayton, 1993)

$$L = -\frac{1}{2}\log|V| - \frac{1}{2}\log|X'V^{-1}X| - \frac{1}{2}(Y - X\hat{\alpha})'V^{-1}(Y - X\hat{\alpha}),$$

where Y is the adjusted dependent variable given by (3.1), V is its approximate covariance matrix defined as in (3.2), and $\hat{\alpha}$ is the current estimate of the fixed effect parameters. In computing derivatives of L, $\hat{\alpha}$, and hence $\hat{W}$ in (3.2), are treated as being constant. Simplification of the computations is achieved by writing the third term in L as $-\frac{1}{2}Y'PY$, where $P = V^{-1} - V^{-1}X(X'V^{-1}X)^{-1}X'V^{-1}$. Letting $\theta' = (\theta_1, \theta_2) = (\sigma, \lambda)$, the elements of the score, observed information, and expected information are given by

$$s_i = \frac{\partial L}{\partial \theta_i} = \frac{1}{2}Y'P\frac{\partial V}{\partial \theta_i}PY - \frac{1}{2}\text{tr}\left(P\frac{\partial V}{\partial \theta_i}\right),$$

$$I_{ij}^{obs} = -\frac{\partial^2 L}{\partial \theta_i \partial \theta_j} = \frac{1}{2}\text{tr}\left[P\left(\frac{\partial^2 V}{\partial \theta_i \partial \theta_j} - \frac{\partial V}{\partial \theta_i}P\frac{\partial V}{\partial \theta_j}\right)\right]$$

$$-\frac{1}{2}Y'P\left(\frac{\partial^2 V}{\partial \theta_i \partial \theta_j} - 2\frac{\partial V}{\partial \theta_i}P\frac{\partial V}{\partial \theta_j}\right)PY,$$

and

$$I_{ij}^{exp} = -E\left[\frac{\partial^2 L}{\partial \theta_i \partial \theta_j}\right] = \frac{1}{2}\text{tr}\left(P\frac{\partial V}{\partial \theta_i}P\frac{\partial V}{\partial \theta_j}\right).$$

The derivatives of V for $\sigma > 0$ and $0 < \lambda < 1$ are given below:

$$\frac{\partial V}{\partial \sigma} = 2\sigma R_\lambda^{-1},$$

$$\frac{\partial V}{\partial \lambda} = -\sigma^2 R_\lambda^{-1}(R - I)R_\lambda^{-1},$$

$$\frac{\partial^2 V}{\partial\sigma\partial\sigma} = 2R_\lambda^{-1},$$

$$\frac{\partial^2 V}{\partial\sigma\partial\lambda} = -2\sigma R_\lambda^{-1}(R-I)R_\lambda^{-1},$$

and

$$\frac{\partial^2 V}{\partial\lambda\partial\lambda} = 2\sigma^2 R_\lambda^{-1}(R-I)R_\lambda^{-1}(R-I)R_\lambda^{-1},$$

where $R_\lambda = (1-\lambda)I + \lambda R$ and R is the matrix defined in section 2.

REFERENCES

[1] BESAG, J., *Spatial interaction and the statistical analysis of lattice systems (with discussion)*, Journal of the Royal Statistical Society, Series B, **36**, (1974), pp. 192–236.

[2] BESAG, J., YORK, J. AND MOLLIÉ, A., *Bayesian image restoration, with two applications in spatial statistics*, Annals of the Institute of Statistical Mathematics, **43**, (1991), pp. 1–20.

[3] BRESLOW, N.E. AND CLAYTON, D.G., *Approximate inference in generalized linear mixed models*, Journal of the American Statistical Association, **88** (1993), pp. 9–25.

[4] CLAYTON, D. AND KALDOR, J., *Empirical Bayes estimates of age-standardized relative risks for use in desease mapping*, Biometrics, **43**, (1987), pp. 671–681.

[5] CRESSIE, N., *Statistics for spatial data*, Wiley, New York, 1991, pp. 900.

[6] KEMP, I., BOYLE, P., SMANS, M. AND MUIR, C. *Atlas of Cancer in Scotland, 1975–1980. Incidence and Epidemiologic Perspective. IARC Scientific Publication No. 72*, International Agency for Research on Cancer, Lyon, 1985.

[7] SINGH, B.B. AND SHUKLA, G.K., *A test of autoregression in Gaussian spatial processes*, Biometrika, **70**, (1983), pp. 523–527.

[8] YASUI, Y. AND LELE, S., *A regression method for spatial disease rates: an estimating function approach*, Journal of the American Statistical Association, **92**, (1997), pp. 21–32.

[9] ZEGER, S.L., LIANG, K.-Y., AND ALBERT, P.S., *Models for longitudinal data: a generalized estimating equation approach*, Biometrics, **44**, (1988), pp. 1049–1060.

MARKOV CHAIN MONTE CARLO METHODS FOR CLUSTERING IN CASE EVENT AND COUNT DATA IN SPATIAL EPIDEMIOLOGY

ANDREW B. LAWSON AND ALLAN B. CLARK*

Abstract. The analysis of clustering in small area data in epidemiology is considered. A modelling paradigm which is based on point process models is proposed for both case event and count data observed in arbitrary regions. Use is made of combinations of Markov Chain Monte Carlo (MCMC) methods, including forms of data augmentation, to provide a common approach. Examples of case event and count data are provided.

1. Introduction. The analysis of clustering in small area health data has attracted increased interest in recent years, see Lawson et al. [29]. Both public concern for the existence of 'clusters' of disease and growing interest in the causes of clustering, per se, are partly responsible for this increase. A growing interest in environmental issues both in the general public and the scientific community, has led to interest in clusters related to environmental hazards, e.g. power stations, incinerators, electro-magnetic fields or toxic waste dumping sites. The analysis of clustering in small area health data can be approached in a variety of ways, depending on the purpose of the study.

Two fundamental considerations should first be assessed:

1) Is the clustering in the data of primary interest?
2) Is the clustering of secondary interest, and hence, a nuisance feature?

In the first case, some detailed aspects of clustering may be of interest, e.g. How likely are n clusters? What is the marginal posterior distribution of the centres of clustering, given n clusters? Are there different scales of clustering supported by the data?

In the second case, clustering tendency is to be estimated, perhaps as part of a background feature of the process, but other aspects of the disease process are of major interest. For example, some diseases are known to form clusters at certain scales (e.g. Leukaemias [10]), but the relation of the disease incidence to putative sources of hazard may be of prime interest. Hence, in this case, clustering is a 'nuisance' background characteristic. A review of these is provided in Lawson and Kulldorff [34].

In this paper, an approach to the analysis of clustering in small area health data is proposed, which can accommodate both of the above cases, via direct modelling of clustering within a more general model framework. The methods used are primarily Bayesian, as considerable use is made of

*Department of Mathematical Sciences, King's College, University of Aberdeen, Aberdeen AB24 3UE, UK.

MCMC methods. The methods have considerable generality and can be applied to both case event and counts of cases in arbitrarily-defined regions.

2. Model development. The data $\mathbf{y}$ and cluster centres $\mathbf{x}$ are spatial point patterns:

$$\mathbf{y} = \{y_1, \ldots\ldots\ldots y_m\}, \qquad m > 0 , \qquad y_i \in T ,$$
$$\mathbf{x} = \{x_1, \ldots\ldots\ldots x_n\}, \qquad n \geq 0 , \qquad x_i \in U$$

where T is the study window and U is a region which encloses T. By allowing U to differ from T, we allow the possibility of locating putative cluster centres outside the window of observation of the data. This makes some allowance for the edge effect where data could appear in the window but a centre lies outside, i.e. the boundary splits a cluster so that some part of the form is censored. The observed data $\mathbf{y}$ in this paper are address locations of cases of disease, observed within T and a fixed time period. Diseases of interest could be leukaemias, which are thought to cluster weakly [10], or possibly, respiratory disease, such as respiratory cancer, larynx cancer or bronchitis, which could relate to one or more sources of health hazard (e.g. incinerators, waste dump sites etc.). In either case, unobserved heterogeneity in the environment and/or population experiencing the disease events could lead to clustered disease incidence over the window T.

In any analysis of $\mathbf{y}$, the population experiencing the disease events must be considered. The variation of population over space, in its density *and* its propensity to contract a disease (its 'at-risk' structure) can lead to apparent 'clustering' or 'heterogeneity' in $\mathbf{y}$. Hence, to properly assess clustering in such data it is important to account for the spatial variation in the 'at-risk' structure of the population. To achieve this, a variety of approaches can be adopted. The commonest approach is to estimate the 'at-risk' surface either, from the known features of the population, such as age-sex structure or measurements of deprivation or lifestyle information. These data are usually available for small areas, from national censuses. Or alternatively to use a 'control' disease. The first approach is often termed 'standardisation', when applied to count data in census tracts (see, e.g. [21]). It has been applied to the assessment of a single 'cluster' of case event data (see [23]). The second approach can be applied where a 'control' disease can be chosen which has a similar 'at-risk' structure to the case disease, but is not known to display clustering. This approach has been used by a variety of workers [13, 15, 23], to examine possible 'clusters' around putative sources of health hazard. In these cases, the control should not be known to be affected by the hazard, and hence should not 'cluster' near possible sources. In the general clustering case, where no specific environmental cause or factor is hypothesised and can be measured, then the 'control' disease should be known to be free from a clustering tendency.

In what follows we represent this modelling approach by using the first order intensity of the process, with suitable parameterisation for particular applications:

$$\lambda(\mathbf{y}|\mathbf{x}) = g(\mathbf{y}) \cdot f(\mathbf{y}, \mathbf{x}; \theta) \ . \tag{1}$$

In all the applications we examine, $g(\mathbf{y})$ is considered to represent the background 'at-risk' process, and $f(.)$ is defined as a function of $\mathbf{y}$, $\mathbf{x}$ and a parameter vector θ. The exact form of $f(.)$ will be determined by the application, and will be discussed further in section 2.2 and 2.3.

Note that we assume a multiplicative link between the population background and $f(.)$ which implies that any spatial structure modelled in $f(.)$ will be directly modified by variations in $g(\mathbf{y})$. The alternative of a pure additive link (see , e.g. [6, p.142]), would imply that spatial structures modelled in $f(.)$ (e.g. clusters) were of fixed size and hence unaffected by the population structure. This would appear to be inappropriate for spatial epidemiological data.

In what follows the definitions of Besag and Newell [4], concerning cluster studies, are adopted. The term 'focussed' is used to imply that the clustering of interest is around *known* foci (centre) locations. The term 'non-focussed' is used for the situation where foci (centre) locations are unknown. The analysis of putative sources of hazard are usually 'focussed', even though the data around foci may not form conventional clusters (e.g. electro-magnetic fields). The estimation of the locations of cluster foci, as in the Geographical Analysis Machine (see e.g. [35]) and extensions [4], are examples of 'non-focussed' clustering. A review of methods for 'focussed' clustering is available [31]. The general approach of this paper encompasses both approaches as special cases. While this paper solely concerns model-based approaches to clustering, the development of a general approach to hypothesis testing in cluster studies has been proposed by Tango [39].

2.1. Case event models. Where case event locations are to be modelled, it is possible to define a general point process model. Assume that, conditional on the $\mathbf{x}$, the case events are independently distributed as a modulated heterogeneous Poisson Process (hepp) with intensity given by (1). In the case of focussed clustering, the $\mathbf{x}$ are known and no conditioning is required. In the case of non-focussed clustering, we condition on the realisation of a spatial stochastic process governing the $\mathbf{x}$ locations. Hence, for this case, we require a 'prior' spatial distribution to describe the $\mathbf{x}$ behaviour. In both cases, however, the general model of conditional independence of cases is assumed.

Some examples of this approach are:

a) *Focussed clustering*

$$\lambda(\mathbf{y}|\mathbf{x}) = g(\mathbf{y}) \cdot \prod_{i=1}^{n} (1 + f(\mathbf{y} - x_i)) \ , \tag{2}$$

where n is the number of known foci [13, 15, 23].

b) *Non-Focussed clustering*

$$\lambda(\mathbf{y}|\mathbf{x}) = g(\mathbf{y}) \cdot \left(1 + \sum_{j=1}^{n_x} h(\mathbf{y} - x_j)\right) \tag{3}$$

where n_x is the unknown number of clusters, $\{x_j\}$ are the cluster foci locations and $h(\mathbf{y} - \mathbf{x})$ is a defined cluster distribution function [25]. Such functions are defined as for those standard cluster point process models (see e.g. [12]).

c) *Clustered background-Focussed clustering*

$$\lambda(\mathbf{y}|\mathbf{x}) = g(\mathbf{y}) \cdot \left(1 + \sum_{j=1}^{n_x} h(\mathbf{y} - x_j)\right) \cdot \prod_{i=n_x+1}^{n} (1 + f(\mathbf{y} - x_i)) \tag{4}$$

where the disease is known to cluster, but the analysis is 'focussed' on known foci [26].

In these examples, the cluster link is defined as a multiplicative *relative* risk.

2.2. Prior distributions and cluster structure. In the case of non-focussed clustering, prior distributions must be provided for the components n_x, $\mathbf{x}$ and parameters in $h(\mathbf{y} - \mathbf{x})$. Typically, the number of centres is assumed to have a Poisson (ρ) distribution, while $\mathbf{x}$ could follow a homogeneous Poisson process. The author and coworkers [2, 27] discuss the theoretical justification for this in non-modulated cluster processes and Cox processes. Alternative specifications for the $\mathbf{x}$ prior distribution (e.g. a Markov inhibition process) can be suggested based on algorithmic considerations (see section 4). The cluster distribution function can take a variety of forms. A commonly used form is

$$h(y - x) = \frac{\mu}{2\pi\kappa} e^{-[\|y-x\|]^2/2\kappa} \tag{5}$$

a radially isotropic Gaussian form with parameters μ and κ, the cluster variance. However, alternative forms are possible, including non-parametric versions. For example,

$$h(y - x) = \frac{1}{n_x m s_1 s_2} \sum_{i=1}^{m} k\left(\frac{y - y_i}{s_1}\right) \cdot \sum_{j=1}^{n_x} k\left(\frac{y - x_j}{s_2}\right) \tag{6}$$

where $k(.)$ is a kernel function (see, e.g. [37]), provides a nonparametric estimator for h.

The possibility of allowing a flexible cluster shape, via density estimation, may be attractive in situations where the exact form of clusters cannot be parameterised. This allows a considerable latitude in the definition of the cluster form while retaining a general model paradigm.

2.3. Applications in count modelling. Small area data is often available only as counts of cases within arbitrary regions (usually census tracts). Hence, a considerable literature has grown around the analysis of clustering of such data. While methods have been developed to test for global clustering (e.g. [36, 41]), and focussed clustering of counts (e.g. [5, 20, 22, 38]), there has been little attention paid to the examination of non-focussed clustering of count data. The methods applied to case event data can be applied here also. Given the conditional independence assumption, then counts in disjoint regions are independent Poisson random variables with mean $\int_A \lambda(\mathbf{u}|\mathbf{x})d\mathbf{u}$, where A is an arbitrary region. It is therefore possible to recover the intensity function $\lambda(\mathbf{y}|\mathbf{x})$, suitably parameterised as in (2),(3), and (4) based on count data.

3. Algorithms. The development of Markov Chain Monte Carlo methods and other iterative simulation tools [3, 40], has allowed the implementation of algorithms which can explore posterior distributions of the spatial problems identified above. Note that for both case and count data, if foci are known then straightforward likelihood models, or conventional spatial Bayesian models can be applied (see, e.g. [8, 24, 25]). If the locations of foci are unknown, then spatial prior distributions must be invoked.

3.1. Incorporation of background risk. Before considering the detail of basic algorithms, it is important to examine the issue of how the background risk surface ($g(\mathbf{y})$), can be incorporated in these problems. So far two basic approaches have been proposed:

3.1.1. Profile likelihood. In early work on case events [13, 23], the function $g(\mathbf{y})$ was estimated nonparametrically, and inference was made conditional on the fixed value of $\widehat{g}(\mathbf{y})$, without regard to estimation errors inherent in $\widehat{g}(\mathbf{y})$. Diggle [13] proposed the use of a control disease case event map to provide a density estimate of $g(\mathbf{y})$, while Lawson and Williams [23] compared the use of a control disease, and expected deaths, to estimate $g(\mathbf{y})$. Both approaches require smoothing of the background risk based on *external* data. An alternative hybrid model which used expected deaths in regions directly was also proposed by [23]. The use of control disease event maps has a number of disadvantages. In particular, the matching of a control disease to the 'at-risk' group of the cases, while being unrelated to the effect under study, can be difficult. Indeed, Diggle [13] provides an example of a control disease (respiratory cancer) which is related to the effect under study (air pollution). The use of expected deaths does not suffer from this problem but is usually only available at an aggregated level (e.g.census tract). Other background factors should also be incorporated where known, e.g. deprivation indices. However, these are usually only available at tract level also.

3.1.2. Label modelling. For the special case where a control disease is used, it is possible to use a *bivariate* point process model which directly incorporates the control event locations in the model. By conditioning on the locations of cases and controls, then it is possible to directly model the mark labels on the events (see e.g. [1]), and thereby the window (T) becomes irrelevant to the inference. In addition, this conditioning can be used to avoid estimation of $g(\mathbf{y})$. Diggle and Rowlingson [15] (DR) suggested the use of this approach in focussed clustering problems. This leads to a logistic regression formulation of the problem. Note, also that, as a special case of a Markov point process, conditional on the locations, the labels form a binary markov random field [1] and the auto-logistic model results. Assuming an Ising model, standard logistic regression methods apply.

3.1.3. A Bayesian smoothing model. The label modelling approach above, is only applicable when an appropriate control disease is available. To keep the model approach general, it is important to pursue methods which are not limited to such a specific case. An alternative approach is to regard the smoothing operator in $\widehat{g}(\mathbf{y})$ as a sample realisation of possible smoothing values which have a prior distribution. This both allows the incorporation of $\widehat{g}(\mathbf{y})$ within the estimation process and allows the exploration of the variation in $\widehat{g}(\mathbf{y})$ *in relation* to the other parameter dimensions. This is discussed further in the next section.

3.2. Basic point event algorithm. In the most general Bayesian formulation of the cluster model (from (2),(3),and (4)), we define the joint posterior distribution of $\{\mathbf{x}, \theta\}$ as

$$P(\mathbf{x}, \theta|\mathbf{y}) \propto L(\mathbf{y}|\mathbf{x}) \cdot p(\mathbf{x}) \cdot g(\theta) \tag{7}$$

where

$$L(\mathbf{y}|\mathbf{x}) = \left\{ \prod_{i=1}^{m} \lambda(y_i|\mathbf{x}) \right\} \cdot \exp\left\{ - \int_T \lambda(\mathbf{u}|\mathbf{x}) d\mathbf{u} \right\} \tag{8}$$

$p(\mathbf{x}) \equiv$ prior distribution for $\mathbf{x}$ (Markov inhibition or Uniform) and n_x (Poisson (ρ)),

$g(\theta) \equiv$ prior distributions for cluster function parameters.

$$\lambda(y_i|\mathbf{x}) = g(y_i) \cdot \left(1 + \sum_{j=1}^{n_x} h(y_i - x_j)\right) \cdot \prod_{k=n_x+1}^{n} (1 + f(y_i - x_k)) \tag{9}$$

where there are n_x unknown and n known foci. Note that the final fixed-foci term of (9) could also be dependent on covariates related to the individual observations $\{y_i\}$ or random effects.

3.3. Algorithm I. It is convenient to define three sets of parameters for the purpose of the algorithm steps. These sets can be considered as separate components of the sampler design. A two stage sampler proceeds by considering spatial cluster parameters within an inner iterative sampler conditional on current values of other parameters. The three nested sampling schemes are:

1) spatial cluster (**sc**) parameters: $\mathbf{x}, n_x$
2) non-spatial (**nc**) parameters: for example ρ, κ and μ (assuming a Gaussian cluster distribution is used)
3) smoothing parameter(s): for example $\widehat{g}(\mathbf{y})$ may depend on s (a smoothing parameter).

3.3.1. SC parameters. The derivation and properties of the following algorithm are discussed in [27] and [28]. The posterior distribution (7) could be explored by conventional iterative simulation methods, except for the cluster term, where a summation with a random upper limit occurs. This is essentially a mixture problem, and the **sc** parameters in this problem are best explored by a reversible jump Metropolis-Hastings (MH) sampler [17, 18], involving a mixture kernel. Essentially the joint distribution of $\mathbf{x}$ and n_x must be explored during iteration. This can be achieved by a spatial-birth-death-shift (SBDS) algorithm, where centres are added, deleted or shifted with given probability. A sequence of likelihood ratios can be specified for each case. In general, for a new configuration $\mathbf{x}'$, the posterior density ratio is, conditional on **nc** and h parameters:

$$PR(x, x') = \frac{L(\mathbf{y}|\mathbf{x}')}{L(\mathbf{y}|\mathbf{x})} \cdot \frac{p(\mathbf{x}')}{p(\mathbf{x})} \,. \tag{10}$$

This ratio is evaluated for $\mathbf{x}'$ within the SBDS algorithm based on an MH criterion. A proposal configuration $\mathbf{x}'$ is accepted with probability

$$A(\mathbf{x}, \mathbf{x}') = \min\left\{1, PR(x, x') \cdot \frac{q(\mathbf{x}', \mathbf{x})}{q(\mathbf{x}, \mathbf{x}')}\right\} \tag{11}$$

where $q(\mathbf{x}', \mathbf{x})$ is the proposal distribution for the new state. Often the proposal distribution for a point $\mathbf{u}$ is defined as a function of $h(\mathbf{y} - \mathbf{u})$ itself (e.g. $\frac{1}{m}\sum_{i=1}^{m} h(y_i - \mathbf{u})$) as simpler uniform proposals can lead to high rejection rates. We use Markov inhibition priors for $\mathbf{x}$, as the peaked nature of the likelihood surface can lead to multiple response, and it is important to propose spatially-separate new $\mathbf{x}$ values to avoid this problem. To this end, the Strauss prior can be used, and is defined for the proposed addition of a point $\mathbf{u}$ as

$$\frac{p(\mathbf{x} \cup \mathbf{u})}{p(\mathbf{x})} = \beta\gamma^{n_R(\mathbf{u})} \tag{12}$$

where β and $0 < \gamma < 1$ are parameters and $n_R(\mathbf{u})$ counts the number of $\mathbf{x}$ within a distance R of $\mathbf{u}$. Similar ratios can be defined for deaths and shifts.

For the likelihood, (8), the likelihood ratios are:
for addition:

$$\prod_{i=1}^{m}\left[1+\frac{h(y_i-\mathbf{u})}{1+\sum_{j=1}^{n_x}h(y_i-x_j)}\right]\cdot e^{-\Lambda(T|\mathbf{u})} \tag{13}$$

for deletion:

$$\prod_{i=1}^{m}\left[1-\frac{h(y_i-\mathbf{x}_d)}{1+\sum_{j=1}^{n_x}h(y_i-x_j)}\right]\cdot e^{\Lambda(T|\mathbf{x}_d)} \tag{14}$$

where $\mathbf{x}_d$ is the point to be deleted;
for shifting:

$$\prod_{i=1}^{m}\left[1+\frac{h(y_i-\mathbf{u})-h(y_i-\mathbf{x}_d)}{1+\sum_{j=1}^{n_x}h(y_i-x_j)}\right]\cdot e^{[\Lambda(T|\mathbf{x}_d)-\Lambda(T|\mathbf{u})]} \tag{15}$$

where

$$\Lambda(T|\mathbf{x})=\int_T \lambda(\mathbf{u}|\mathbf{x})d\mathbf{u}\ . \tag{16}$$

Note also that it is usual to include a constant rate scale parameter in $\lambda(\mathbf{u}|\mathbf{x})$ (δ say). However, it is possible to condition out δ from the analysis, and this can reduce the parameter dimensionality of the algorithm. To do this the likelihood ratio in (10), can be written in the form, conditional on m:

$$\prod_{i=1}^{m}\left\{\frac{1+\sum^{\mathbf{x}'}h(y_i;\mathbf{x}')}{1+\sum^{\mathbf{x}}h(y_i;\mathbf{x})}\right\}\cdot\left\{\frac{\Lambda_{\mathbf{x}}(T|\mathbf{x})}{\Lambda_{\mathbf{x}'}(T|\mathbf{x}')}\right\}^m, \tag{17}$$

where δ is removed from $\lambda(\mathbf{u}|\mathbf{x})$ and $\Lambda(.)$. It is straightforward to derive the equivalent ratios to (13)–(15), for this case.

3.3.2. NC parameters. The parameters of the cluster distribution function, and other prior distributions can be treated conventionally. In most cases here, we assume that n_x has a Poisson(ρ) prior distribution. This parallels the assumptions which specify a Poisson Cluster Process in ordinary point process models [12, 25] . It is also possible to assume a prior distribution for ρ, and a Gamma distribution is often used. We have no strong prior reason to assume any other distribution than a uniform indifference prior on a suitable range (usually $\leq m$).

The cluster distribution parameters (μ,κ), based on model (5), are also assumed to have uniform indifference priors. The sampler steps used for ρ,μ and κ differ depending on whether a Gibbs or MH step is simple to implement. A Gibbs step is straightforward for ρ, whereas to implement a Gibbs step for κ or μ requires an optimisation step (to obtain ml estimates), and in these cases an MH step is used.

3.3.3. Smoothing parameters.

The function $g(\mathbf{y})$. In previous work $g(y)$ has been estimated nonparametrically, or has been conditioned out of the analysis (see section 3.1). It is possible to incorporate the estimation of $g(y)$ within the MCMC algorithm. We regard the smoothing parameter (s) of a smoothing operation which estimates $g(y)$, as a random quantity. We can update the parameter s just like any other parameter in the MCMC algorithm. In order to specify the Bayesian model completely we need to define a prior distribution for s. A natural choice, motivated by work on Gaussian Mixtures [11], is the inverse gamma distribution.

$$p(s|\alpha,\beta) = \frac{\alpha^{\beta}}{\Gamma(\beta)} s^{-\beta-1} \exp\Big(-\frac{\alpha}{s}\Big) .$$

The hyperparameters (α, β) can be assigned non-informative hyperpriors. This approach discussed further in Lawson and Clark [30].

Cluster distribution smoothing. If the cluster distribution function is estimated non-parametrically as in (6), then the appropriate smoothing constants (s_1, s_2) must also be included in the iterative estimation scheme. A procedure similar to that above can be used and replaces the steps for μ and κ.

3.4. The label modelling algorithm (Algorithm II). The alternative to direct estimation of $g(\mathbf{y})$ in profile likelihood or the Bayesian smoothing model, is the label modelling (DR) approach. In this case we can define a conditional probability of a case event at $\mathbf{y}$, out of a case/control disease bivariate realisation, as:

$$(18)\qquad \begin{aligned} P(\mathbf{y}) &= \frac{g(y)\cdot f(y,x;\theta)}{g(y) + g(y)\cdot f(y,x;\theta)} \\ &= \frac{\delta\cdot(1+\sum_{j=1}^{n_x} h(\mathbf{y}-x_j))\cdot\prod_{i=n_x+1}^{n}(1+f(y-x_i))}{1+\delta\cdot(1+\sum_{j=1}^{n_x} h(\mathbf{y}-x_j))\cdot\prod_{i=n_x+1}^{n}(1+f(y-x_i))} .\end{aligned}$$

Note that this conditional model can be derived from a full bivariate competing risk model for cases and controls, i.e.

$$\begin{aligned}\Pr(\text{case at } \mathbf{y}) &= \lambda_1(\mathbf{y}|\mathbf{x}).e^{-\int_T \sum_l^2 \lambda_l(\mathbf{u}|\mathbf{x})d\mathbf{u}} \\ \Pr(\text{event at } \mathbf{y}) &= \sum_l^2 \lambda_l(\mathbf{y}|\mathbf{x}).e^{-\int_T \sum_l^2 \lambda_l(\mathbf{u}|\mathbf{x})d\mathbf{u}}\end{aligned}$$

where λ_l is the intensity of the relevant effect (λ_1 for cases)(see e.g. [33]). The likelihood of m_1 cases and m_2 controls is

$$(19)\qquad L = \prod_{i=1}^{m_1} P(y_i)\cdot\prod_{j=m_1+1}^{m_1+m_2}(1-P(y_j)) .$$

This conditional approach can also be used to replace $L(\mathbf{y}|\mathbf{x})$ in (8) by (19) within the main cluster algorithm. This leads to the following ratios for the SBDS algorithm:

addition:

$$(20)\quad \prod_{i=1}^{m_1}\left[\frac{H_i+h(y_i-\mathbf{u})}{H_i\cdot\left\{1+\frac{f(d_i).h(y_i-\mathbf{u})}{1+f(d_i)\cdot H_i}\right\}}\right]\cdot\prod_{j=m_1+1}^{m_1+m_2}\left[\left(1+\frac{f(d_j)\cdot h(y_j-\mathbf{u})}{1+f(d_j)\cdot H_j}\right)^{-1}\right]$$

deletion:

$$(21)\quad \prod_{i=1}^{m_1}\left[\frac{H_i-h(y_i-\mathbf{x}_d)}{H_i\cdot\left\{1-\frac{f(d_i)\cdot h(y_i-\mathbf{x}_d)}{1+f(d_i)\cdot H_i}\right\}}\right]\cdot\prod_{j=m_1+1}^{m_1+m_2}\left[\left(1-\frac{f(d_j)\cdot h(y_j-\mathbf{x}_d)}{1+f(d_j)\cdot H_j}\right)^{-1}\right]$$

shifting:

$$(22)\quad \begin{aligned}&\prod_{i=1}^{m_1}\left[\frac{H_i+h(y_i-\mathbf{u})-h(y_i-\mathbf{x}_d)}{H_i\cdot\left\{1+\frac{f(d_i))\cdot(h(y_i-\mathbf{u})-h(y_i-\mathbf{x}_d))}{1+f(d_i)\cdot H_i}\right\}}\right]\\&\cdot\prod_{j=m_1+1}^{m_1+m_2}\left[\left(1+\frac{f(d_j)\cdot(h(y_j-\mathbf{u})-h(y_j-\mathbf{x}_d))}{1+f(d_j)\cdot H_j}\right)^{-1}\right]\end{aligned}$$

where $H_i\equiv 1+\sum_{l=1}^{n_x}h(y_i-x_l)$, and $f(d_i)$ is a function representing covariates and known foci terms (with their current parameter values), and d_i is the distance to a known foci for the ith event .

The **nc** parameter sampler can be constructed as for the basic algorithm and it is also possible to use a non-parametric estimate of $h(\mathbf{y}-\mathbf{x})$ in this situation.

3.5. Extensions to count cluster modelling. It is possible to extend these basic point event algorithms to the case where only counts of the case disease are observed within arbitrary regions. This application of the algorithms is of considerable importance given the ready availability of such data and level of interest in its analysis.

We assume that conditional on the $\mathbf{x}$, the process is a regionalised hepp governed by $\lambda(\mathbf{y}|\mathbf{x})$ and

$$(23)\qquad E(n_i)=\int_{A_i}\lambda(\mathbf{u}|\mathbf{x})d\mathbf{u}\equiv\mathbf{\Lambda}(A_i|\mathbf{x})$$

where A_i denotes the ith region, and n_i the disease count in the region. As disjoint regions are independent under conditioning, then the $\{n_i\}$ are Poisson distributed with rates $\mathbf{\Lambda}(A_i|\mathbf{x})$. Conditional on N, the total number of cases (i.e. $N=\sum_{i=1}^{p}n_i$), the likelihood for p regions is

$$(24)\qquad L(\mathbf{n}|\mathbf{x},\theta)=\prod_{i=1}^{p}\left[\frac{\mathbf{\Lambda}(A_i|\mathbf{x})}{\sum_{l=1}^{p}\mathbf{\Lambda}(A_l|\mathbf{x})}\right]^{n_i}.$$

Now in this case we do not observe the point case events but only know their region totals. At this point it is possible to use conventional likelihood-based inference concerning parameters relating to *fixed* foci or covariates, or to include conventional Bayesian methods incorporating prior distributions. However, for unknown foci locations ($\mathbf{x}$) we can use directly the basic point process algorithms and replace the likelihood ratios with those based on (24). Note that if expected death variation is known for the ith region, then the likelihood (24) can be written

$$L(\mathbf{n}|\mathbf{x},\theta) = \prod_{i=1}^{p} \left[\frac{\int_{A_i} E(\mathbf{u}) \cdot \lambda(\mathbf{u}|\mathbf{x}) d\mathbf{u}}{\sum_{l=1}^{p} \int_{A_l} E(\mathbf{u}) \cdot \lambda(\mathbf{u}|\mathbf{x}) d\mathbf{u}} \right]^{n_i} . \tag{25}$$

Often this can be reduced to :

$$\prod_{i=1}^{p} \left[\frac{E_i \cdot \mathbf{\Lambda}(A_i|\mathbf{x})}{\sum_{l=1}^{p} E_l \cdot \mathbf{\Lambda}(A_l|\mathbf{x})} \right]^{n_i}$$

and a further reduction to constant region rate (λ_i) would allow the use of GLM software for fixed foci or covariate models. The $E(\mathbf{u})$ function plays the role of $g(\mathbf{y})$ in the case event process situation. Note that the use of (25) requires integration over arbitrary regions. Hence this approach utilises the counts directly in the cluster algorithm.

Another approach extends this count algorithm by exploiting ideas based on data augmentation. Tanner [40] discusses the different algorithmic approaches to data augmentation. In our approach we use the ideas of data augmentation but implement them within conventional Gibbs or MH steps. In particular we exploit the idea that censoring of observations leads to missing data and hence can be modelled by iterative augmentation of the missing portion. This can be applied in a variety of ways in point process modelling. For example the use of an external border (U) which encloses T allows the iterative simulation of cluster centres outside the observation window. In addition it could be possible to also simulate *data events* within U or indeed to simulate into internal areas of the window where events are censored (holes). In application to count modelling it is possible to regard the point process underlying the counts as a censored event set. In this way we could conditionally simulate the point events within our count event model. This could lead to many realisations which were of comparable likelihood, due to the inherent smoothness of the aggregated data. However, this does allow the reconstruction of the appropriate underlying point process intensity which is not available when constant region rate models are fitted. In addition spatially-continuous covariates can be correctly incorporated in the model.

Define $\{z_{ij}\}$, $j = 1, 2, ..., n_i$, the point locations of case events within the ith region. In each region, the conditional distribution of $\mathbf{z}$ given $\{\mathbf{n}, \theta\}$ is given by:

$$(\mathbf{z}|\mathbf{n},\theta) \sim \frac{\lambda(\mathbf{z})}{\sum_{i=1}^{p}\int_{A_i}\lambda(\mathbf{u})d\mathbf{u}}\,. \tag{26}$$

Hence, within the ith region, the joint distribution of $\{z_{ij}\}$ is

$$\frac{\prod_{j=1}^{n_i}\lambda(z_{ij})}{\left\{\sum_{i=1}^{p}\int_{A_i}\lambda(\mathbf{u})d\mathbf{u}\right\}^{n_i}}\,. \tag{27}$$

This suggests the following iterative algorithm:

Algorithm III

- initialise with $\theta^l, \mathbf{z}^l \quad (l = 0)$
- generate z_{ij}^{l+1} from $\left[\lambda(\mathbf{z}^l)/\lambda_{\max}(\mathbf{z}^l)\right]$ for each region up to n_i where max is the maximum over all the regions.
- either generate θ^{l+1} from the $(\theta|n_{i,}z_{ij}^{l+1})$ distribution or use a M-H update, or maximise the likelihood

$$l = \frac{\prod_{j=1}^{n_i}\prod_{i=1}^{p}\lambda(z_{ij}^{l+1})}{\left\{\sum_{i=1}^{p}\int_{A_i}\lambda(\mathbf{u})d\mathbf{u}\right\}^{N}}\,. \tag{28}$$

After initialisation the steps are repeated to convergence. Note that the method described is defined only for a likelihood-based model. This can be straightforwardly extended to accommodate prior distributions for components of the parameter vectors.

The important result of this algorithm is that the likelihood (or full posterior distribution) is now a function of the 'pseudo-data' and hence point process modelling can be used via augmentation to model count data. The extension of this algorithm to the cluster models described earlier is relatively straightforward. Assuming that it is required to estimate cluster centres $\{\mathbf{x}\}$ from the count data, as in the point process case, then suitable parameterisation of $\lambda(\mathbf{z})$ with cluster terms and the inclusion of an inner MH iteration for $\{\mathbf{x}, n_x\}$, prior to the θ^{l+1} step, provides a cluster version of Algorithm III.

3.6. Data examples.

3.6.1. Humberside Leukaemia and Lymphoma data. Cuzick and Edwards [9] first presented an analysis of a realisation of 62 cases of childhood leukaemia and lymphoma in the North Humberside area for the period 1974 to 1986. In addition to these data, the locations of a random selection of 141 births from the register for the same period is available. This data set was regarded as a spatial 'control' for the case data set. Figure 1 displays these data and the study window. Further analysis of this data set was made by Diggle and Chetwynd [14], who assessed second-moment properties via K-function methods. Both of these analyses attempted to test *random labelling* between cases and controls as a null hypothesis [14]

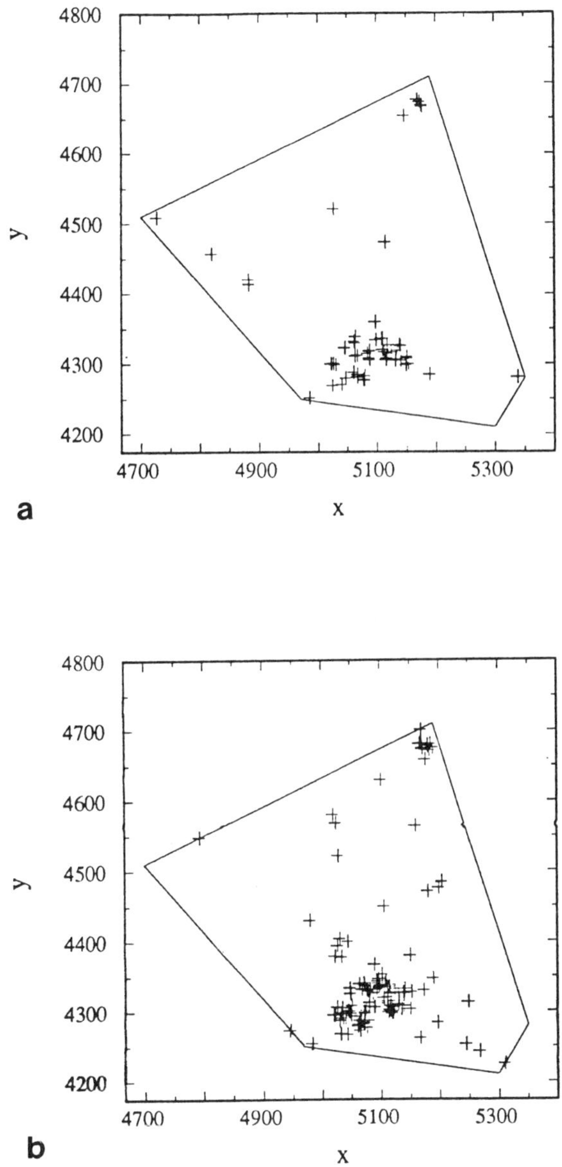

FIG. 1. *Humberside example: a) case data location map, b) control data location map.*

also assessed the spatial scale of clustering. However, both analyses were restricted to the assumption of stationarity in the processes considered and do not provide estimates of cluster centre locations. Here, our aim is to model the clustering tendency of the case events given the local population structure. Hence, we assume n_x and $\mathbf{x}$ are unknown and we are interested in the joint posterior marginal distribution and conditional distribution of $\mathbf{x}$ given n_x. This distribution is useful when conditioning on the modal posterior value of n_x.

We assume that the case locations have occurred within a heterogeneous population, and that given the local population structure then clusters will follow a cluster process. In this case the realisation of the intensity process consists of a background process, $g(y)$, which represents the 'at-risk' population, and a cluster distribution $h(.)$, as defined in (5).The intensity of cases is assumed to be governed by (9). Initially, inference concerning cluster parameters was made conditionally on $\widehat{g}(\mathbf{y})$, separately estimated from the birth register sample. Cross-validation(cv) has been used to provide an 'optimal' choice of bandwidth. Likelihood cv yielded a constant of 0.05 (on the unit square). The results of this analysis are presented in Figure 2. To make allowance for the possible dependence of inference on the smoothing constant, a range of values have been used. These have covered a range around the cv value. Label modelling can also be used here and the results of fitting a label modelling cluster algorithm are also presented in Figure 3.

In all the example runs we have assumed U=T to allow for the problem of seaward boundaries and have used $p = 1$,$q = 0.5$, death rate of $1/n_x$ and uniform birth rate in a disc of radius 0.01. The Strauss prior parameters are $\log\beta = \log\gamma$ =-10 and interaction distance (R) =0.084. These parameter values have been found to yield enough inhibition of centres to prevent multiple response in the sampler. A Gibbs step is used for ρ while a M-H step is used for μ and κ. The SBDS algorithm was run for 400 iterations conditional on each parameter realisation of the **nc** sampler, which itself was run to convergence. This usually took place by 5000 iterations.

The results of both approaches appear to suggest that there is little evidence of clustering, although label modelling supports a higher modal number of cluster centres than the ordinary profile method. However, the conditioning inherent in $\widehat{g}(\mathbf{y})$ estimation, does not support a strong difference in model preference. More research is required to assess which models are to be preferred in specific situations.

3.6.2. Respiratory cancer in central Scotland. A study of respiratory cancer incidence in Central Scotland has been initiated. The purpose of the study is to examine the clustering tendency of a variety of diseases in Falkirk, a town formerly associated with a variety of heavy industries during the early to mid 20th century. The famous Carron steel foundry operated in this area, and a number of mines were active in the vicinity up to the 1980s.

For the purposes of this example, respiratory cancer (ICD code: 162) incidence in a subset of 26 contiguous Falkirk enumeration districts (eds) has been recorded for a five year period 1978-1983. The total cancer count, expected count based on 16 age $\times$ sex strata and external (Scottish) rates for the period, and digitised ed boundaries are available for this example. Deprivation indices [7] have not been utilised in this example, although they could be included in any case applications. Figure 4 displays the location map and outline ed map.

As part of a larger study the clustering tendency of respiratory cancer is to be assessed. While such cancer is closely related to environmental health hazards such as air pollution, it is also related to lifestyle (e.g. smoking behaviours) [32]. At the large scale of this study it was not possible to obtain measurements of smoking behaviour. Deprivation indices do notprovide a perfect matchof smoking lifestyle to deprivation status and in this case were not available. The intention in the following analysis is to demonstrate the application of the of the count data algorithm to the estimation of cluster structure in this example.

We have applied algorithm III, including augmentation of point events, with the following conditions.We initialise $\mathbf{z}$ with completely spatially random (CSR) events in $A_T = \sum_{i=1}^{p} A_i$. New values of $\mathbf{z}$ are rejection sampled from $\lambda(\mathbf{z}^l)$. M-H updates are used for μ, whereas a Gibbs step is straightforward for ρ (the cluster rate parameter) and κ. These steps are based on the likelihood (28), with E_i assumed constant across regions and $\lambda(\mathbf{z}_{ij}) = E_{i.}C(\mathbf{z}_{ij})$, where $C(\mathbf{z}_{ij})$ represents the cluster model terms. We have only included the unknown foci term for this example. A Markov (Strauss) prior has been included with parameters defined as for the Humberside example. Figure 5 displays the results of augmentation applied to this data set. Convergence occurred relatively quickly (< 200 iterations of main algorithm). There is some evidence that the number of centres lies in the range of 1 to 3, although the parent rate mode is 1.12. The posterior marginal distribution of centres is relatively uniform.

4. Conclusions and further work. The main conclusion of this work is that it demonstrates the flexibility of reversible jump MCMC algorithms in the analysis of point process models with heterogeneous backgrounds. Further wc have demonstrated a method which allows the analysis of aggregated count data based on the underlying point process models and hence avoiding the so-called ecological fallacy inherent in Markov Random Field models [29].

Future development of this work lies in three important areas

1. The modelling of general cluster situations with additional (non-specific) random effects (correlated or uncorrelated); see Lawson and Clark [30] for details.

2. The extension to space-time is, in principal, straightforward but portends a wide application area.
3. The analysis of goodness-of-fit of point process models in spatial epidemiology.

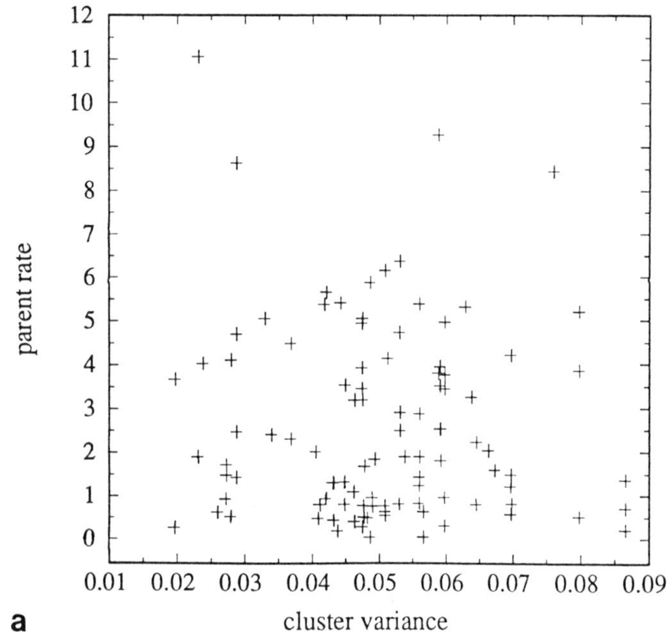

FIG. 2. *Humberside: Ordinary model: a) Posterior marginal distribution of parent rate and cluster variance.*

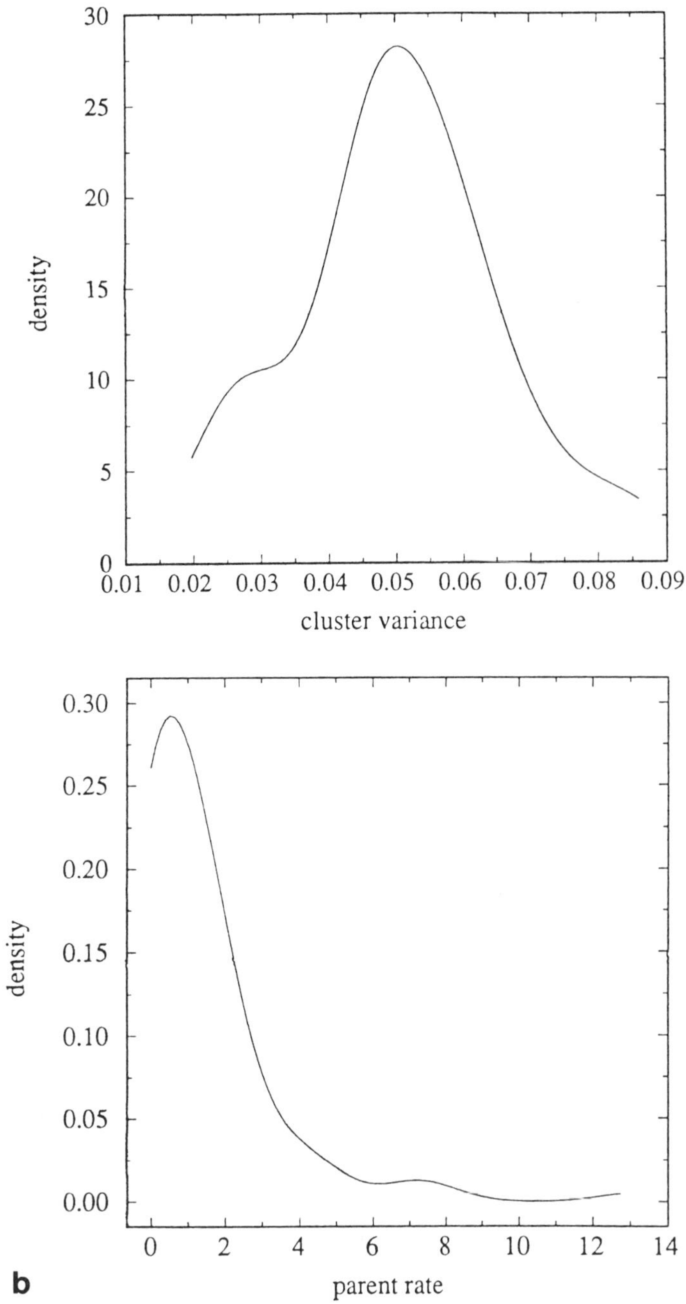

FIG. 2. *Humberside: Ordinary model: b) parent rate and cluster variance marginal densities.*

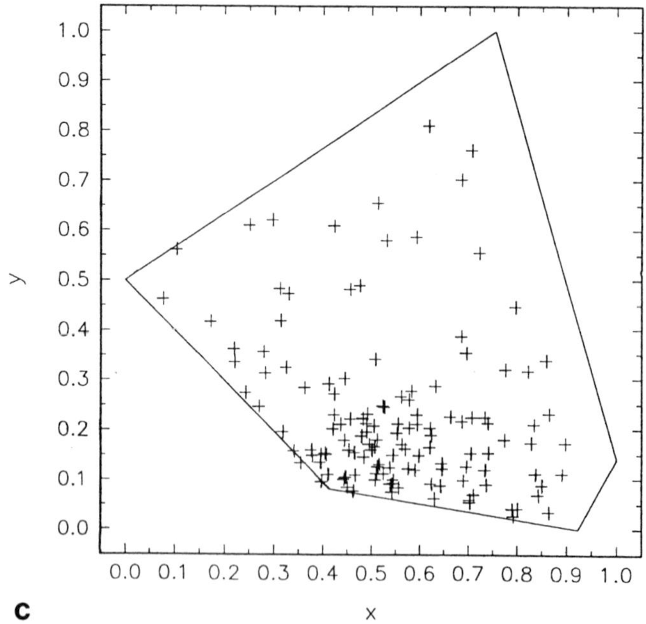

FIG. 2. *Humberside: Ordinary model: c) cluster center posterior marginal distribution.*

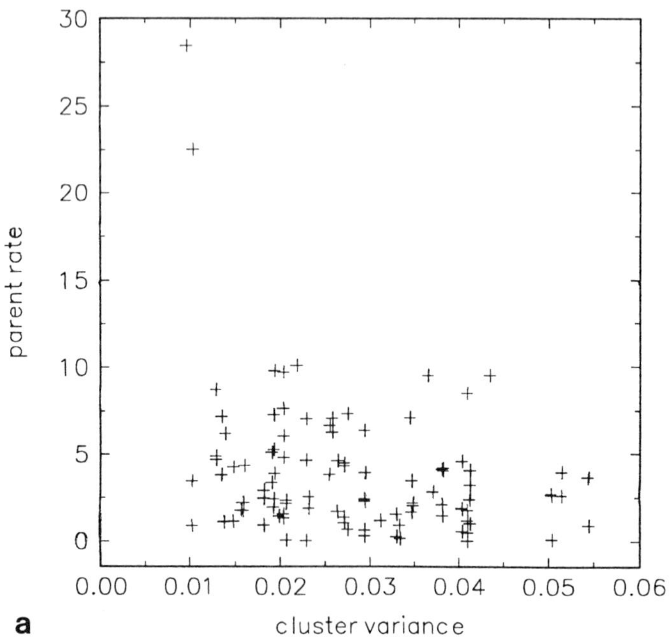

FIG. 3. *Humberside: D&R model: a) Posterior marginal distribution of parent rate and cluster variance.*

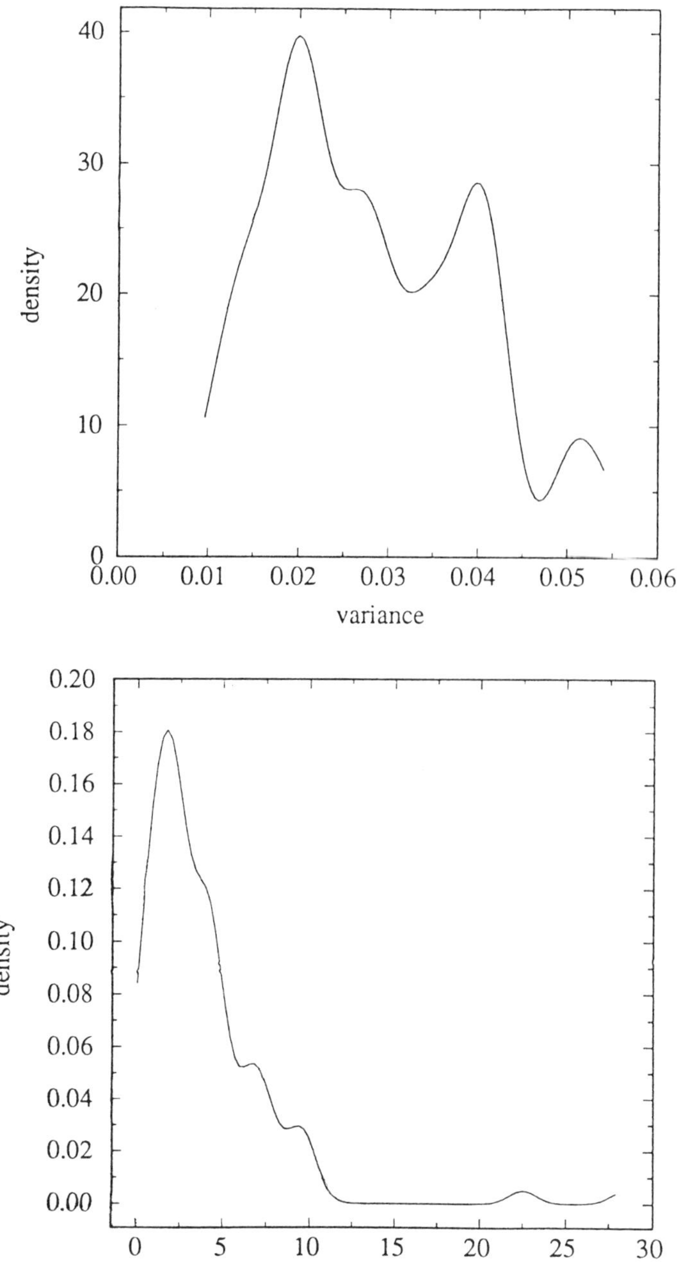

b

FIG. 3. *Humberside: D&R model: b) parent rate and cluster variance marginal densities.*

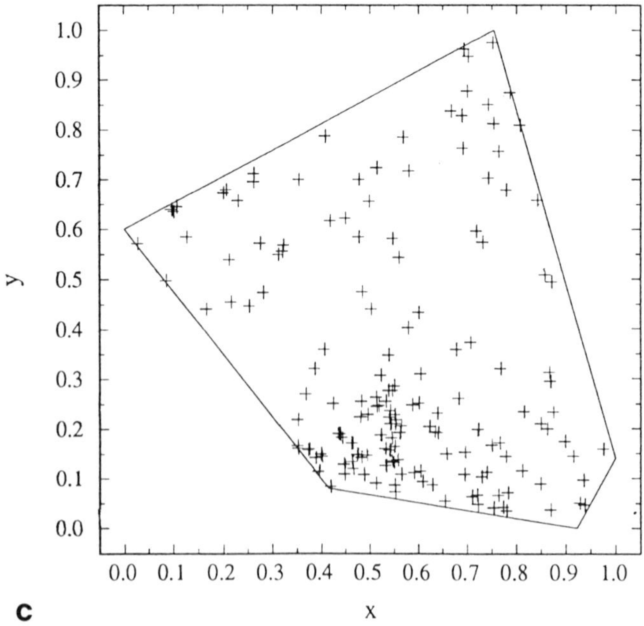

FIG. 3. *Humberside: D&R model: c) cluster centre posterior marginal distribution.*

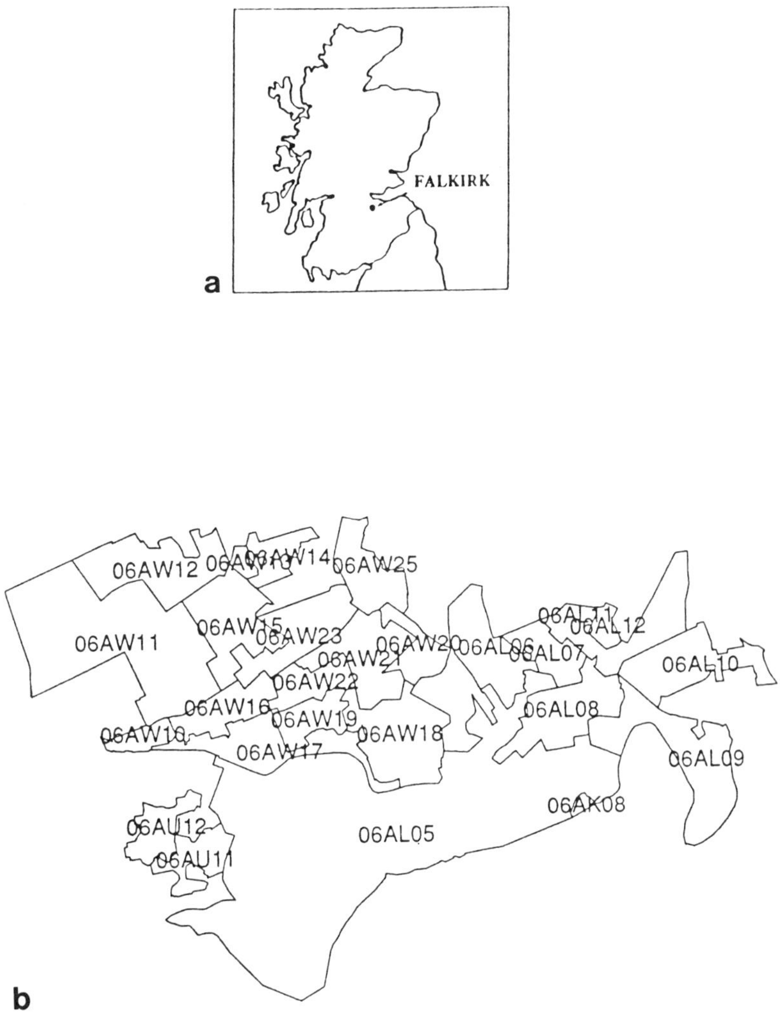

FIG. 4. *Falkirk example: a) location map, b) enumeration district (ed) map.*

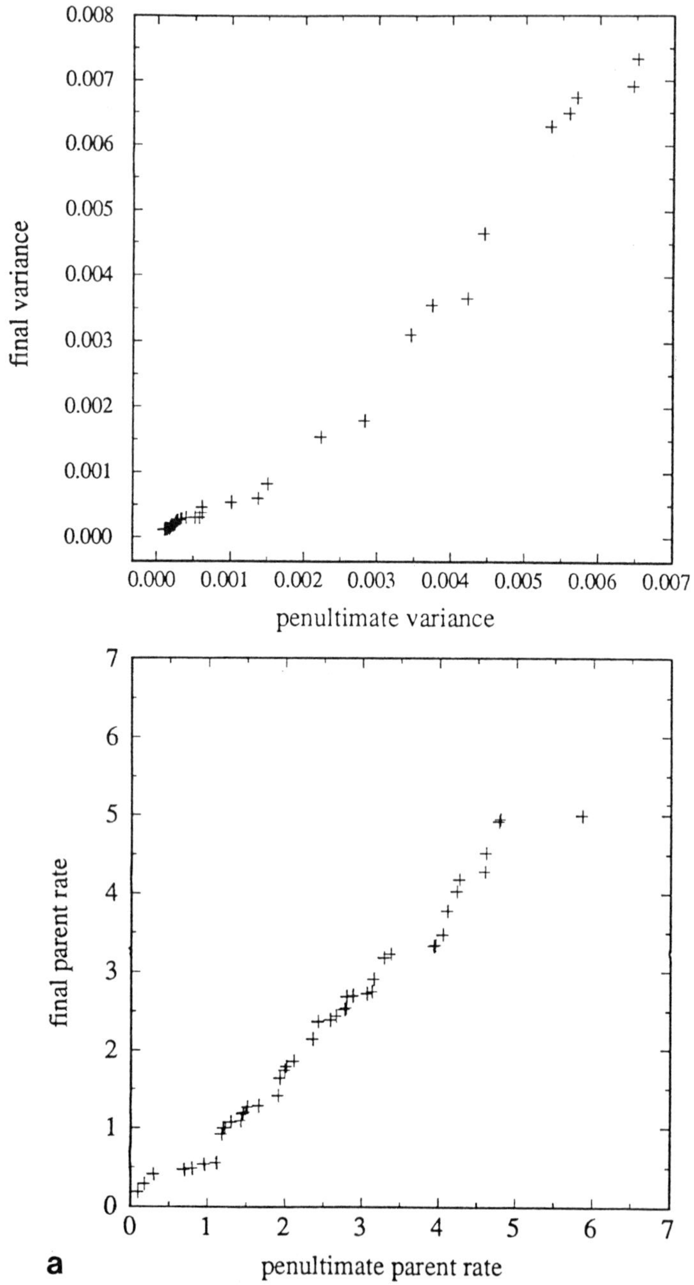

FIG. 5. *Falkirk example: a) parent rate and cluster variance qq plots (last 50-50 iterations.*

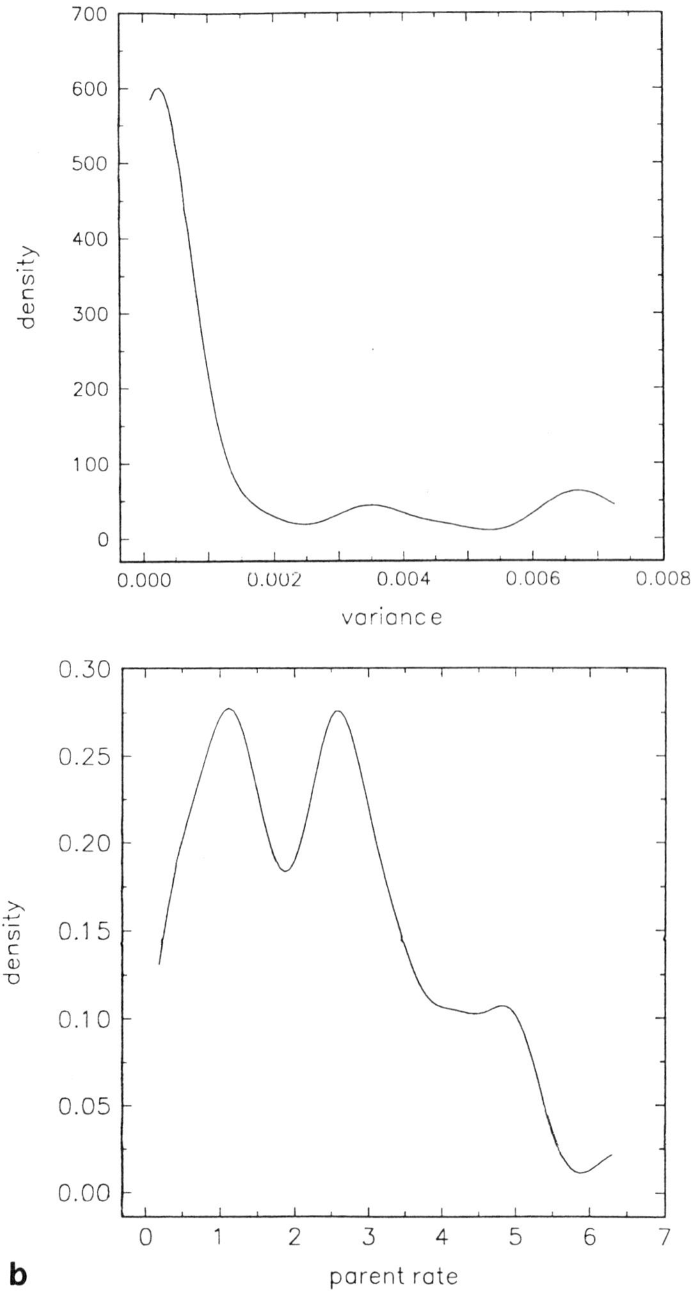

FIG. 5. *Falkirk example: b) posterior marginal densities of parent rate and cluster variance.*

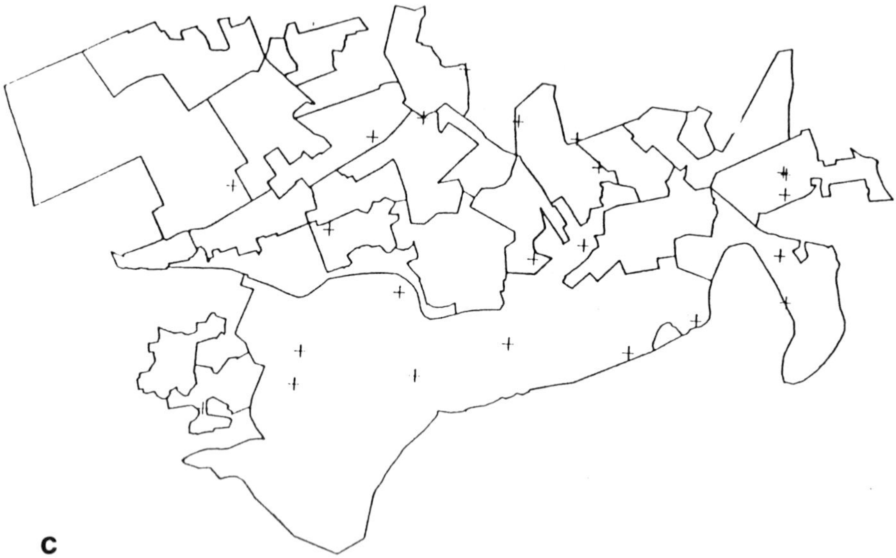

c

FIG. 5. *Falkirk example: c) cluster centre posterior marginal distribution.*

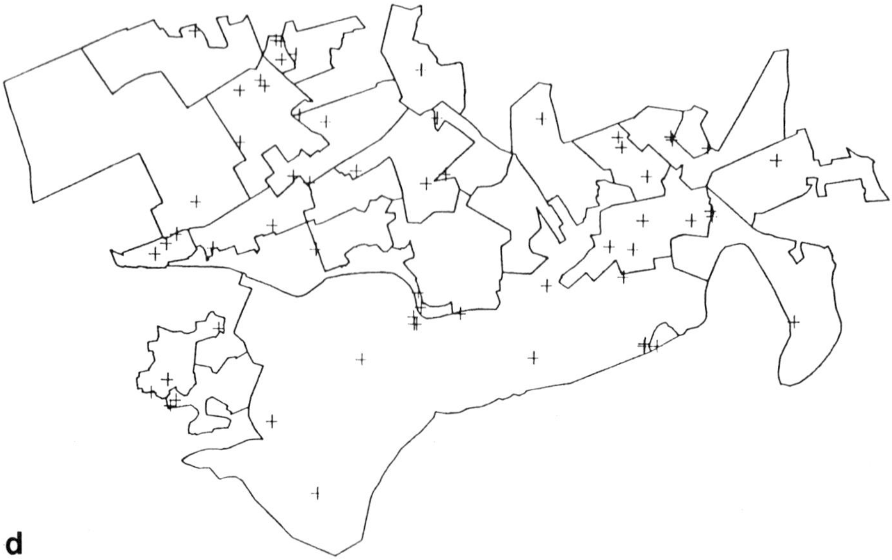

d

FIG. 5. *Falkirk example: d) final iteration z distribution realisation.*

REFERENCES

[1] A. Baddeley and J. Møller. Nearest-neighbour Markov point processes and random sets. *International Statistical Review*, **57**:89–121, 1989.

[2] A.J. Baddeley, H.Y.W. Cheng, A.B. Lawson, M.N.M. van Lieshout, and N.I. Fisher. Extrapolating and interpolating spatial patterns. *submitted*, 1996.

[3] J. Besag and P.J. Green. Spatial statistics and Bayesian computation. *Journal of the Royal Statistical Society, Series B*, **55**:25–37, 1993.

[4] J. Besag and J. Newell. The detection of clusters in rare diseases. *Journal of the Royal Statistical Society, Series A*, **154**:143–155, 1991.

[5] J. Bithell and R. Stone. On statistical methods for analysing the geographical distribution of cancer cases near nuclear installations. *Journal of Epidemiology and Community Health*, **43**:79–85, 1989.

[6] N. Breslow and N. Day. *Statistical Methods in Cancer Research, Volume* **2**: *The design and analysis of Cohort Studies*. International Agency for Research on Cancer, Lyon, 1987.

[7] V. Carstairs. Small area analysis and health service research. *Community Medicine*, **3**:131–139, 1981.

[8] D. Clayton and L. Bernardinelli. Bayesian methods for mapping disease risk. In P. Elliott, J. Cuzick, D. English, and R. Stern, editors, *Geographical and Environmental Epidemiology: Methods for Small-Area Studies*. Oxford University Press, 1992.

[9] J. Cuzick and R. Edwards. Spatial clustering for inhomogeneous populations (with discussion). *Journal of the Royal Statistical Society, series B*, **52**:73–104, 1990.

[10] J. Cuzick and M. Hills. Clustering and clusters-summary. In G. Draper, editor, *Geographical epidemiology of childhood leukaemia and non-hodgkin lymphomas in Great Britain 1966–1983*, pages 123–125. HMSO, London, 1991.

[11] J. Diebolt and C.P. Robert. Estimation of Finite Mixture Distributions through Bayesian Sampling. *Journal of the Royal Statistical Society, series B*, **56**:363–375, 1994.

[12] P. Diggle. *Statistical Analysis of Spatial Point Patterns*. Academic Press, London, 1983.

[13] P. Diggle. A point process modelling approach to raised incidence of a rare phenomenon in the vicinity of a prespecified point. *Journal of the Royal Statistical Society, series A*, **153**:349–362, 1990.

[14] P. Diggle and A. Chetwynd. Second-order analysis of spatial clustering for inhomogeneous populations. *Biom.*, **47**:1155–1163, 1991.

[15] P. Diggle and B. Rowlingson. A conditional approach to point process modelling of elevated risk. *Journal of the Royal Statistical Society, series A*, **157**:433–440, 1994.

[16] P. George. *Automatic Mesh Generation: Applications to Finite Element Methods*. Wiley, New York, 1991.

[17] C. Geyer and J. Møller. Simulation procedures and likelihood inference for spatial point processes. *Scandinavian Jour Statist.*, **21**:84–88, 1994.

[18] P.J. Green. Reversible jump MCMC computation and Bayesian model determination. *Biometrika*, **82**:711–732, 1995.

[19] W. Härdle. *Smoothing Techniques: With Implementation in S*. Springer-Verlag, New York, 1991.

[20] M. Hills and F. Alexander. Statistical methods used in assessing the risk of disease near a source of possible environmental pollution: A review. *Journal of the Royal Statistical Society A*, **152**:353–363, 1989.

[21] H. Inskip, V. Beral, P. Fraser, and P. Haskey. Methods for age-adjustment of rates. *Statistics in Medicine*, **2**:483–493, 1983.

[22] A. Lawson. On the analysis of mortality events around a prespecified fixed point. *Journal of the Royal Statistical Society, series A*, **156(3)**:363–377, 1993.

[23] A. Lawson and F. Williams. Armadale: A case study in environmental epidemiology. *Journal of the Royal Statistical Society, series A*, **157**:285–298, 1994.

[24] A.B. Lawson. On using spatial Gaussian priors to model heterogeneity in environmental epidemiology. *The Statistician*, **43**:69–76, 1994. Proceedings of the Practical Bayesian Statistics Conference.

[25] A.B. Lawson. Markov chain Monte Carlo methods for putative pollution source problems in environmental epidemiology. *Statistics in Medicine*, **14**:2473–2486, 1995.

[26] A.B. Lawson. The analysis of putative sources of hazard in clustered small area data via mcmc methods. *Statistics in Medicine*, 1996, submitted.

[27] A.B. Lawson. Markov chain Monte Carlo methods for spatial cluster processes. In *Computer Science and Statistics: Proceedings of the Interface*, Volume **27**, pages 314–319, 1996.

[28] A.B. Lawson. Cluster Modelling for Small area health data via MCMC methods *Journal of Statistical Planning and Inference (to appear)*, (1999).

[29] A. Lawson, A. Biggeri, D Boehning, E. Lesaffre, J.F. Viel and R Bertollini, editors, *Disease Mapping and Risk Assessment for Public health Decision Making.* Wiley, 1998, to appear.

[30] A.B. Lawson and A.B. Clark. Markov chain Monte Carlo methods for putative sources of hazard and general clustering. In A. Lawson, A. Biggeri, D Boehning, E. Lesaffre, J.F. Viel and R Bertollini, editors, *Disease Mapping and Risk Assessment for Public health Decision Making.* Wiley, 1998, to appear.

[31] A.B. Lawson and L. Waller. A review of point pattern methods for spatial modelling of events around sources of pollution. *Environmetrics*, **7**:471–488, 1996.

[32] A.B. Lawson and F. Williams. Armadale: A case study in environmental epidemiology. *Journal of the Royal Statistical Society A*, **157**:285–298, 1994.

[33] A.B. Lawson and F.L.R. Williams. Spatial competing risk modelling, *submitted*, 1999.

[34] A.B. Lawson and M. Kulldorff. A review of cluster detection methods. In A. Lawson, A. Biggeri, D. Boehning, E. Lesaffre, J.F. Viel and R. Bertollini, editors, *Disease Mapping and Risk Assessment for Public health Decision Making.* Wiley, 1998, to appear.

[35] S. Openshaw, M. Charlton, C. Wymer, and A. Craft. A mark I geographical analysis machine for the automated analysis of point data sets. *International Journal of Geographical Information Systems*, **1**:335–358, 1987.

[36] R.F. Raubertas. Spatial and temporal analysis of disease occurrence for detection of clustering. *Biometrics*, **44**:1121–1129, 1988.

[37] K. Roeder. Density estimation with confidence sets exemplified by superclusters and voids in the galaxies. *Journal of the American Statistical Association*, **85(411)**:617–624, 1990.

[38] R. Stone. Investigations of excess environmental risks around putative sources: Statistical problems and a proposed test. *Statist. Med.*, **7**:649–660, 1988.

[39] T. Tango. A class of tests for detecting 'general' and 'focussed' clustering of rare diseases. *Statistics in Medicine*, **14**:2323–2334, 1995.

[40] M. Tanner. *Tools for Statistical Inference.* Springer Series in Statistics. Springer Verlag, New York, 1996.

[41] A. Whittemore, N. Friend, B. Brown, and E. Holly. A test to detect clusters of disease. *Biometrika*, **74**:631–635, 1987.

A SIMULATION STUDY OF THE EPIDEMIOLOGICAL IMPACT OF AIR POLLUTION: DIAGNOSTICS OF THE CONFOUNDING EFFECTS FOR GENERALIZED LINEAR MODELS

COLIN CHEN*, DAVID P. CHOCK†, AND SANDRA L. WINKLER†

Abstract. Using synthetic data sets, the present study shows the impact of confounding on the estimated coefficients of the covariates and the significance of the estimated coefficients in a generalized linear model. The study also shows how this impact changes with the ranges of the covariates and the sample size. There is qualitative agreement between the study results and the corresponding expressions for the large-sample limit in the ordinary linear models. Modeling bias or misfit is a likely occurrence when regression models are used in an effort to identify the causes of a health outcome in an uncontrolled environment. This occurrence can lead to seriously erroneous conclusions when confounding between the relevant variates or covariates exists. The main effect of confounding for model overfit is a reduction in the significance of the estimated coefficients. The effect of model underfit or misfit, on the other hand, leads to not only erroneous estimated coefficients, but a misguided confidence that the estimated coefficients are significant.

Key words. Generalized linear model, confounding effects.

AMS(MOS) subject classifications. 32E30, 65D05, 93B55, 93C35, 14M15.

1. Introduction. The epidemiological studies in the past few years associating particulate matter (PM, primarily as total suspended particulate or PM_{10} , whose aerodynamic diameter is 10 microns or less) with daily mortality and morbidity (based on hospital admissions and emergency-room visits) have played a key role in shaping the National Ambient Air Quality Standards for particulate matter (including both PM_{10} and $PM_{2.5}$) recently promulgated by the US Environmental Protection Agency. The studies are almost exclusively ecologic time series studies regressing the daily mortality against the ambient air quality for given urban areas (See Ref. [1]). While there are serious and legitimate questions regarding whether outdoor pollutant concentrations and speciations can represent those indoors where individuals spend typically more than 90 percent of their time, and whether they represent actual exposure by an individual, there are other issues pertaining to the validity of the conclusions based on the methodology and the statistical property of the data alone. For example, the choice of covariates, the effect of confounding among the covariates, the sample size, etc., all have a major impact on the conclusion. Analyses and re-analyses of the same or similar data sets for identical urban areas often lead to different or contradictory conclusions [2–11].

*Presently with Department of Statistics, Purdue University, West Lafayette, IN 47907.

†Ford Research Laboratory, P.O. Box 2053, MD-3083, Dearborn, MI 48121-2053.

A typical pairwise scatter plot for the daily ambient air quality and weather data and the daily mortality data is shown in Figure 1. These data are for Pittsburgh (Allegheny County) for all seasons during the period of 1989–1991. The pollutants are all daily-maximum 1h concentrations, with the exception of PM_{10} which is a daily-averaged concentration. The meteorological variables are for the hour of the day when the dry-bulb temperature reaches the maximum. The same-day correlation coefficients between all possible pairs of the variables in Figure 1 are shown in Table 1.

Even though the Table averages out the seasonal effects, there is a strong seasonal dependence in the correlation between several pollutant concentrations. For example, the correlation between ozone (O_3) and PM_{10} is high in the summer (0.66) but very low in the winter (-0.06), as is the O_3 - NO_2 correlation (0.56 in the summer, 0.11 in the winter). On the other hand, the correlation between CO and PM_{10} is moderately high (0.44) in the summer and quite high (0.72) in the winter. The correlations between NO_2 and CO, and between NO_2 and SO_2 do not strongly depend on the season. Also, both O_3 and PM_{10} are well correlated with dry-bulb temperature (0.70 and 0.58, respectively) in the summer but less well correlated (0.34 and 0.30, respectively) in the winter. However, the above information is not critical to our discussion here. What is important is that, because of the high correlation between pairs of several of the potentially important variables, confounding definitely plays a key role in dictating the results of the ecologic time-series studies.

The functional relation between the ambient pollutant concentrations and a health endpoint such as mortality or morbidity is often not clear because of a lack of clinical or animal model studies. This is particularly true in regard to PM. Consequently, a constructed model is likely to have the problem of bias due to underfitting, overfitting or misfitting of the covariates. The impact of this bias on the estimated coefficients of the chosen covariates in an ordinary least squares (OLS) linear model was briefly described by Seber [12]. The large-sample limits of this impact for an OLS model has been provided by Chen and Zhang [13]. In the case of mortality where the counts are discrete integers, most investigators assume a log-linear relation between mortality and the ambient pollutant concentrations. The coefficients of the pollutant concentrations are then estimated by Poisson regression [14] and represent the rates of change of mortality per unit of species concentrations. However, no closed form is available to describe the impact of bias due to underfitting, overfitting and misfitting of covariates on the estimated coefficients of a generalized linear model [14] (GLM). This knowledge has great theoretical and practical importance in view of the role of Poisson regression in the PM epidemiological studies. The purpose of this paper is to investigate how model bias impacts the estimated coefficients, and, more important, how covariate confounding and sample size affect this impact in a Poisson regression. Our approach is, first, to construct synthetic data sets of a Poisson variate whose mean is

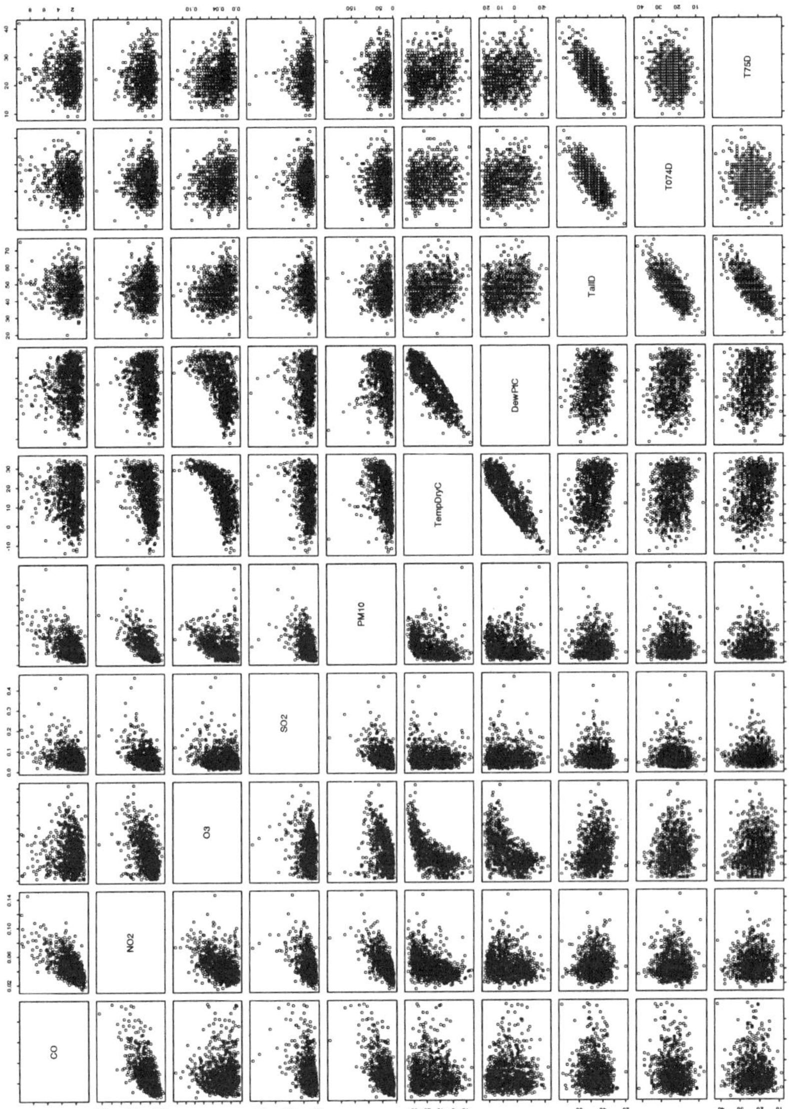

FIG. 1. *Pairwise scatter plots for the daily-maximum hourly concentrations of CO,* NO_2, O_3, SO_2 *(all in ppmV), daily* PM_{10} *(in* $\mu g/m^3$*), daily-maximum dry-bulb temperature and dew point at the time of maximum temperature (both in* $°C$ *), daily mortality from all causes except accidental (TallD), daily mortality for people under 75 (T074D), and daily mortality for people 75 and over (T75D) for Pittsburgh (Allegheny County, PA) during 1989–1991.*

Table 1

	CO	NO_2	O_3	SO_2	PM_{10}	TempDryC	DewPtC	TallD	T074D	T75D
CO	1.0000	0.6213	0.0108	0.3809	0.5910	0.0666	-0.0368	0.1148	0.1198	0.0543
NO_2	0.6213	1.0000	0.4540	0.4395	0.6932	0.4504	0.2109	-0.0560	-0.0279	-0.0559
O_3	0.0108	0.4540	1.0000	0.1745	0.3303	0.7058	0.5197	-0.2113	-0.1286	-0.1886
SO_2	0.3809	0.4395	0.1745	1.0000	0.4653	0.1302	-0.0071	0.0157	0.0224	0.0015
PM_{10}	0.5910	0.6932	0.3303	0.4653	1.0000	0.3766	0.2205	0.0362	0.0378	0.0171
TempDryC	0.0666	0.4504	0.7058	0.1302	0.3766	1.0000	0.8532	-0.2789	-0.1812	-0.2379
DewPtC	-0.0368	0.2109	0.5197	-0.0071	0.2205	0.8532	1.0000	-0.2301	-0.1588	-0.1873
TallD	0.1148	-0.0560	-0.2113	0.0157	0.0362	-0.2789	-0.2301	1.0000	0.7427	0.7634
T074D	0.1198	-0.0279	-0.1286	0.0224	0.0378	-0.1812	-0.1588	0.7427	1.0000	0.1345
T75D	0.0543	-0.0559	-0.1886	0.0015	0.0171	-0.2379	-0.1873	0.7634	0.1345	1.0000

determined by an exact linear model containing no more than two covariates having a range of correlation, and then, to estimate the coefficients of the covariates for a biased Poisson regression model applied to the synthetic data sets. In addition, the sample size will also be varied to see how it influences the t value of the estimated coefficients. Section 2 describes the closed form results for the OLS models. Section 3 describes the protocol for the construction of the synthetic data sets. Section 4 describes the results of different Poisson regressions applied to the data sets. And Section 5 describes our conclusions.

2. Confounding and random effects of covariates for linear models. Before the simulation study of GLM, let's first show some theoretical results for the linear models. Here we only give the results instead of detailed proofs. Interested readers can refer to Chen and Zhang [13]. Consider a linear regression model

$$y = \sum_{j-1}^{p} \beta_j x_j + \epsilon. \tag{2.1}$$

Let $X = (x_1, ..., x_p)^\tau$; ϵ and X are random variable and vector, mutually independent; $E(X) = \underline{\mu}$, $E(\epsilon) = 0$; $var(\epsilon) = \sigma^2$, $\mathrm{VAR}(X) = \Sigma > 0$; β_j, $j = 1, ..., p$ are parameters. Now we get a group of data $(X_i, y_i), i = 1, ..., n, iid$. Suppose that the joint distribution of (X, y) is $F(X, y)$, then $(X_1, y_1) \sim F(X, y)$. The OLS estimator of $\underline{\beta} = (\beta_1, ..., \beta_p)^\tau$ is

$$\hat{\underline{\beta}} = [\mathbf{X}^\tau \mathbf{X}]^{-1} \mathbf{X}^\tau \mathbf{Y}, \tag{2.2}$$

where $\mathbf{Y} = (y_1, ..., y_n)^\tau; \mathbf{X} = (x_{ij})_{n \times p}$.

2.1. Unbiased. If the data are actually generated from a model identical to (2.1), we call (2.1) unbiased for the data. With these assumptions we have in the large-sample limit

$$E(\hat{\underline{\beta}}) = \underline{\beta}, \tag{2.3}$$

$$V(\hat{\underline{\beta}}) \sim \frac{\sigma^2}{n} (\Sigma + \underline{\mu \mu^\tau})^{-1}. \tag{2.4}$$

As a special case with the simple linear model,

$$y = \alpha + \beta x + \epsilon, \tag{2.5}$$

we have

$$E(\hat{\alpha}) = \alpha \ , \qquad E(\hat{\beta}) = \beta, \tag{2.6}$$

$$var(\hat{\alpha}) \sim \frac{\sigma^2}{n}(1+\frac{\mu^2}{\eta^2}), \qquad var(\hat{\beta}) \sim \frac{\sigma^2}{n}\frac{1}{\eta^2}, \tag{2.7}$$

where $E(x) = \mu$ and $var(x) = \eta^2$.

For the case of two covariates without an intercept,

$$y = \beta_1 x_1 + \beta_2 x_2 + \epsilon, \tag{2.8}$$

we have

$$E(\hat{\beta}_1) = \beta_1, \qquad E(\hat{\beta}_2) = \beta_2, \tag{2.9}$$

$$var(\hat{\beta}_1) \sim \frac{\sigma^2}{n}\frac{(\eta_2^2+\mu_2^2)}{((1-\rho^2)\eta_1^2\eta_2^2 + (\eta_1^2\mu_2^2 + \eta_2^2\mu_1^2 - 2\rho\eta_1\eta_2\mu_1\mu_2))}, \tag{2.10}$$

$$var(\hat{\beta}_2) \sim \frac{\sigma^2}{n}\frac{(\eta_1^2+\mu_1^2)}{((1-\rho^2)\eta_1^2\eta_2^2 + (\eta_1^2\mu_2^2 + \eta_2^2\mu_1^2 - 2\rho\eta_1\eta_2\mu_1\mu_2))}, \tag{2.11}$$

where $E(x_1) = \mu_1$, $E(x_2) = \mu_2$, $var(x_1) = \eta_1^2$, $var(x_2) = \eta_2^2$ and $cov(x_1, x_2) = \rho\eta_1\eta_2$.

2.2. Biased. If the data are generated from the model

$$y = \sum_{j=1}^{t} \beta_j x_j + \epsilon \tag{2.12}$$

with $t \neq p$, we call the model (2.1) biased for the data.
Consider the following two biased cases.

For $t > p$, underfit, we have in the large-sample limit,

$$E(\hat{\underline{\beta}}) \sim \underline{\beta} + V_X{}^{-1} V_{XZ}\underline{\gamma}, \tag{2.13}$$

$$V(\hat{\underline{\beta}}) \sim \frac{1}{n}[\sigma^2 + tr(V_Z - V_{ZX}V_X{}^{-1}V_{XZ})(\underline{\gamma}^\tau\underline{\gamma})]V_X^{-1}, \tag{2.14}$$

where $V_X = E(XX^\tau)$, $V_Z = E(ZZ^\tau)$, $V_{ZX} = E(ZX^\tau)$ and $V_{XZ} = E(XZ^\tau)$ with $Z = (x_{p+1}, ..., x_t)^\tau$ and $\underline{\gamma} = (\beta_{p+1}, ..., \beta_t)^\tau$.

For $t = 2$ and $p = 1$, X and Z are both one dimensional random variables. We have

$$E(\hat{\beta}) \sim \beta + \frac{\rho\eta_x\eta_z + \mu_x\mu_z}{\eta_x^2 + \mu_x^2}\gamma, \tag{2.15}$$

$$var(\hat{\beta}) \sim \frac{1}{n}\frac{(\sigma^2 + (\eta_z^2 + \mu_z^2 - (\rho\eta_x\eta_z + \mu_x\mu_z)^2(\eta_x^2+\mu_x^2)^{-1})\gamma^2)}{(\eta_x^2+\mu_x^2)}, \tag{2.16}$$

where $E(x) = \mu_x$, $E(z) = \mu_z$, $var(x) = \eta_x^2$, $var(z) = \eta_z^2$ and $cov(x, z) = \rho\eta_x\eta_z$.

For $t < p$, overfit, we have in the large-sample limit,

$$E(\underline{\hat{\beta}}) = (\beta_{1\times t}, 0_{1\times(p-t)})^{\tau}, \tag{2.17}$$

$$V(\underline{\hat{\beta}}) \sim \frac{\sigma^2}{n} V_X^{-1}. \tag{2.18}$$

For $t = 1$ and $p = 2$, we have

$$E(\hat{\beta}_1) = \beta, \qquad E(\hat{\beta}_2) = 0. \tag{2.19}$$

For variances we have the same results as in (2.10) and (2.11),

$$var(\hat{\beta}_1) \sim \frac{\sigma^2}{n} \frac{(\eta_2^2 + \mu_2^2)}{((1-\rho^2)\eta_1^2\eta_2^2 + (\eta_1^2\mu_2^2 + \eta_2^2\mu_1^2 - 2\rho\eta_1\eta_2\mu_1\mu_2))},$$

$$var(\hat{\beta}_2) \sim \frac{\sigma^2}{n} \frac{(\eta_1^2 + \mu_1^2)}{((1-\rho^2)\eta_1^2\eta_2^2 + (\eta_1^2\mu_2^2 + \eta_2^2\mu_1^2 - 2\rho\eta_1\eta_2\mu_1\mu_2))},$$

where $E(x_1) = \mu_1$, $E(x_2) = \mu_2$, $var(x_1) = \eta_1^2$, $var(x_2) = \eta_2^2$ and $cov(x_1, x_2) = \rho\eta_1\eta_2$.

2.3. Misfit. If the data are generated by covariates X_1 but we fit the model using X_2, then we have in the large-sample limit,

$$E(\underline{\hat{\beta}}) = V_{X_2}^{-1} V_{X_2X_1} \underline{\beta_1}, \tag{2.20}$$

$$V(\underline{\hat{\beta}}) \sim \frac{1}{n}\left[\sigma^2 + tr(V_{X_1} - V_{X_1X_2} V_{X_2}{}^{-1} V_{X_2X_1})(\underline{\beta_1}^{\tau}\underline{\beta_1})\right] V_{X_2}^{-1}, \tag{2.21}$$

where $V_{X_1} = E(X_1X_1^{\tau})$, $V_{X_2} = E(X_2X_2^{\tau})$, $V_{X_1X_2} = E(X_1X_2^{\tau})$ and $V_{X_2X_1} = E(X_2X_1^{\tau})$.

If X_1 and X_2 are one dimensional variables, we have

$$E(\hat{\beta}) = \frac{\rho\eta_1\eta_2 + \mu_1\mu_2}{\eta_2^2 + \mu_2^2}, \tag{2.22}$$

$$V(\hat{\beta}) \sim \frac{1}{n} \frac{(\sigma^2 + (\eta_1^2 + \mu_1^2 - (\rho\eta_2\eta_1 + \mu_2\mu_1)^2(\eta_2^2 + \mu_2^2)^{-1})\beta_1^2)}{(\eta_2^2 + \mu_2^2)}, \tag{2.23}$$

where $E(x_1) = \mu_1$, $E(x_2) = \mu_2$, $var(x_1) = \eta_1^2$, $var(x_2) = \eta_2^2$ and $cov(x_1, x_2) = \rho\eta_1\eta_2$.

3. Protocol for the construction of synthetic data sets. In the simulations, no more than two covariates were considered. The two covariates, x_1 and x_2, could be considered as corresponding to, say, PM_{10} and CO, respectively. The dependent variable, y, could be considered as the daily mortality. In generating the synthetic data, we assumed an exact log-linear relationship between y and x_i, with the coefficients for x_i being $\beta_1 = 0.0005$ and $\beta_2 = 0.005$. If we assumed the units of $\mu g/m^3$and ppmV, respectively, for x_1 and x_2, then these coefficients are approximately the estimated coefficients from the Poisson regression of the daily mortality of people at age 75 or over against PM_{10} and CO in Pittsburgh during 1989–1991 [15]. The average daily mortality for this age group was 22.93. We assumed this number to represent the intercept, α, being equal to 3.132446 in the exact log-linear model. The chosen coefficients above should be considered hypothetical since they themselves were estimated in the presence of confounding and the significance of the estimates is highly model dependent [15].

Both x_1 and x_2 were assumed to follow a bivariate lognormal distribution with means and standard deviations extracted from the logarithmically transformed PM_{10} and CO data for Pittsburgh during 1989–1991. In the logarithmic space, the corresponding means were 3.5 and 0.87, and the corresponding standard deviations were 0.619 and 0.475 for x_1 and x_2, respectively. In the concentration space, the above information essentially recovers the observed means of 40.22 $\mu g/m^3$and 2.68 ppmV, and the observed standard deviations of 26.25 $\mu g/m^3$and 1.41 ppmV for PM_{10} and CO, respectively. In the generation of the synthetic data sets, the standard deviation of x_1 in the logarithmic space , denoted η_1, was held fixed at 0.6 while that of x_2, denoted η_2, was allowed to vary from 0.2 to 1.0. With both η_1 and η_2 being ≤ 1, the corresponding standard deviations in the concentration space are roughly proportional to η_1 and η_2, respectively. As a measure of confounding between two variates, the correlation coefficient, ρ, between the variates in the logarithmic space was also allowed to vary. Again, because of the small (but realistic) values chosen for both η_1 and η_2, the correlation coefficients between the two variates in the concentration space are typically no more than 10 percent less than ρ when $\rho = 0.5$ or 0.9 and are essentially 0 when $\rho = 0$. Since the correlation coefficients between any two explanatory variables in Table 1 are generally positive, only positive ρs were considered in our simulations. For each realization, the values of x_1 and x_2 in the logarithmic space were generated using an S-Plus random number generator for a bivariate normal distribution on an IBM RS6000 computer. The antilogarithms of these values were used to determine the value, m, of an exact model, $log(m) = \alpha + \beta_1 x_1 + \beta_2 x_2$. In fact, m plays the role of the daily mortality. It serves as the mean of the Poisson variate, y, which was generated using the S-Plus random number generator for the Poisson distribution. A collection of y values with a sample size, n, constitutes the synthetic data set to be used for Poisson regression:

$$log(E(y)) = \alpha + \beta_1 x_1 + \beta_2 x_2. \tag{3.1}$$

The sample size was also allowed to vary from 365 to 7 times 365, corresponding to a period of 1 to 7 years. Note also that seasonal behavior and long-term trends were not considered in the data sets. To assure that the results of the Poisson regressions were stable, the procedure for each synthetic data set generation and the subsequent regression was performed for a total of 100 times. The means of the 100 repetitions are reported in the Results section. No significant differences were found between the means with 100 repetitions and those with 1000 repetitions.

To study the impact of model underfit, the synthetic data set was constructed using the exact model for x_1 and x_2, while the regression model assumed only x_1 as the covariate. For model overfit, the synthetic data set was constructed from an exact model using only x_1 while the regression model assumed both x_1 and x_2 to be the covariates. For model misfit, two cases were considered. First, the synthetic data set was based on only x_1 while the regression model contained only x_2 as the covariate. Second, only x_2 was used in the synthetic data set while only x_1 was the covariate in the regression. The latter is not equivalent to the former because we always allowed only the range of x_2 to vary.

4. Results. The impact of (1) confounding or correlation between x_1 and x_2, (2) the data range or standard deviation of x_2, and (3) the sample size, on the outcome of the Poisson regression will be presented in the same order as in Section 2 above. The outcome is represented by the estimates of the coefficients, $E(\hat{\beta}_i)$, and their respective t values. A t value ≥ 2 is considered significant. In all cases, the overdispersion parameter, estimated as the residual deviance divided by the model degrees of freedom, is within 1 percent of 1.

4.1. Unbiased. Both $E(\hat{\beta}_1)$ and $E(\hat{\beta}_2)$ are not impacted by the correlation between the two covariates. The estimates are not significantly different from the coefficients of the exact model. This is consistent with (2.9) for the ordinary linear models. However, both $t(\hat{\beta}_1)$ and $t(\hat{\beta}_2)$ decrease with increasing ρ. This is qualitatively consistent with the increasing variance of the estimated coefficients when ρ increases in (2.10) and (2.11) for the ordinary linear models. Also, for the parameters used in the exact model, (2.10) indicates a weak dependence of $t(\hat{\beta}_1)$ on η_2 (the range of x_2) while (2.11) indicates an essentially linear dependence of $t(\hat{\beta}_2)$ on η_2. Figure 2 shows both $t(\hat{\beta}_1)$ and $t(\hat{\beta}_2)$ as a function of n, ρ and η_2. From the Figure, one sees that the dependence of $t(\hat{\beta}_2)$ on η_2 is not linear.

There is no major qualitative difference in the behavior of the estimated coefficients between the ordinary linear model and the Poisson

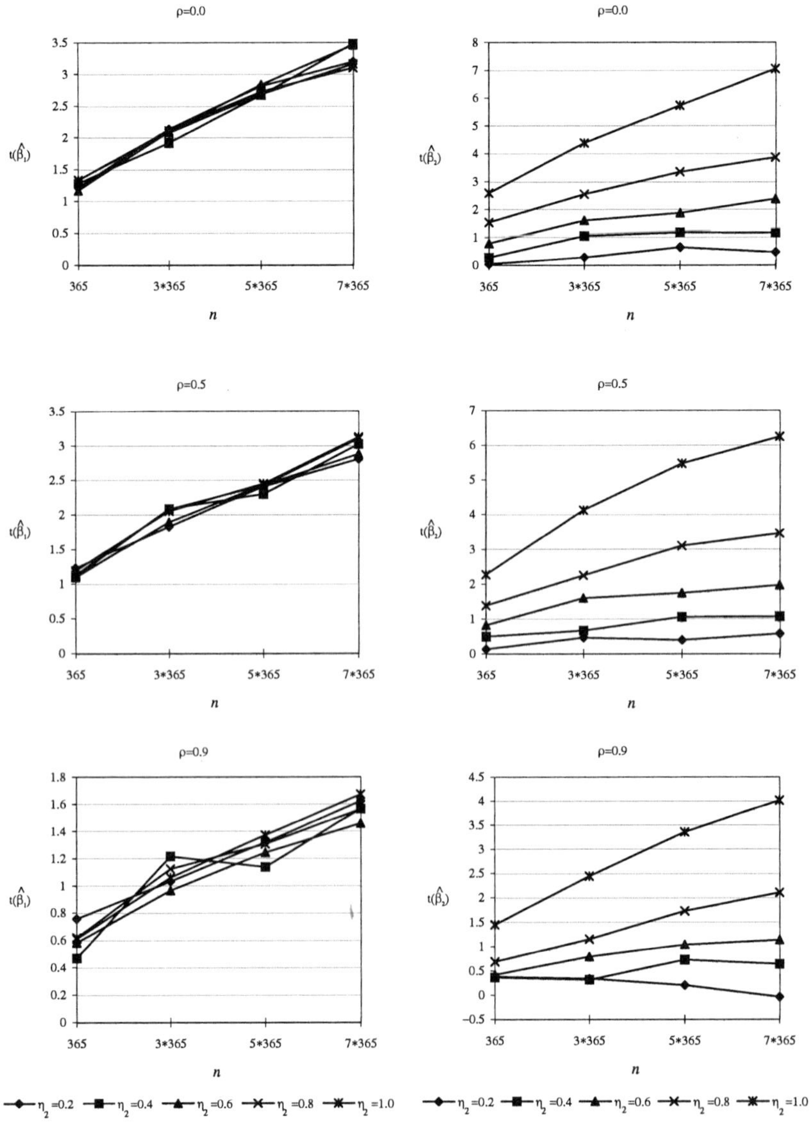

FIG. 2. *Behavior of $t(\hat{\beta}_1)$ and $t(\hat{\beta}_2)$ as a function of n, η_2, and ρ for an unbiased Poisson regression using the same covariates as the exact model.*

regression when all causal variates are covariates in the regression model. An unbiased regression model can recover the estimated coefficients of the covariates. But if the correlation among the covariates increases, the significance of the estimated coefficients decreases.

4.2. Biased. In the underfit case, the synthetic data sets contain the effect of both x_1 and x_2 while the regression model contains only x_1 as the covariate. In the ordinary linear regression, (2.15) indicates that $E(\hat{\beta}_1)$ increases with ρ and η_2, or more precisely, $E(\hat{\beta}_1)$ is asymptotically linearly related to $\rho\eta_2$. This is qualitatively consistent with a nearly linear relation observed in the Poisson regression (See Fig. 3). The estimated coefficient departs significantly from the β_1 of the exact model as ρ and η_2 increase. The variance of $\hat{\beta}_1$ decreases with ρ in the asymptotic expression (2.16) for the ordinary linear model. This is again consistent with the simulation result that $t(\hat{\beta}_1)$ increases with ρ. In addition, $t(\hat{\beta}_1)$ also increases with η_2, as expected, and this increase is enhanced by an increasing ρ (See Fig. 3). As the sample size increases, $t(\hat{\beta}_1)$ increases as well (See Figs. 3 and 4). If x_2 were used in the regression model, then, based on (2.15) and (2.16) and the parameters of the exact model, one would expect $E(\hat{\beta}_2)$ to be essentially proportional to ρ/η_2 and $t(\hat{\beta}_2)$ to again increase with ρ.

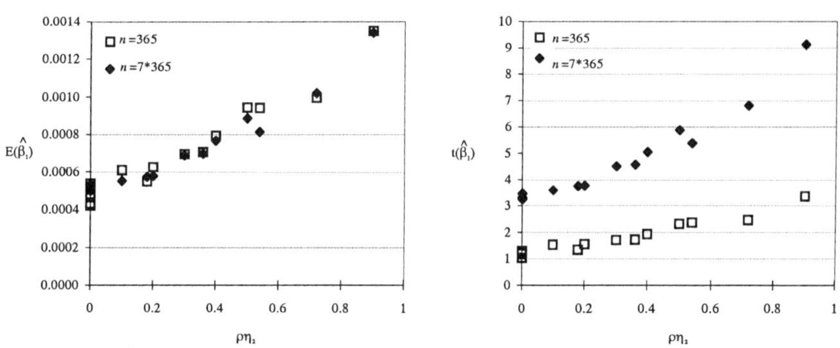

FIG. 3. *Behavior of* $E(\hat{\beta}_1)$ *and* $t(\hat{\beta}_1)$ *as a function of* $\rho\eta_2$, *and* n *for an underfitting Poisson regression containing* x_1 *as the covariate to describe data created from an exact model containing* x_1 *and* x_2.

The above result has a profound implication insofar as the PM mortality studies are concerned. Underfitting is very likely when the number of covariates used is small. If a causal variate is missing in the regression model and the variate is highly correlated with a covariate in the regression model, then the regression model will indicate a strong but erroneous association of the dependent variable or effect (say, daily mortality) with the covariate. In fact, the estimated coefficient of the covariate will be compromised by the size of the actual coefficient of the missing variate, the range of the missing variate, as well as the magnitude of the correlation coefficient between the covariate and the missing variate. In addition, a large sample size (say, several years of data) actually makes the erroneous association appear more convincing.

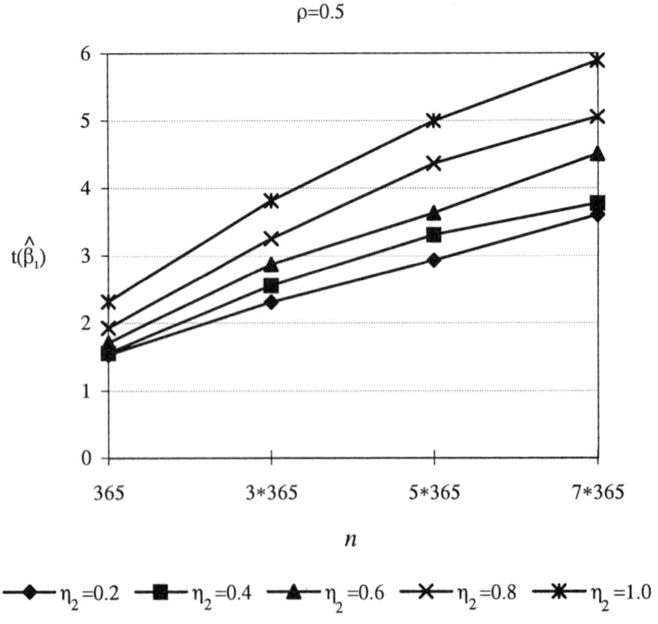

FIG. 4. *Behavior of* $t(\hat{\beta}_1)$ *as a function of* n *and* η_2*, given* $\rho = 0.5$*, for an underfitting Poisson regression containing* x_1 *as the covariate to describe data created from an exact model containing* x_1 *and* x_2*.*

In the overfit case, the synthetic data sets were constructed using only x_1 while the regression model contains both x_1 and x_2 as the covariates. In agreement with (2.19) for the ordinary linear regression, the estimated coefficients of both covariates are not significantly different from their exact values, being zero for $E(\hat{\beta}_2)$. They are not affected by the correlation coefficient between the two covariates. The $t(\hat{\beta}_1)$, on the other hand, decreases with increasing ρ, and does not depend strongly on η_2. Figure 5 shows $t(\hat{\beta}_1)$ as a function of ρ and n, with η_2 held constant at 0.2. As expected, $t(\hat{\beta}_2)$ is essentially zero. If the exact model contains only x_2 , one expects $t(\hat{\beta}_1)$ to be unaffected by η_2, $t(\hat{\beta}_2)$ to be increasing with η_2 and both to be decreasing with ρ.

The above result indicates that overfitting should not lead to a serious bias in the estimated coefficients of the covariates; but the correlation between the causal and redundant covariates will reduce the significance of the estimates of both types of covariates.

4.3. Misfit. In the first misfit case, x_1 was used in the exact model and x_2 was the covariate in the regression model. Even though x_2 plays no role in the dependent variable of the synthetic data sets, in the regression model, x_2 influences $E(\hat{\beta}_2)$ and $t(\hat{\beta}_2)$ through ρ. For the ordinary linear regression, (2.22) shows that $E(\hat{\beta}_2)$ increases with increasing ρ and decreases with increasing η_2. Figure 6 shows $E(\hat{\beta}_2)$ as a function of ρ/η_2. The magnitude of the estimated coefficient is linked to the values of x_2 and y, though the linkage has no causal implication. The significance of the estimate, $t(\hat{\beta}_2)$, increases with ρ and n, but not clearly with η_2 (See Fig. 7).

In the second misfit case, x_2 was used in the exact model and x_1 was the covariate in the regression model. In this case, the variation in η_2 directly impacts the dependent variable in the synthetic data sets. Figure 8 shows a plot of $E(\hat{\beta}_1)$ as a function of $\rho\eta_2$. The departure from linearity is somewhat at variance with the linear relation indicated in (2.22) for the parameters of the exact model. Again, no causal meaning can be attached to the magnitude of the estimated coefficient. Even so, Figure 9 shows that $t(\hat{\beta}_1)$ can be large and increase with ρ and η_2, in contrast with $t(\hat{\beta}_2)$ above, which has little or no dependence on η_2.

Model misfit is again a likely common occurrence. The result of the misfit is a set of totally meaningless estimated coefficients, yet with increasing significance as the sample size increases and as the correlation between the covariates and the true causal variates increases. The potential for misleading inference in model misfit in epidemiological studies cannot be overemphasized.

5. Conclusion. Using synthetic data sets, the present study shows the impact of confounding on the estimated coefficients of the covariates and the significance of the estimated coefficients in a generalized linear model. The study also shows how this impact changes with the ranges of the covariates and the sample size. There is qualitative agreement between the study results and the expressions for the large-sample limit in the ordinary linear models. The study results are highly relevant to the present active investigations of an association between ambient air pollutant concentrations, especially PM, and daily mortality and morbidity.

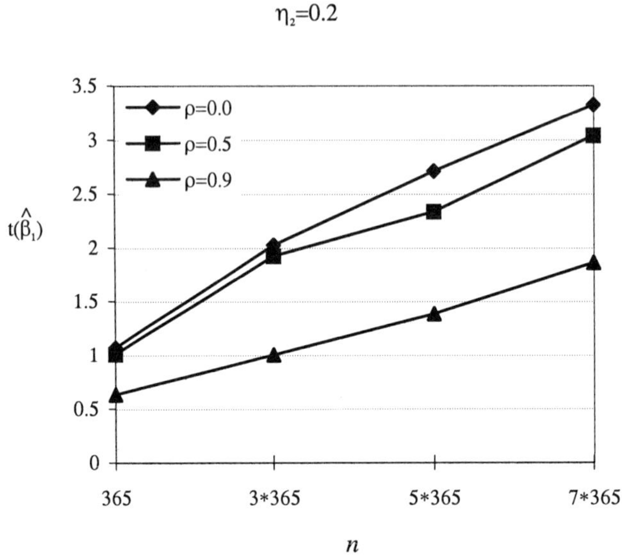

FIG. 5. *Behavior of $t(\hat{\beta}_1)$ as a function of n and ρ, given $\eta_2 = 0.2$, for an overfitting Poisson regression containing x_1 and x_2 as the covariates to describe data created from an exact model containing x_1.*

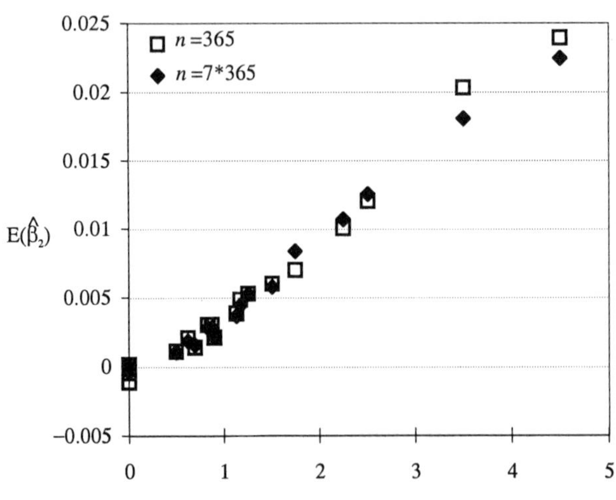

FIG. 6. *Behavior of $E(\hat{\beta}_2)$ as a function of n and ρ/η_2 for a misfitting Poisson regression containing x_2 as the covariate to describe data created from an exact model containing x_1.*

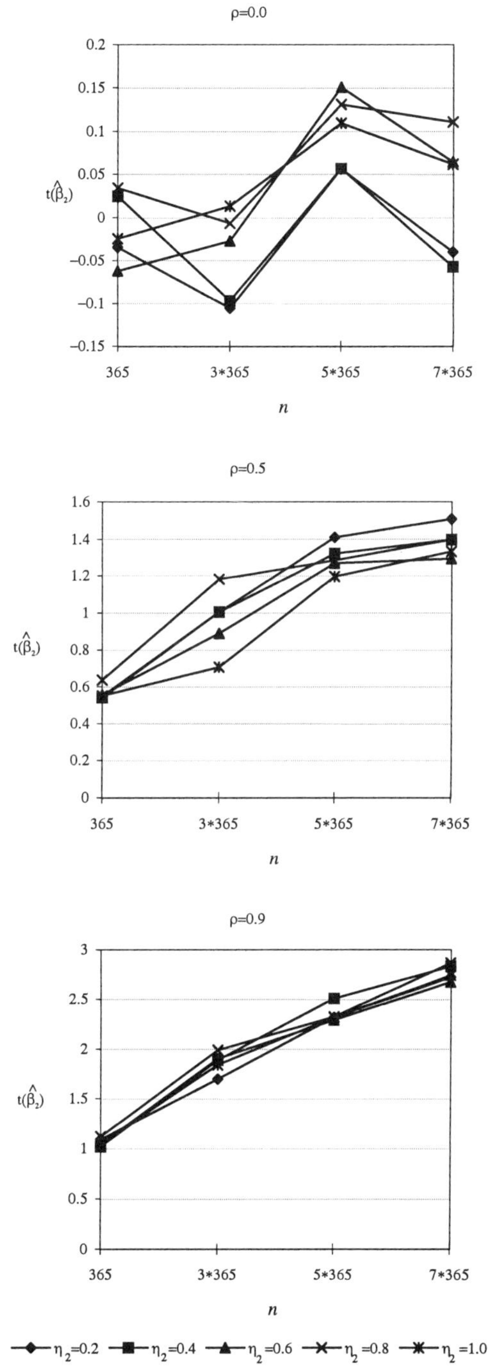

FIG. 7. *Behavior of* $t(\hat{\beta}_2)$ *as a function of* n, η_2 *and* ρ *for a misfitting Poisson regression containing* x_2 *as the covariate to describe data created from an exact model containing* x_1.

Modeling bias or misfit is a likely occurrence when regression models are used in an effort to identify the likely causes of a health outcome in an uncontrolled environment. This occurrence can lead to seriously erroneous conclusions when confounding between the relevant variates or covariates exists. The main effect of confounding for model overfit is a reduction of the significance of the estimated coefficients. The effect of model underfit or misfit — a more common occurrence, on the other hand, leads to not only erroneous estimated coefficients, but a misguided confidence that the estimated coefficients are significant.

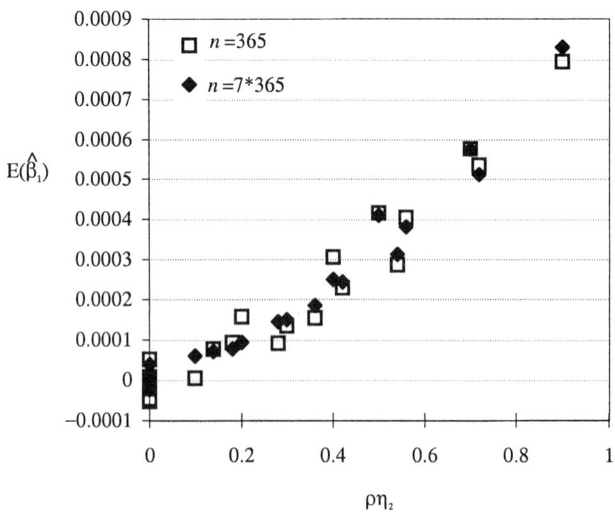

FIG. 8. *Behavior of* $E(\hat{\beta}_1)$ *as a function of* $\rho\eta_2$ *and* n *for a misfitting Poisson regression containing* x_1 *as the covariate to describe data created from an exact model containing* x_2.

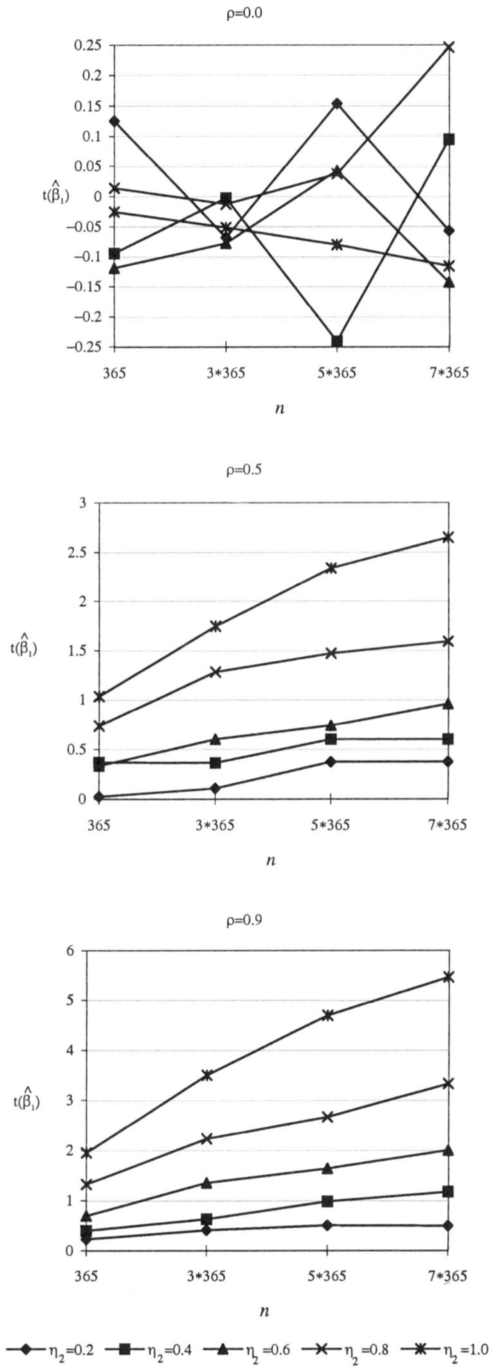

FIG. 9. *Behavior of $t(\hat{\beta}_1)$ as a function of n, η_2 and ρ for a misfitting Poisson regression containing x_1 as the covariate to describe data created from an exact model containing x_2.*

REFERENCES

[1] VEDAL, S., *Ambient particulates and health: Lines that divide*, J. Air and Waste Manage. Assoc., 1997, **47**, 551–581.

[2] SCHWARTZ, J. AND DOCKERY, D.W., *Increased mortality in Philadelphia associated with daily air pollution concentrations*, Am. Rev. Respir. Dis., 1992, **145**, 600–604.

[3] MOOLGAVKAR, S.H.; LUEBECK, E.G AND HALL, T.A. ANDERSON, *Air pollution and daily mortality in Philadelphia*, Epidemiology, 1995, **6**, 476–484.

[4] SAMET, J.M.; ZEGER, S.L. AND BERHANE, K., *The association of mortality and particulate air pollution,* In *Particulate Air Pollution and Daily Mortality: Replication and Validation of Selected Studies. The Phase I Report of the Particle Epidemiology Evaluation Project,* Health Effects Institute, August 1995.

[5] MOOLGAVKAR, S.H. AND LUEBECK, E.G., *A critical review of the evidence on particulate air pollution and mortality*, Epidemiology, 1996, **7**, 420–428.

[6] SAMET, J.M.; ZEGER, S.L.; KELSALL, J.E.; XU, J. AND KALKSTEIN, L.S., *Air pollution, weather, and mortality in Philadelphia 1973–1988,* In *Particulate Air Pollution and Daily Mortality: Analyses of the Effects of Weather and Multiple Air Pollutants. The Phase I.B Report of the Particle Epidemiology Evaluation Project,* Health Effects Institute, March 1997.

[7] SCHWARTZ, J. AND DOCKERY, D.W., *Particulate air pollution and daily mortality in Steubenville, Ohio*, Am. J. Epidemiology, 1992, **135**, 12–19.

[8] SCHWARTZ, J., *Air pollution and daily mortality in Birmingham, Alabama*, Am. J. Epidemiology, 1993, **137**, 1136–1147.

[9] DAVIS, J.M.; SACKS, J.; SALTZMAN, N.; SMITH, R.L. AND STYER, P., *Airborne particulate matter and daily mortality in Birmingham, Alabama,* National Institute of Statistical Science, Tech. Rept. #**55**, 1996.

[10] MOOLGAVKAR, S.H.; LUEBECK, E.G.; HALL, T.A. AND ANDERSON, E.L., *Particulate air pollution, sulfur dioxide, and daily mortality: a reanalysis of the Steubenville data*, Inhalation Toxicol., 1995, **7**, 35–44.

[11] LIPFERT, F.W. AND WYZGA, R.E., *Air pollution and mortality: issues and uncertainties,* J. Air and Waste Manage. Assoc., 1995, **45**, 949–966.

[12] SEBER, G.A.F., *Linear Regression Analysis*, John Wiley & Sons, Inc., New York, 1977.

[13] CHEN C. AND ZHANG, Y.G., *Large Sample Properties of A Series Estimators of Cross-Validation in Linear Regression Models*, Purdue University, Dept. of Stat., Tech. Rept. #**96-19**, 1996.

[14] MCCULLAGH, P. AND NELDER, J.A., *Generalized Linear Models.*, Second Ed. Chapman & Hall, London., 1989.

[15] CHOCK, D.P.; CHEN, C. AND WINKLER, S.L., *A Study of the Association between Daily Mortality and Air Pollutant Concentrations in Pittsburgh*, 1989–1991, In Preparation for publication.

THE USE OF REFERENCE PRIORS AND BAYES FACTORS IN THE ANALYSIS OF CLINICAL TRIALS

DALENE STANGL*

1. Introduction. This paper was motivated by foundational issues that underlie the application of Bayesian methods. Advances in numerical methods and computation make applying Bayesian methods relatively easy, so now as a discipline we can step back and contemplate what these new tools will allow us to do with respect to the theoretical foundations of our work, and if desired, adjust our actions accordingly. The foundational issues that this paper will address are the use of reference priors and the use of Bayes factors in the analysis of clinical trials. The question that merges these two foundational issues is "Should data analysis and decision-making be approached as two separate tasks or should there be a seamless integration with each stage of the clinical trial being viewed as a subsequent step in a sequential decision-making problem?"

A clinical trial is an experiment on humans to evaluate one or more interventions or therapies. We categorize clinical trials into three groups. Phase I trials seek an acceptable dose and schedule with respect to toxicity for a new treatment being tried on humans for the first time. Phase II trials determine if the therapy has any beneficial effect. Phase III trials compare one or more experimental therapies with the best standard therapy or competitive therapies. Each of these phases is structured to address a set of sequential questions: whether to start, how to proceed, what to conclude, and what to do with the results. Each question asks for a decision and requires an assessment of utilities on competing actions. Movement to the next phase cannot ensue without decisions being made at the previous. From the Bayesian viewpoint decisions require incorporating all previous information along with information in the current trial within a decision theoretic framework. Yet a persistent view, even within the set of statistician who are avowedly Bayesian, is that the results the statistician should provide are only those represented by the current data and that any conclusions drawn from those results should correspond to the implicit conventional utilities passed on from the frequentist paradigm. More simply, current data results should be presented distinctly and separately from decision making. In applying Bayesian methods to the analysis of clinical trials, this view has encouraged the use of reference priors and focused attention towards model fitting while diverting efforts away from amalgamating what we know and using it in a coherent fashion to help decision making. This paper argues that by adopting the commonplace use

*Institute of Statistics and Decision Sciences, Duke University, Durham, NC 27708–0251.

of reference priors and Bayes' factors the Bayesian community has moved too much in accord with the separatist view.

This paper begins with a discussion of reference priors and methods for checking sensitivity to priors. The discussion of reference priors will be followed by a discussion of Bayes factors for model fitting and testing of parameters. The paper examines what these methods offer and where they fall short, and suggests alternatives. It will be argued that these alternatives do better at integrating data analysis with decision making, and that this is the direction that the analysis of clinical trials should move.

2. Reference priors. In this paper the label 'reference prior' will be used to describe any prior other than those based on someone's beliefs or past data. This includes any prior that helps the statistician get through Bayes theorem while absolving anyone from the responsibility of quantifying what previous and often conflicting evidence suggests while allowing research participants and consumers to set aside the notion that the probabilities calculated are still subjective belief.

Some of the most commonly used 'reference' priors are described here. Jeffreys' priors arise from the principle that any rule for defining prior densities should yield an equivalent result if applied to a transformed parameter. To get such priors we take the prior proportional to the square root of the Fisher information for the parameter of interest. Flat, constant or uniform priors entail picking a plausible range for the parameter and placing uniform probability across this range. The skeptical/enthusiastic continuum of priors developed by Spiegelhalter and colleagues generates a set of priors; ranging from those that represent the belief of a person that would be hard to convince of a treatment effect, to those that represent the belief of a person that is already pretty sure that there is a treatment effect. A fourth type of reference prior is the point-mass prior. These priors place a point mass on the null hypothesis of no treatment effect and are an attempt to make the prior more conservative to prevent rejecting the null hypothesis too hastily. Point-mass priors also allow us to get positive posterior probability on the point null hypothesis. The last type of reference prior to be mentioned here include all the current-data-dependent priors. These priors use the current data to define priors. For example, the data is used to make the central location of the prior consistent with the likelihood and then variance is added. These methods adapt the empirical Bayes methods that simply use method-of-moments or maximum likelihood methods to give estimates of prior parameters, but they improve upon them by including uncertainty about the prior parameters. This type of prior includes the unit information priors that center the prior near the maximum likelihood estimate and set the concentration about the same as the concentration of the likelihood after one observation.

In perusing journals and attending conference presentations, it is apparent that reference priors are being used to the exclusion of modeling anything known apriori. Indeed one of the greatest advantages to a Bayesian approach is its ability to model what is known going into a clinical trial. Yet this advantage is not being realized. Most analysis is in the opposite direction, sometimes to the point of putting a reference prior on the whole real line when noncontroversial evidence exists that the effect is positive. So why are we so unwilling to make use of prior information?

One major reason for the use of reference priors rather than making use of prior information is the pressure to present Bayesian analysis analogous to frequentist methods. It is hard to break convention. A second reason is that specifying well thought out prior distributions is a time-consuming task for which there are no agreed upon conventions to guide us. Who's beliefs should be elicited and which historical data should be included are open to debate. Even some of the more informative reference priors are met with hesitation. Quoting Gail, (1995)

> "...Obtaining consensus on what constitutes a skeptical prior... will depend on the context and application. Unless some conventions become widely acceptable, these requirements may inhibit widespread use of these methods."

Beyond time and convention constraints, informative priors are easy targets for reviewer critique regardless how much care and thought goes into them. The search for automatic procedures obviating the need for priors on parameters is a less-risky proposition. Hence we turn to reference priors that allow us to make inferences without quantifying what past evidence tells us.

Another justification put forth in an ASA invited talk on Bayesian methods in clinical trials (Greenhouse and Wasserman, 1995b) put forth the following rationale for reference priors:

> "Even die-hard subjectivists who dislike the idea of using reference priors can still find it useful to begin an analysis with the reference priors. The reference prior analysis together with simple sensitivity tools leads to an understanding of which priors are important in the problem".

This argument is specious. Most often we do not need to do any analysis at all to know that our data will have less information about certain parameters and that conclusions about particular parameters will be more sensitive to the prior. We only needed thought, not reference prior analysis to tell us this.

A final justification relies on sensitivity analysis and argues that for inferences to be convincing they must hold across a range of priors. This is the argument applied by Spiegelhalter to support the skeptic/enthusiastic continuum. This argument is convincing and hard to argue against. Yet, if this is true, why do we allow such superficial sensitivity analysis, and why are we not equally rigorous in demanding sensitivity analysis for the utilities that guide our conclusions?

Sensitivity analysis is being used as a substitute for carefully thinking through and justifying priors. Somehow we have developed the attitude that adjusting a few priors one at a time should give us a sense of security in our answers. Are we providing a false sense of security? Typically the assumption that is altered is the variance in the prior for each parameter. We increase the variance, giving more or less weight to the data, to see whether this changes our results. However, we ignore many other model assumptions. Rarely do sensitivity analysis check other assumptions such as the central location, the presence of symmetry, and the dependence between parameters? Only a very limited area in the parameter space is checked, but then it is argued that results are robust to the prior specification. With this tack, sensitivity analysis can not serve as an effective substitute for careful thought and modeling of what is know apriori.

Several other tacks being promoted to get around the specification of priors are the methods that allow one to judge the sensitivity of results by looking at classes of priors (Berger, 1990, Wasserman, 1992, and Greenhouse and Wasserman, 1995b) and partitioning priors into subspaces which either support or do not support the null hypothesis (Carlin et al., 1995, Carlin and Louis, 1996, Sargent and Carlin, 1996). Greenhouse and Wasserman (1995b) demonstrate replacing a single prior with a class of epsilon-contaminated priors in monitoring a phase II safety trial and in an analysis of an ECMO trial. This class is defined by

$$\Gamma_\epsilon = \{\pi = (1-\epsilon)\pi_0 + \epsilon q; q \in Q\}$$

where $\epsilon \in [0,1]$ reflects the amount of uncertainty concerning the accuracy of π_0, and Q is the class of all prior distributions. Upper and lower bounds for the posterior expectation of quantities of interest are calculated with reference to the entire class of priors. These bounds are computed for all values of ϵ, and the results are plotted versus ϵ. The authors indicate that if ϵ is small, and the interval between the upper and lower bounds is large, then the inferences are sensitive to the choice of the prior. In this circumstance one must either refine the specification of the prior distribution, collect more data, or recognize that the existing results are not definitive.

Carlin et al. (1995) give a partial characterization of the class of priors that leads to a given decision, conditionally on the observed data. They demonstrate their method in the analysis of a trial design to determine the effect of two drugs to prevent toxoplasmosis in patients with AIDS. The decision of concern is whether to stop the trial. They focus on the sensitivity of the stopping decision to the elicited prior distribution for the treatment effect. Extensions of this approach appear in Sargent and Carlin (1996) and are reviewed in Carlin and Louis (1996).

So, what alternatives are there to reference priors? This paper will explore two: clinical-expert priors, and previous-data priors. Acceptance of the use of clinical experts ranges from 'never trust the expert', to 'experts underestimate uncertainty', to 'experts are the best we can do and hence should be trusted'. There are many cases where most of the medical community was convinced of some 'untruth'; however, most of the time experts do have information. The following is a quote from Breslow (1990):

(in reference to various stages of clinical trials) "*...each of these areas involves the explicit use of scientific data for decision-making or regulatory purposes where the introduction of prior beliefs is both natural and unavoidable. It is perfectly appropriate in a democratic society that a carefully quantified measure of expert opinion be used ....*"

Research on elicitation of experts has been led by Chaloner. In a recent work, Chaloner (1996) presents an example of eliciting prior distributions from experts. The setting is a clinical trial aimed at determining the appropriate dosage of trimethoprim/sulfamethoxazole for fighting pneumocystis carinii pneumonia (PCP) in patients with AIDS. Using graphical methods as described in Chaloner et al. (1993) beliefs were elicited from three experts: two infectious disease MDs and another investigator. Chaloner (1996) presents the entire script used in the elicitation process. After responding to questions, the expert is presented with a parametric distribution that approximates his/her beliefs and is allowed to use slide-dialogs to adjust the curve to more accurately represent their beliefs. This method does not restrict beliefs to parametric families. Chaloner indicates that a high quality elicitation process provides elicitees with interactive feedback, a scripted interview, and a systematic literature review. She encourages using percentiles (rather than, for example, means and standard deviations) and suggests involving as many experts from as many sources of expertise as practically feasible.

Another example of eliciting expert opinions is presented in Kadane and Wolfson (1996, 1997). They elicit quantiles of a predictive distribution, arguing that experts can more accurately and comfortably express opinions about an observable quantity than about parameters. Their example demonstrates elicitation for a normal linear regression model, and their methodology can handle up to 4 covariates. Approaches demonstrating the elicitation of expert beliefs outside the medical setting include O'Hagan (1997) and Craig et al. (1997).

The second alternative to reference priors, empirically-based priors derived from past studies, is exemplified by James Brophy and Lawrence Joseph. In their "Placing Trials in Context Using Bayesian Analysis", published in the *Journal of the American Medical Association*, (1995), they use Bayesian methods and empirically based priors to reexamine the conclusions from what was to be the definitive trial comparing tissue plasminogen activator and streptokinase in acute myocardial infarction. The trial under review is called "Global Utilization of Streptokinase and Tissue Plasminogen Activator for Occluded Coronary Arteries" or 'GUSTO' for short. (The GUSTO Investigators, 1993) The GUSTO investigators concluded

> "The findings of this large-scale trial indicate that accelerated t-PA given with intravenous heparin provides a

> survival benefit over previous standard thrombolytic regimens.

Joseph and Brophy thought through the strengths and weaknesses of several previous trials to come up with empirically-based priors for their analysis of the GUSTO trial. They used various discounting schemes to assess the sensitivity of conclusions to the incorporation of this previous data. Their conclusion:

> "This analysis suggests that the clinical superiority of tissue-type plasminogen activator over streptokinase remains uncertain."

The question this example raises is: why aren't results from previous trials used more often for developing empirically-based priors? Researchers verbalize several arguments against using empirically-based priors. Publication bias is one reason. Studies with positive results are more likely to be published than those with negative results. Hence positive study results will be more accessible and empirically based priors will be biased towards finding a treatment effect. This problem is likely to become less problematic as computerization takes over publishing. Electronic journals will make journal space less scarce, and researchers will have the ability to make public what journals will not. A second barrier to using empirically-based priors boils down to time and responsibility. Who does the extrication of data and assimilates it into a prior? This job requires expert knowledge of the subject area as well as statistics. Finally, incompatibility of studies is also a problem. In the editorial debate following Brophy and Joseph's analysis several researchers made claims that the trials should not be analyzed through formal Bayesian methods because the studies did not have uniform patient entry criteria, t-PA dosages, and treatment delivery mechanisms. The popular science magazine *Discover*, picked up on this debate and ran an article entitled "The Mathematics of Making Up Your Mind" (May, 1996). It clearly describes the debate between the GUSTO investigators and Brophy and Joseph and more generally between Bayesian and frequentist statistics. This series of articles clearly explicates how information can and should be amalgamated across studies using Bayesian methods.

3. Bayes factors. Bayes factors are being promoted by the Bayesian community on par with reference priors. This section will begin by briefly reviewing Bayes factors and outlining some problems associated with their use.

Suppose the researcher is considering K sub-models mk indexed by:

prior probabilities	π_k,	
parameters	θ_k,	
likelihoods	$f_k(x\|\theta_k)$	
priors	$g_k(\theta_k)$,	for $k = 1, ...K$.

Then the posterior on model k, M_k and θ_k, is proportional to

$$f_k(x|\theta_k)g_k(\theta_k)\pi_k,$$

and the posterior probability of M is

$$P(M = m_k) = \frac{\pi_k \int f_k(x|\theta_k)g_k(\theta_k)d\theta_k}{\sum_{j=1}^{k} \pi_j \int f_j(x|\theta_j)g_j(\theta_j)d\theta_j}$$

and the posterior odds on M are

$$\begin{aligned} O(k) &= P(M = m_k)/1 - P(M = m_k) \\ &= \frac{\pi_k \int f_k(x|\theta_k)g_k(\theta_k)d\theta_k}{\pi_j \int_{j \neq k} f_j(x|\theta_j)g_j(\theta_j)d\theta_j} \end{aligned}$$

When $K = 2$, i.e. there are only 2 competing models k and k' then

$$\begin{aligned} O(k) &= \frac{\pi_k \int f_k(x|\theta_k)g_k(\theta_k)d\theta_k}{\pi_{k'} \int f_{k'}(x|\theta_{k'})g_{k'}(\theta_{k'})d\theta_{k'}} \\ \text{or} & \\ &= \frac{\pi_k}{\pi_{k'}} \times \frac{\int f_k(x|\theta_k)g_k(\theta_k)d\theta_k}{\int f_{k'}(x|\theta_{k'})g_{k'}(\theta_{k'})d\theta_{k'}} \\ &= \text{Prior Odds} \times \text{Bayes Factor} \\ &= \text{Prior Odds} \times B(k, k') \end{aligned}$$

The Bayes Factor tells us, of the models we are considering, which does the current data support most. If we consider only ill fitting models, one of them will still come out the best, and the probabilities will sum to 1. Relating this to clinical trials, the two models we may consider correspond to whether the parameter measuring treatment effect is equal to 0. This looks at Bayes factors as the Bayesian analogue of frequentist hypothesis testing. We can arrive at the posterior odds that the parameter is 0 versus some other value.

When $K > 2$, then the odds for model k become

$$0(k) \qquad = P(M = m_k)/1 - P(M = m_k)$$

The odds for model k is a function of the Bayes Factor of that model with every other model. In this case the prior probabilities do not factor out.

An example of the use of Bayes factors in clinical trials was presented by Greenhouse (1992). He demonstrated the use of Bayes factors in model checking in an analysis of the data from the North Central Cancer Treatment Group clinical trial of the relative efficacy of six different chemotherapy regimens in the treatment of advanced colorectal carcinoma. He used Bayes' factors to test whether the shape parameter of a Weibull distribution equaled 1 indicating a constant hazard rate model.

What is the meaning of $P(M_k)$? Most authors side-step the issue but imply that $P(M_k)$ is the probability that M_k is the correct model? This is a strong and questionable interpretation. The Bayes Factor approach requires model probabilities to sum to 1, and it implies that a 'correct' model exists, and that the 'correct' model is one of the K models under consideration. Unless our set of K models is exhaustive, it is not clear what $P(M_k)$ means. Perhaps, that M_k is the 'best' among the set of K models considered? Even with this interpretation question aside, a more detrimental influence of Bayes factors is that they place the focus of our analysis on the models and parameters instead of on prediction and decisions.

In general, the Bayes Factor approach provides a focus that has led us astray from a more important focus. Bayes factors lead our thinking into the accept/reject mode of hypothesis testing. For the Greenhouse example, the primary concern became the model, and the goal appeared to be generating a model that is a good representation of the real-world processes involved. Indeed this goal is consistent with how many scientists think and following this line can lead to improvements in models and advances in science. However, clinical trials are designed to inform us about making the best treatment decision. The bottom line is 'will the next patient that comes through the door experience a better outcome if I give him/her the drug'. We want to make the best decision we can, and to do that our interest is in trying to make good predictions. Our primary focus should be a probability distribution on the outcome or outcomes of interest. Predictions should rely on all available information and should reflect as much of the uncertainty as possible. Hence combining models rather than choosing one particular model seems a more appropriate mind set. Prediction must take precedence over discrimination among models. The models themselves are not of primary interest, but of secondary interest in the sense that they are helpful in coming up with a distribution of the outcome that reflects the available information. This does not mean that the models are not important. They are crucial in improving our predictions about the outcome, and it is important to evaluate models. The focus on predicting the outcome, does not remove the importance of such evaluation and of trying to improve models, it does suggest that Bayes Factors lead us to thinking about questions of secondary importance.

So why are Bayes factors attractive? Bayes factors are attractive for many of the same reasons that reference priors are attractive. They provide a Bayesian analogue to a frequentist method, hypothesis testing. At the extreme, adherents of these methods would like to have "Bayesian" procedures that would make decisions without the necessity of a loss or utility function (or without calling attention to it). However the assumptions needed to make the use of Bayes Factors a logically coherent exercise are quite special.

Bayes factors are useful when 1) it is required to choose a particular model, and 2) there is a $0-1$ loss for the decision being made. Kadane and Dickey (1980) show sufficiency of Bayes factors if and only if a $0-1$ loss obtains. A $0-1$ loss function implies that if we choose the wrong decision then it matters not whether we pick an alternative that is close or far from the correct one. This is clearly not the case in clinical trials. Similarly, Lavine and Schervish (1997) argue that Bayes factors should not be used for quantifying the degree to which observed data support or counterindicate particular models because of logical incoherencies. They investigate the reasons for these incoherencies and offer more appropriate interpretations of Bayes factors.

So what are the alternatives to using Bayes factors? For model selection problems there are three alternatives: theoretically justified models, embedding models into super-models, and model averaging. For making decisions about whether a treatment is effective or more effective than its competitors there is one alternative, decision theoretic frameworks.

When it comes to selecting models, ideally we would be able to choose between models based upon some theoretical justification. However, this is a bit like choosing the right expert for a prior elicitation. There will always be competing theoretically justifiable models. We are forced to choose between three options: choosing a model based on measures of goodness-of-fit, embedding competing models into super-models, or using model-averaging techniques. Gelman et al. (1995) offers methods for goodness-of-fit in a Bayesian context. Depending on the measures and utilities we choose, these answers can mimic the solution and suffer the same problems as Bayes factors. Embedding models into super-models can be a daunting task if the submodels are already complex. Model averaging, unlike these other options, allows us to take into account the uncertainty about model choice in our conclusions. Model averaging is the best option as it more accurately represents the uncertainty that goes into our estimates. The question that arises in model averaging is what are the most appropriate weights, and here Bayes factors may be useful.

When it comes to Bayes factors summarizing our support for whether there is a treatment effect, the only alternative is decision-theoretic frameworks. Full decision-theoretic frameworks are not only an improvement on Bayes factors, but they also move us away from the separatist view of statistics and decision making. By seeking automatic priors and automatic decision conventions, we are ignoring a critical part of the problem and the part to which Bayesian methods are extremely well suited, the decision theoretic part. The decision theoretic part makes explicit the utilities we hold, and combines them with the data analysis results, to help us choose between actions. There are 2 prevailing attitudes both of which serve to perpetuate the avoidance of adopting decision theoretic frameworks in clinical trials. The first is the separatist attitude that clinical trials are not decision problems. In a paper that I reviewed several years ago, the authors (taking Anscombe out of context) stated:

"*We are informal having no notion of a loss function hence*

> *no notion of an optimal, e.g., Bayes decision rule. In fact we do not specify a decision rule at all. As Anscombe (1963) notes, 'a medical trial is not, in any clear-cut fashion, a decision procedure."*

The second attitude which reflects less of the separatist attitude but more of a 'first things first' attitude is that decision theory is more difficult than the rest of Bayesian analysis. While eliciting utilities is as hard as eliciting priors, is calculating expected utilities really any harder than implementing the rest of the Bayesian paradigm? Now that calculating predictive distributions is routine, the only difficulty in calculating expected utility really is the elicitation. While elicitation is hard, how difficult is it to be more sophisticated than a $0-1$ loss function? Requiring that all articles make explicit the implicit loss function embedded in their analysis, by requiring public display of our simplicity, more pressure would be applied to getting it right, or at least making some effort at not getting it wrong. The following quote from Dennis Lindley's discussion of the Spiegelhalter et al (1995) paper states the problem eloquently:

> "*The authors dismiss the use of expected utility as being unrealistic....It must be recognized that clinical trials are not there for inference but to reach a decision, and the omission of their raison d'etre is serious. In the long term, expected utility is realistic, and indeed, necessary... We should use Bayesian concepts firstly because they work and secondly because only with them is it possible to be coherent. To appreciate this, contemplate the situation when you have just been given some data. Why not just look at them and express an opinion about the parameter? Why go through elaborate calculations, whether frequentist or Bayesian? If we can assess a prior directly, why not a posterior? The answer is: to achieve coherence, to make all our beliefs cohere: in particular, to make our final beliefs cohere with those that went into our likelihood. This is why frequentist p-values, interpreted as beliefs in the null hypothesis, are unsound; they do not cohere. The same reasoning applies to decisions as to beliefs. It is only by using expected utility that we can be sure that our actions will fit together sensibly. I suspect that the procedure of continuing with the trial until a tail area probability in the posterior is small, is just as incoherent as a belief based on the tail area, p-value. Or if it is coherent, it implies an inept utility, such as one taking only values 0 and 1.*"

Spiegelhalter and colleagues have taken a first attempt to incorporate utilities, by setting up regions corresponding to utility. Regions of clinical inferiority, equivalence, and superiority are more realistic than the frequentist dichotomization of the parameter space, but we need to take this further. Simes (1986) and Hilden and Habbema (1990) offered a formal framework for decision analysis as did Stangl (1995). These works demonstrate methods for making utilities explicit. While considering only one outcome, these methods should easily generalize to trials with multiple outcomes that need to be taken into account.

Now that computation has advanced to a point where predictive distributions for outcomes can be calculated even in complex models, we can get more sophisticated in terms of eliciting priors and integrating statistical output with decision making. This will happen with predictive distributions and utilities. We must move from the $0-1$ utilities to utilities that put values on units of the outcome(s) of interest.

Why is it so important to move in this direction? Again Brophy and Joseph's(1995) work highlights the importance. Brophy and Josephs paper did two things. It argued for the use of Bayesian rather than frequentist methods, but more importantly it showed that we should be thinking about clinical trials from a more decision theoretic than hypothesis testing framework. The biggest difference between the frequentist and Bayesian analysis was the implicit utility function. The frequentists concluded t-PA was 'superior' based on a rejected null hypothesis and an observed treatment difference of 1%. The Bayesians analysis did not disagree with the rejection of a treatment difference of zero. They did disagree with the conclusion that t-PA was 'superior', because the posterior probability that the treatment difference was at least 1% was only about 50%. The utility functions implicit in their definitions of 'superior' conflicted.

There are other examples in the literature that make clear the decision making involved in every stage of clinical trials: Berry (1985, 1987, 1988, 1989, 1991, 1993, 1995) and Berry and colleagues' (1985, 1988,1992, 1993, 1994) work on vaccine and clinical trials, Parmigiani and Kamlet's (1993) work on scheduling mammograms, Parmigiani and colleagues (1996) work on clinical guidelines, and Stangl's (1995) work demonstrating the use of predictive distributions within a decision theoretic framework, are but a few. These works show that sensitivity analysis is not just for the priors and models we choose, but also for the utility or loss functions we choose? The utility function will have as much or more impact on the problem as the prior and model, so it is time to recognize and address this issue. We should demand that implied utilities be made explicit whether the analysis is frequentist or Bayesian, and we should demand that sensitivity analysis focus on the utilities as well as the prior distributions.

REFERENCES

[1] BERGER J.O., *Robust Bayesian analysis: sensitivity to the prior*, Journal of Statistical Planning and Inference, **25**, 1990, pp. 303–328.

[2] BERRY D.A., *Interim analysis in clinical trials: classical versus Bayesian approaches*, Statistics in Medicine, **4**, 1985, pp. 521–526.

[3] BERRY, D.A., *Interim analysis in clinical trials: The role of the likelihood principle*, The American Statistician, **41**, 1987, pp. 117–122.

[4] BERRY, D.A., *Interim analysis in clinical research*, Cancer Invest., **5**, (1988a), pp. 469–477.

[5] BERRY, C.A., *Multiple comparisons, multiple tests, and data dredging: A Bayesian perspective with discussion)*. In *Bayesian Statistics 3*, (eds. J.M. Bernardo, M.H. DeGroot, D.V. Lindley, and A.F.M. Smith), Oxford University Press, (1988b), pp. 79–94.

[6] BERRY, D.A., *Monitoring accumulating data in a clinical trial*, Biometrics, **45**, 1989a, pp. 1197–1211.

[7] BERRY, D.A., *Inferential aspects of adaptive allocation rules*, Proceedings of the Pharmaceutical Section of the American Statistical Association, ASA, Washington DC, 1989c, pp. 1-8.

[8] BERRY D.A., *Bayesian methodology in phase III trials*, Drug Information Association Journal, **25**, 1991, pp. 345–368.

[9] BERRY DA, *Experimental design for drug development: A Bayesian approach*, Journal of Biopharmaceutical Statistics, **1**, 1991, pp. 81–101.

[10] BERRY, D.A., *A case for Bayesianism in clinical trials (with discussion)*, Statistics in Medicine, **12**, 1993, pp. 1377–1404.

[11] BERRY, D.A., *Decision analysis and Bayesian methods in clinical trials*, In *Recent Advances in Clinical Trial Design and Analysis*, (ed. P. Thall), Kluwer Press, New York, 1995, pp. 125–154.

[12] BERRY D.A., AND FRISTEDT, B., *Bandit Problems: Sequential Allocation of Experiments*, London: Chapman-Hall, 1985.

[13] BERRY, D.A., AND HARDWICK, J., *Using historical controls in clinical trials: Application to ECMO*, Statistical Decision Theory and Related Topics V, New York: Springer-Verlag. (eds. Berger JO, Gupta S), 1993, pp. 141–156.

[14] BERRY, D.A., AND EICK, S.G., *Adaptive assignment versus balanced randomization in clinical trials: A decision analysis*, Statistics in Medicine, **14**, 1994, pp. 231–246.

[15] BERRY, D.A., AND HO, C.H., *One-sided sequential stopping boundaries for clinical trials: A decision-theoretic approach*, Biometrics, **44**, 1988, pp. 219–227.

[16] BERRY, D.A., WOLFF, M.C., AND SACK, D., *Public health decision making: A sequential vaccine trial (with discussion)*, In *Bayesian Statistics*, (eds. Bernardo JM, Berger JO, Dawid AP, Smith AFM), Oxford, England: Oxford University Press, 1992, pp. 79–96.

[17] BERRY, D.A., WOLFF, M.C., AND SACK, D., *Decision making during a phase III randomized controlled trial*, Controlled Clinical Trials, **15**, 1994, pp. 360–379.

[18] BRESLOW, N., *Biostatistics and Bayes*, Statistical Science, **5**, 1990, pp. 269–284.

[19] BROPHY J.M., AND JOSEPH, L., *Placing trials in context using Bayesian analysis: Gusto revisited by Reverend Bayes*, Journal of the American Medical Association, **273(11)**, 1995, pp. 871–875.

[20] CARLIN, B.P., AND LOUIS, T.A., *Bayes and Empirical Bayes Methods for Data Analysis*, Chapman and Hall, 1996.

[21] CARLIN, B.P., CHALONER, K. M., LOUIS, T.A., AND RHAME, F.S., *Elicitation, monitoring, and analysis for an AIDS clinical trial*, In *Case Studies in Bayesian Statistics: Volume II*, (eds. C. Gatsonis, J. Hodges, R. Kass, and N. Singpurwalla), Springer, 1995, pp. 48–84.

[22] CHALONER, K., *Elicitation of Prior Distributions*, In *Bayesian Biostatistics*, (eds. D.A. Berry and D.K. Stangl), Marcel Dekker, 1996, pp. 141–156.

[23] CHALONER, K., CHURCH, T., MATTS, J.P., AND LOUIS, T.A., *Graphical elicitation of a prior distribution for an AIDS clinical trial*, The Statistician, **42**, 1993, pp. 341–353.

[24] CRAIG, P.S., GOLDSTEIN, M., SEHEULT, A.H., AND SMITH, J.A., *Constructing partial prior specifications for models of complex physical systems*, The Statistician, **47(1)**, 1998, pp. 37–53.

[25] GAIL, M., *A discussion of: Bayesian approaches to randomized trials*, J. Royal Statistical Soc. Ser. A, **157**, 1995, pp. 357–416.

[26] GELMAN, A., CARLIN, J.B., STERN, H.S., AND RUBIN, D. B., *Bayesian Data Analysis*, Chapman & Hall, London, 1995.

[27] GREENHOUSE J.B., AND WASSERMAN, L., *A practical, robust method for Bayesian model selection: A case study in the analysis of clinical trials*, Paper presented at the American Statistical Association Meetings, Carnegie-Mellon Technical Report #626, 1995a.

[28] GREENHOUSE, J.B., AND WASSERMAN, L., *Robust Bayesian methods for monitoring clinical trials*, Statistics in Medicine, **14**, 1995b, pp. 1379–1391.

[29] GREENHOUSE, J.B., *On some applications of Bayesian methods in cancer clinical trials*, Statistics in Medicine, **11**, 1992, pp. 37–53.

[30] HILDEN, J. AND HABBEMA, J., *The marriage of clinical trials and clinical decision science*, Statistics in Medicine, **9**, 1990, pp. 1243–1257.

[31] HIVELY, W., *The mathematics of making up your mind*, Discover, May 1996.

[32] KADANE, J.B., AND WOLFSON, L. J., *Priors for the design and analysis of clinical trials*, In *Bayesian Biostatistics*, D. Berry and D. Stangl (eds.), Marcel Dekker, New York 1996.

[33] KADANE, J.B., AND WOLFSON, L. J., *Experiences in elicitation*, The Statistician, **47(1)**, 1998, pp. 3–19.

[34] KADANE, J.B., AND DICKEY, J.M., *Bayesian decision theory and the simplification of models*, In *Evaluation of Econometric Models*, (eds. J. Kmenta and J. Ramsey), Academic Press, 1980, pp. 245–268.

[35] LAVINE, M., AND SCHERVISH, M., *Bayes factors: What they are and what they are not*, The Statistician, 1999, to appear.

[36] LINDLEY, D., *A discussion of: Bayesian approaches to randomized trials*, J. Royal Statistical Soc. Ser. A, **157**, 1995, pp. 357–416

[37] O'HAGAN, A., *Eliciting expert beliefs in substantial practical applications*, The Statistician, **47(1)**, 1998, pp. 21–35.

[38] PARMIGIANI, G., ANCUKIEWICZ, M. AND MATCHAR, D., *Decision models in clinical recommendations development: The stroke prevention policy model*, In *Bayesian Biostatistics*, ed. D.A. Berry and D.K. Stangl, Marcel Dekker, 1996, pp. 207–233.

[39] PARMIGIANI, G. AND KAMLET, M.S., *A cost-utility analysis of alternative strategies in screening for breast cancer*, In *Case Studies in Bayesian Statistics*, (eds. C. Gatsonis, J. Hodges, R. Kass, and N. Singpurwalla, Springer-Verlag, 1993, pp. 390–402.

[40] SARGENT, D. AND CARLIN, B.P., *Robust Bayesian design and analysis of clinical trials via prior partitioning (with discussion)*, IMS Lecture Note Series: Second International Workshop on Bayesian Robustness, 1996.

[41] SIMES, R.J., *Application of statistical decision theory to treatment choices: Implications for the design and analysis of clinical trials*, Statistics in Medicine, **5**, 1986, pp. 411–420.

[42] SPIEGELHALTER , D.J., FREEDMAN, L.S., AND PARMAR, M.K., *Bayesian approaches to randomized trials*, J. Royal Statistical Soc. Ser. A, **157**, 1994, pp. 357–416.

[43] STANGL, D., *Prediction and decision making using Bayesian hierarchical models*, Statistics in Medicine, **14**, 1995, pp. 2173–2190.

[44] THE GUSTO INVESTIGATORS, *An international randomized trial comparing four thrombolytic strategies for acute myocardial infarction*, N. Engl. J. Med., **329**, 1993, pp. 673–682.

[45] WASSERMAN, L., *Recent methodological advances in robust Bayesian inference*, In *Bayesian Statistics IV*, (eds. J.M. Bernardo, M.H. DeGroot, D.V. Lindley, and A.F.M. Smith), Oxford University Press, 1992, pp. 483–502.

SURROGATE ENDPOINTS IN CANCER CLINICAL TRIALS

STEPHEN L. GEORGE*

Abstract. Cancer is a major public health problem in the United States and worldwide. In the U.S. in 1996, an estimated 1,360,000 new cases of cancer were diagnosed, and an estimated 555,000 cancer patients died of their disease [1]. The current estimated lifetime risk of developing an invasive cancer is one in three for woman and an amazing one in two for men. The disease "cancer" is a diverse set of diseases, with the common characteristics of invasion of normal tissues by cancer cells and the propensity of these cells to spread, or metastasize, beyond the site of origin. All cancers also share the potential to cause significant morbidity and death. However, the natural history, epidemiology, biology, prevention, detection, and treatment of cancer varies widely by the specific type of cancer. Among other things, these differences necessitate different approaches for each type of cancer in the design and analysis of cancer clinical trials.

Although the field with the largest literature and interest in surrogate endpoints is perhaps AIDS research [2–6], this topic has received increasing attention in recent years in cancer research as well [7–9]. The purpose of this paper is to discuss the role of surrogate endpoints in cancer clinical trials, including prevention, screening, and therapeutic trials. Examples of trials in prostate cancer, breast cancer, and lung cancer will be used to illustrate the key points.

1. General comments on the concepts of surrogate and true endpoints. The concept of a surrogate endpoint includes, of necessity, the concept of an endpoint, often referred to as the true endpoint, for which the surrogate is a substitute or replacement although there are often references in the literature to a surrogate endpoint variable without any obvious true endpoint. Temple [10] defined true and surrogate endpoints as follows: "A true endpoint is a clinically meaningful endpoint that measures how a patient feels, functions, or survives. A surrogate endpoint is a laboratory measurement or a physical sign used as a substitute for a clinically meaningful endpoint. Changes induced by a therapy on a surrogate endpoint are expected to reflect changes in a clinically meaningful endpoint." The potential benefits of using surrogates are that results may be determined earlier, smaller sample sizes are required, they may be measured frequently, and may be used when the true endpoint is infeasible because of costs or ethics. The adjectives "true" and "surrogate" are, themselves, relative to the circumstances of the particular trial and disease under study. In some settings, an endpoint (e.g., initial response to therapy) may be treated as a surrogate endpoint for, say, overall survival, while in other settings (e.g., phase II therapeutic trials), the same endpoint may be the true endpoint.

The terminology of true and surrogate endpoints may obscure some important issues in the proper choice of endpoints in clinical trials. The proper evaluation of a treatment for cancer generally includes an assessment of a wide range of endpoints, including overall survival, disease-free survival, the initial clinical response to therapy, toxicity, quality of life,

*Division of Biometry, Duke University Medical Center, Durham, NC 27710.

and costs. Overall survival is certainly a key endpoint in any phase III therapeutic trial, but it is wrong to assume that overall survival is always the "true" endpoint, or that all other endpoints need to be assessed with respect to how well they are surrogates for overall survival. This makes little or no sense for endpoints such as quality of life and costs, and, for clinical response or disease-free survival, misses the point that valuable information about the biological activity of treatment can be gained from some endpoints, regardless of their ability to serve as surrogates for the "true" endpoint of overall survival. In addition, in some cancers, there are treatments that can be given after a relapse or disease progression and that greatly prolong survival in some patients. Since the range of possible treatments after initial failure from a study-specified treatment cannot usually be controlled either ethically or practically, the interpretation of treatment effects from a clinical trial in such a setting is quite problematic. This does not mean that overall survival is not of major importance, but that the attempt to distinguish between "true" and "surrogate" endpoints is overly restrictive and often not very helpful. What is needed is a careful discussion of all appropriate endpoints and a thoughtful integration of these endpoints into an overall evaluation of the treatments.

Prentice [11] has given a formal definition of a surrogate endpoint that involves two criteria. First, the surrogate S must correlate with the true endpoint T. That is, S must be prognostic for T. Second, S must fully capture the effect of treatment X on the true endpoint T. This latter criteria means that after adjustment for the surrogate S, there is no effect of treatment on outcome. Note that this second criteria depends explicitly on a given treatment X so that it is meaningless to talk of a surrogate without reference to a specific treatment. Because of this, the search for surrogate endpoints for overall survival can perhaps be dismissed as a futile one. The a priori probability that some putative surrogate endpoint that can be measured early enough to make a difference in reducing the size or length of the trial and that truly meets the stringent statistical requirements of this definition is small. Even if such a surrogate could be found and validated, its dependence on the therapy under study would require revalidation for a new therapy with a different mode of action. Also, there are frightening examples of using plausible surrogates as replacements for more definitive clinical endpoints. Two of these are the Cardiac Arrhythmia Suppression Trials (CAST I and CAST II), [12, 13] in which patients taking drugs effective in preventing arrhythmias led to a higher mortality rate than that for patients on placebo. In prostate cancer, the drug diethylstilbestrol (DES), despite its tumor shrinkage capability, was associated with higher mortality than placebo, presumably due to its cardiotoxicity [14].

The primary difficulty with the surrogate endpoint framework is that a true surrogate must meet such stringent validation requirements [15]. Freedman, et al., [16] conclude that unless the unadjusted standardized treatment effect is quite large (effect/se > 4), we are likely to be able to conclude at most that the data are inconsistent with the surrogate criteria [11]. Even when the standardized treatment effect is large, we can usually estimate only that some putative surrogate explains some percentage of the treatment effect, not that it explains 100 % as required by the strict criteria of surrogacy. Based on these considerations, Freedman, et al., [16] proposed a stepwise validation procedure for a potential surrogate S. First, test for interaction between S and the treatment X with respect to the effect on the true outcome T. If significant, stop and conclude no surrogacy. If not significant, adopt a no interaction model relating the true outcome to S and X. Test for a treatment effect. If significant, conclude against surrogacy. If not significant, estimate the proportion of the treatment effect explained by the surrogate and calculate confidence limits on this estimate. This procedure has the advantage of rejecting a potential surrogate S as well as providing an estimate of the 'percentage of surrogacy' rather than requiring 100%.

Despite these objections to the semantics of surrogacy, the potential value of biologically relevant markers of disease process and intermediate outcome variables, even if they fail the strict tests of surrogacy, should not be minimized. In the epidemiology literature, the term 'intermediate endpoint' is often used synonymously with 'surrogate endpoint' [17], but here it is used more loosely to refer to some observable variable that may or may not be a surrogate. These markers may be useful in accelerating the evaluation of interventions in early phase clinical trials, and they provide insights into disease mechanisms. To my knowledge, there are no adequately validated surrogate markers in cancer, but there are many biomarkers that have proved helpful in the elucidation of biological effects of drugs. Thus, objection to the language of surrogacy and the likely futility of the search for surrogate endpoints is not an objection to the study of biomarkers or intermediate endpoints. The fact that an endpoint is not a surrogate for some primary clinical endpoint does not mean that it is not useful, only that it cannot fully replace the clinical endpoint.

In cancer, a disease with many biomarkers, a more fruitful approach than the search for true surrogate endpoints is the development of models and analyses relating the marker process to the true endpoint with treatment as a covariate [18]. This allows us to supplement information on censored survival time, for example, with the additional information available on the marker process up to the time of censoring. The work of Fleming, et al., [19], on 'auxiliary' endpoints is relevant in this respect.

In summary, the concept of a surrogate endpoint for some true endpoint has limited value in most cancer studies. There is a continuing need for a thoughtful synthesis of multiple endpoints, of varying degrees of importance, and of varying strengths of surrogacy. However, the terminology of surrogacy is by now firmly established and unlikely to change because of these objections. The remainder of the paper will focus on some issues arising from consideration of surrogate endpoints in the design and analysis of cancer prevention, screening, and therapeutic trials.

2. Types of cancer clinical trials. Cancer clinical trials can be classified into prevention, screening, or therapeutic trials:

- Prevention - trials designed to assess procedures for preventing the development of cancer. These trials can be divided further into 'primary' prevention trials involving the reduction of exposure to carcinogens or other risk factors, and chemoprevention trials, involving the administration of chemical agents or drugs. These latter trials are similar to the large cardiovascular trials.
- Screening - trials designed to assess techniques for detecting asymptomatic or latent cancer. These trials are sometimes misleadingly labeled as secondary prevention trials.
- Therapeutic - trials designed to assess therapeutic interventions for patients with a diagnosis of cancer.

Prevention, screening, and therapeutic trials differ in many respects including eligibility criteria, complexity, size, allowable toxicity, and primary objectives. There are conventions of classifications of the trials into "phases" (generally, I, II, III, etc.) of development of the technique or agent under study. The usual endpoints of these studies are given in Table 1.

TABLE 1
Endpoints in cancer trials.

TYPE OF TRIAL	DEFINITIVE ENDPOINTS	INTERMEDIATE ENDPOINTS
Prevention	Cancer incidence and mortality	Biomarkers
Screening	Cancer-specific mortality	Cancer stage at diagnosis Resectability of tumor Survival after diagnosis
Therapeutic	Overall survival	Biomarkers Response rate Length of response Disease-free survival

A biomarker is a biologically-based measurement (molecular, biochemical, histologic) that has a theoretical relevance to cancer initiation, promotion, progression, invasion, or metastasis [20]. As tumor cells develop and die, products may be released into tissue or serum which can be detected by an appropriate biological assay. Change in the marker value is thus theoretically related to some stage in the cancer process, although most such markers are highly variable and seriously deficient in both sensitivity and specificity. A treatment may have a biologic effect, as measured by some biomarker, without any beneficial clinical effect. Conversely, even in the absence of a biological effect, as measured by the biomarker, the treatment may have a beneficial clinical effect. Validation of the efficacy of these biomarkers is thus of utmost importance.

3. Chemoprevention trials. The fundamental aim of chemoprevention is to give chemical agents or drugs that interrupt the carcinogenic processes leading to the development of invasive cancer [21]. Thus, the primary endpoints of clinical trials of putative chemopreventive agents are cancer incidence and cancer mortality. Unlike cancer therapeutic trials in which the subjects have been previously diagnosed with cancer, chemoprevention trials are carried out in subjects initially without cancer but who are assessed as being at increased risk of developing cancer. Even in subjects at high risk, the annual event rate (i.e., rate of diagnosed cancer) in chemoprevention trials is usually quite low compared to the relevant event rate in therapeutic trials, resulting in the need for very large and very long trials. In such a setting, any intermediate endpoint or combination of endpoints, particularly biomarkers observed early in the carcinogenic process, that could serve as a surrogate for cancer incidence or mortality would be invaluable [22–26].

3.1. Prostate cancer prevention trial. Prostate cancer is the most common cancer in American men and is second only to lung cancer in death rate. An estimated 317,000 new cases of prostate cancer and 41,000 deaths due to prostate cancer occurred in the US in 1996. Risk increases with age, and is higher among black men than white men. There is a large percentage of latent prostate cancer (one study estimates this percentage to exceed 30% in men over 50 years old [27]), but only about 3% of men die of the disease. Several potential biomarkers have been identified in prostate cancer, with the suggestion that some combination of markers may prove useful as a surrogate endpoint for prostate cancer incidence in prevention trials. Some of these markers are prostate specific antigen (PSA), nuclear DNA content (ploidy), oncogene c-erbB-2 expression, angiogenesis, and high-grade prostatic intraepithelial neoplasia (PIN) [28].

The Prostate Cancer Prevention Trial (PCPT) is a randomized double-blinded placebo-controlled trial designed to test the effectiveness of oral finasteride (5 mg/day) in reducing the incidence of prostate cancer [29]. Finasteride inhibits the synthesis of dihydrotestosterone, a hormone necessary for the development of prostate cancer. The design requires 18,000 healthy men at least 55 years of age to be randomized equally between finasteride (5 mg/day) and placebo. Treatment will last for 7 years, at which time all subjects will receive a prostate biopsy. The primary endpoint is biopsy verified prostate cancer at 7 years or earlier (i.e., the 7-year period prevalence). The trial opened in October 1993, and closed in December 1996. Approximately 18,900 subjects were randomized.

There are at least two concerns in using all-stage prostate cancer diagnosis as the primary endpoint in this trial. One is that some of the early stage cancers detected may not be clinically important. It is known that some prostate cancers do not progress or metastasize, but unfortunately, there is no current method to assess this as diagnosis. The second concern is that finasteride is known to reduce the levels of serum PSA so that there might be a differential ascertainment bias (less cancers diagnosed in the finasteride group because of lower PSA values). With the planned 7-year biopsies, this latter problem perhaps would not be serious, except for the drop-outs and inevitable missed 7-year biopsies.

There is still a serious question about whether the 7-year prostate prevalence is a surrogate for prostate cancer mortality, the most relevant clinical endpoint. In fact, such an endpoint was explicitly considered by the trial organizers, but rejected primarily because of the excessive size and duration of a study designed to test for treatment effect on mortality (estimated to require randomization of 51,000 men and a 15-year study).

3.2. Breast cancer prevention trial. Breast cancer is the most common cancer in American women and is second only to lung cancer in death rate. An estimated 186,000 new cases of breast cancer and 45,000 deaths due to breast cancer occurred in the US in 1996.

Tamoxifen is a nonsteroidal antiestrogen that has proven highly effective in treating both advanced and early stage breast cancer and is widely used for this purpose. There has been good compliance in patients taking tamoxifen (a daily oral dose), in part because of its minimal short-term side effects. Reports of some relatively rare but serious long-term adverse effects, especially endometrial cancer and thromboembolic events, have raised some concerns about its use in a prevention trial [30]. In February 1996, the International Agency for Research on Cancer (IARC) issued an announcement of an evaluation of tamoxifen as a potential carcinogen. The IARC concluded that there is "sufficient evidence in humans of the carcinogenicity of tamoxifen in increasing the risk of endometrial cancer," but insufficient evidence for other cancers. However, the risk of endometrial cancer is low, certainly lower than the benefit to breast cancer patients in reducing the risk of contralateral breast cancers. The evidence does cause some concern for the use of tamoxifen as a chemopreventive agent in healthy women, but any risk assessment of these rare events must be weighed against the initial estimates of potential benefit.

The Breast Cancer Prevention Trial (BCPT) is a randomized double-blind trial coordinated by the NSABP comparing the efficacy of tamoxifen with that of placebo in reducing the incidence of invasive breast carcinoma in women at increased risk for breast cancer. Sixteen thousand women were expected to be randomized equally to the two treatment groups with treatment lasting for five years and a minimum planned follow-up of at least seven years on all subjects. The BCPT began in May 1992 and closed in May 1997. Approximately 13,200 subjects were randomized.

The BCPT is an example of a prevention trial in which the primary endpoints are unambiguously clinical endpoints. These endpoints include the incidence of invasive breast carcinoma, breast cancer mortality, incidence of myocardial infarctions (fatal and non-fatal), and bone fractures (osteoporosis outcome). Secondary endpoints include measures of toxicity, compliance, and quality of life as well as lipid and lipoprotein values (serum cholesterol, HDL, LDL).

There are no proposed surrogate endpoints for the primary endpoints of cancer incidence, mortality, and myocardial infarctions. However, for bone fractures, there is a separate companion study evaluating the effect of tamoxifen on bone density and biochemical markers of bone turnover (serum osteocalcin, urinary pyridinoline, deoxypyridinoline) in subsets of both premenopausal and postmenopausal women. Bone density is known to be a strong prognostic factor for bone fracture, and changes in the biochemical markers are assumed to precede changes in bone density. Although this sub-study of bone density was not explicitly designed as an evaluation of putative surrogate endpoints (the word 'surrogate' was not used in the clinical protocol), all of the ingredients are in place: A large randomized trial, a careful evaluation of early biomarkers, and continued follow-up for the 'true' clinical endpoints of bone fracture.

3.3. Lung cancer chemoprevention trials. Lung cancer is the second most common cancer in both men and women but has the highest death rate. An estimated 177,000 new cases of lung cancer and 159,000 deaths due to lung cancer occurred in the US in 1996.

There have been two major chemoprevention trials in lung cancer sponsored by the National Cancer Institute primarily involving heavy smokers. One was the Alpha-Tocopherol Beta Carotene Study (ATBC) [31] testing the efficacy of daily supplements of β-carotene and vitamin E in reducing the incidence of lung cancer in a randomized double-blind 2×2 factorial design. The study subjects were approximately $29,000$ middle-aged male smokers from Finland randomized to one of the four possible treatment groups (placebo, beta carotene alone, alpha-tocopherol alone, and beta carotene plush alpha-tocopherol). Treatment lasted for six years. The results after five to eight years of follow-up were reported in 1994, and were both disappointing and surprising: alpha-tocopherol appeared to have no effect on the incidence of lung cancer, but subjects taking beta carotene appeared to have a significantly *higher* incidence of lung cancer [31].

The other study was the Carotene and Retinol Efficacy Trial (CARET), [32] designed to enroll 18,000 heavy smokers or asbestos-exposed workers in a randomized double-blind study. The two treatments were beta carotene plus vitamin A and placebo. As in the ATBC trial, the major endpoint in CARET was lung cancer incidence. This trial was stopped early in 1997, approximately two years earlier than planned, based on a result remarkably similar to the ATBC trial. The patients receiving beta carotene plus vitamin A had a substantially *higher* incidence of lung cancer than the placebo group.

Two other trials testing beta carotene or vitamin E, not focusing on heavy smokers are the Physician's Health Study (PHS), which began in

1982 and ended in late 1995, and the Women's Health Study (WHS), an ongoing trial which began in 1992. In the PHS, 22,000 men were assigned to beta carotene (50 mg every other day) or placebo. This study also included an aspirin-placebo component until 1988, at which time the reduced rate of myocardial infarctions in the aspirin groups led to a termination of this aspect of the study. The preliminary analysis of the beta carotene treatment indicates no effect with respect to lung cancer incidence or mortality. The WHS is designed to enroll 40,000 apparently healthy women health professionals ages 45 and older. The study agents are beta carotene, vitamin E, aspirin, and placebo. Shortly after the announcement of the CARET results, the beta carotene aspect of this trial was terminated.

These results are sobering and reiterative of the importance of conducting randomized clinical trials even when the epidemiologic and observational studies provide seemingly strong evidence on benefits. For our purposes here, it should be noted that these trials, like the BCPT, did not use surrogate endpoints in their design or analysis.

4. Screening trials. The primary endpoint in cancer screening trials is reduction in cancer-specific mortality. The hazards of using putative surrogate endpoints such as lower stage at diagnosis, increased resectability, and survival after diagnosis are known both theoretically and from practical experience. One danger is the length-bias problem leading to the overdiagnosis of indolent or slow-growing cancers, some of which, in the absence of detection by screening, would never become a clinical problem. Prostate cancer is a prime example of a cancer in which over-diagnosis is a very real problem. Another problem is the lead-time bias, which can give a misleading estimate of survival after diagnosis. Use of cancer-specific mortality as the primary endpoint avoids these difficulties.

There is one large, ongoing randomized clinical trial, the Prostate, Lung, Colorectal and Ovarian Screening Trial (PLCO), sponsored by the National Cancer Institute [33]. The PLCO trial which began in November 1993, is designed to enroll 148,000 subjects (74,000 men and 74,000 women) 60 to 74 years old at entry. All subjects will be randomized equally between an annual screening regimen and a control group (routine medical care). Results are not expected to be available until year 16 of the study (i.e., calendar year 2009).

4.1. Prostate cancer screening. Screening of prostate cancer presents some special problems, since there is such a high percentage of latent cancer in older men, many of whom would not experience clinical cancer symptoms in their lifetimes, and the available treatment options (radiotherapy, radical prostatectomy) have serious complications in a large percentage of patients. Widespread use of the prostate specific antigen (PSA) test and digital rectal examination (DRE) has led to sharply increased detection rates in the US, but the value of early detection in reducing cancer mortality remains uncertain. There is little evidence at present that early detection improves outcome in prostate cancer, and virtually no evidence that screening results in reduced mortality.

There have been many observational studies in prostate cancer screening, but no results of any randomized clinical trial have been reported. The screening regimen on the PLCO trial consists of an annual digital rectal exam and serum PSA determination for each of the first 3 years after enrollment. The endpoint is prostate cancer mortality. No surrogate endpoints are discussed in the design, although the value of DRE and PSA as diagnostic tests is one of the secondary objectives of the study.

4.2. Breast cancer screening trials. There have been at least eight major randomized clinical trials of screening for breast cancer [34]. These trials agree substantially on one point [35]: Screening using mammography every 1 to 2 years clearly reduces mortality from breast cancer in women aged 50 to 69 years. The result is not so clear for younger women or older women. In particular, there is little evidence of any mortality benefit for mammography for younger women (40–49 years old), even though there are considerably more cancers detected by mammography, and at early stage of disease. As in the case of the prostate cancer example, early detection and lower stage at diagnosis are not good surrogates for disease-specific or overall mortality.

4.3. Lung cancer screening trials. In addition to the on-going PLCO screening trial, there have been four highly publicized screening trials in lung cancer, three in the U.S. [36] at the Memorial Sloan-Kettering Cancer Center, the Johns Hopkins Medical Institutions, and the Mayo Clinic, and one in the former Czechoslovakia [37]. None of these trials found any difference in lung-cancer mortality. Two trials (Memorial and Johns Hopkins) compared annual radiographic screening with annual screening plus sputum cytology every 4 months. One trial (Mayo) compared 4 month dual screening (radiograph plus sputum cytology) to usual medical care (recommendation for annual screening) in over 10,000 male smokers with 12 years of follow-up. The Czech trial was similar to the Mayo trial in that there was a control group that received no routine screening for 3 years.

In the Mayo and Czech trials, there was evidence of a higher percentage of early stage disease, increased resectability, and survival from diagnosis in the more heavily screened group of subjects. However, there was no difference in disease-specific mortality, suggesting that some of the aforementioned biases were indeed major factors. Once again, use of stage distribution, resectability rates, or survival from diagnosis as surrogate endpoints is clearly not appropriate.

5. Therapeutic trials. Therapeutic trials in cancer, as in other diseases, fall into two broad types [38]: Drug or product-oriented trials and disease-oriented trials. The former are standard in the pharmaceutical industry where product licensing issues are paramount. It is in this setting that the standard drug-development terminology of phase I, II, and III trials was developed. A treatment effect on survival or quality of life is generally required for FDA approval [39]. Traditionally, no surrogate endpoint was acceptable although recently exceptions are becoming common.

Disease-oriented trials are the standard in the cancer clinical cooperative groups and in academic cancer centers. Here, the emphasis is on improving the therapy for different types of cancer, usually through combination therapy (multi-agent and multi-modality), without the major concerns of product licensing. The distinction between drug-oriented trials and disease-oriented trials is not always a sharp one, but the differences can be important.

Many disease-oriented cancer trials use the phase designations of trials from the drug-oriented trials, despite some logical difficulties in the sequence of single-agent phase I (toxicity) and phase II (disease activity) trials followed by multi-agent phase III (comparative efficacy) trials. The problem is that the phase I and phase II trials are quite similar to the standard drug-oriented trials, but for agents successfully completing these early trials, there is then a leap to complex multi-agent phase III trials. That is, there is no definitive efficacy trial solely for the single agent under study. The use of multi-agent therapy is both ethically and practically proper since the successful cancer therapies are all multi-agent therapies, but it does cause a logical problem in how new agents are definitely assessed and how they are to be included as part of an existing regimen.

The early phase cancer trials are nearly always single-agent trials, since documentation of single-agent activity is essential for the development of effective combination therapy. Phase I trials are designed to determine the proper dose or scheduling for a new agent. The primary endpoint is toxicity, usually some type of dose-limiting toxicity. Phase II trials are designed to screen for anti-cancer activity. The primary end-point is objective clinical response, usually restricted to complete responses (no detectable disease) and sometimes partial responses (significant reduction in measured tumor burden, short of complete disappearance). This, of course, implies that the tumor burden is measurable, which is not always the case. In both types of trial, the endpoints are chosen for the specific purpose of the trial, and there is no assumption that these endpoints are in any way surrogates for some other "true" endpoint such as overall survival.

Phase III trials in cancer, on the other hand, are nearly always multi-agent trials with primary endpoints of survival or disease-free survival. Important secondary endpoints are quality of life and costs. In addition, for trials in which it is relevant (e.g., advanced stage solid tumors and leukemia), the clinical response to the initial treatment (complete response, partial response, and so on) is often considered as an endpoint, but never as a surrogate for long-term outcome or survival. Clinical response in cancer may satisfy the necessary (but not sufficient!) criteria for a surrogate endpoint for survival, since it is generally prognostic (responders live longer than non-responders), is well-defined, and can be measured quite early. However, any attempt to use CR in this way would be unintelligible to most cancer investigators. Also, the fact that responders live longer than non-responders does not by itself imply anything about treatment effects. A treatment effect with respect to clinical response may indicate appropriate anti-tumor activity, but it is highly unlikely that this activity would be an appropriate surrogate for overall survival.

Other clinical endpoints often used in phase III clinical trials in cancer include disease-free survival and duration of response or length of remission, the latter endpoint restricted, of course, to those who have a measurable response to therapy or who achieve clinical remission of their disease. The reasons for studying these endpoints are that they are relevant to the primary objective of controlling the growth or spread of the cancer under study and that the therapy given after recurrence or relapse is ordinarily not controlled by the study design. Of course, these endpoints are also usually highly prognostic for overall survival, but may or may not be appropriate surrogates for overall survival. This depends on the disease and therapies under study and the effectiveness of treatment after relapse. For example, there are some diseases (e.g., Hodgkin's Disease) in which highly effective 'salvage' therapy or therapy after relapse exists and others (e.g., lung cancer) in which there is no known effective therapy after relapse. In any case, disease-free survival is often chosen as a primary end-point, not because it is a surrogate for overall survival, but because it is the most appropriate endpoint for the objectives of the trial. Overall survival and quality of life and other endpoints should also be studied, but none should be considered the single "true" endpoint.

The use of biomarkers as surrogate endpoints in therapeutic trials has not been very successful. Prominent attempts include the use of carcinoembryonic antigen (CEA) in lung cancer and colorectal cancer, PSA in prostate cancer, and CA125 in ovarian cancer. Prostate cancer has received the most attention in this regard [40–43]. The problem is that such biomarkers tend to have large intra-patient variability, much missing data, and poor sensitivity and specificity. There is good evidence of the prognostic importance of certain indices based on CEA or PSA or other markers, but this is not sufficient for surrogacy.

Cancer therapeutic agents are also notoriously toxic, and their effect on non-cancer cells is generally the cause of dose-limiting toxicity. This fact strongly suggests that the impact of these agents will go far beyond their impact on the cancer pathway, making a surrogate endpoint that reflects only activity against cancer strongly suspect. One example of an alternative pathway of action is provided by the anthracyclines, a group of antineoplastic antibiotics, including daunorubicin and doxorubicin (Adriamycin), which have proved highly effective in treating certain types of cancers in both adults and children [44]. Unfortunately, these agents can induce significant cardiotoxicity (anthracycline cardiomyopathy), including congestive heart failure, with the risk increasing with increasing cumulative dose. Other cancer chemotherapeutic agents such as 5-fluorouacil (5-FU) [45] and diethylstibestrol (DES) [14] may also induce cardiotoxicity. Any evaluation of the effectiveness of a regimen involving an anthracycline, 5-FU, or DES must take this cardiotoxicity into account. It is at least a possibility that long-term benefits of cancer suppression will be offset by increased cardiovascular mortality.

A second example is provided by those anticancer agents that are themselves known or suspected to be carcinogens. Tamoxifen and the increased risk of endometrial cancer was discussed earlier in connection with the BCPT. There is another class of agents, the alkylating agents, that are widely used in cancer chemotherapy, and that are strongly implicated as carcinogens themselves [46]. These drugs act through DNA damage and interference with cell replication and thus, in principle, would be expected to have effects other than simple anticancer effects. As in the case with the cardiotoxic agents, the choice of appropriate endpoints must consider the alternative adverse events. Control of the primary cancer is not sufficient by itself for an agent to be considered an effective anticancer agent.

5.1. Breast cancer therapeutic trials. Therapy for breast cancer is conventionally divided into therapy for early stage disease, in which interest usually centers on the effectiveness of 'adjuvant' therapy to prevent disease recurrence and prolong survival in patients rendered free of disease by surgery and therapy for advanced stage disease, in which interest centers primarily on prolonging survival. Endpoints other than overall survival that are usually reported include disease-free survival for adjuvant therapies and response rates (complete plus partial), time to disease progression, and time to treatment failure for therapies for advanced breast cancer.

The Cancer and Leukemia Group B (CALGB) is one of the large clinical cooperative groups in cancer sponsored by the National Cancer Institute. In January 1985, the CALGB opened a clinical trial (CALGB 8541) testing three different adjuvant therapies for women with stage II, node-positive breast cancer [47]. These treatments included the same drugs (cyclophosphamide, doxorubicin, and fluorouracil), but in three different dose intensities (low, standard, high). The study was closed in March 1991 after over 1,500 women had been enrolled. The outcome with respect to overall survival is given in Figure 1 where it is evident that patients on the standard and high dose regimens fared better then patients on the low dose regimen. The outcome with respect to disease-free survival (DFS), a potential surrogate for overall survival, is given in Figure 2. The overall conclusion is similar, although there is a suggestion of a difference in DFS between standard and high dose that is not borne out in overall survival. Another problem with DFS as a surrogate for overall survival is that not much time can be gained, since the time between relapse and death is unfortunately fairly short (median less than 2 years) relative to the overall duration of the study. Survival after relapse is virtually identical in the three treatment groups.

5.2. Head and neck cancer therapeutic trials. Striking examples of the failure of clinical response as a surrogate for survival are provided by the results of two separate but similar trials in recurrent or metastatic head and neck cancer. The first of these [48] involved randomization to one of three regimens: cisplatin, 5-FU and cisplatin plus 5-FU (Table 2). The response rate for the combined regiment was much higher than that for either single agent, but overall survival was no different (Figure 3). Similar results occurred in the second trial [49] (Table 3, Figure 4). The use of cisplatin plus 5-FU may produce higher response rates, but it doesn't improve survival. This is a well-known phenomenon [50].

6. Summary. Despite the extensive research efforts in developing cancer biomarkers and other putative surrogate endpoints, no non-clinical endpoint has been convincingly validated as a surrogate for any of the important clinical endpoints in cancer clinical trials. Some of these markers have proved useful in early phase or exploratory studies to demonstrate anti-cancer activity, but these are studies that are not usually large and time-consuming in any case. In addition, the terminology of 'true' and 'surrogate' endpoints has served to obscure the fact that proper evaluation of interventions, particularly therapeutic interventions for patients with cancer, involves a complex evaluation of many endpoints, including but not limited to, overall survival. Quality of life and costs of therapy are two examples of non-clinical, non-biological endpoints of obvious relevance. Nevertheless, the time and expense required to conduct large-scale prevention, screening, or treatment trials in cancer call for continued research on potential surrogate endpoints whose use could reduce this time and expense. It seems unlikely that such research will yield endpoints that can truly replace the longer-term clinical endpoints, but important supplemental information can certainly be gained.

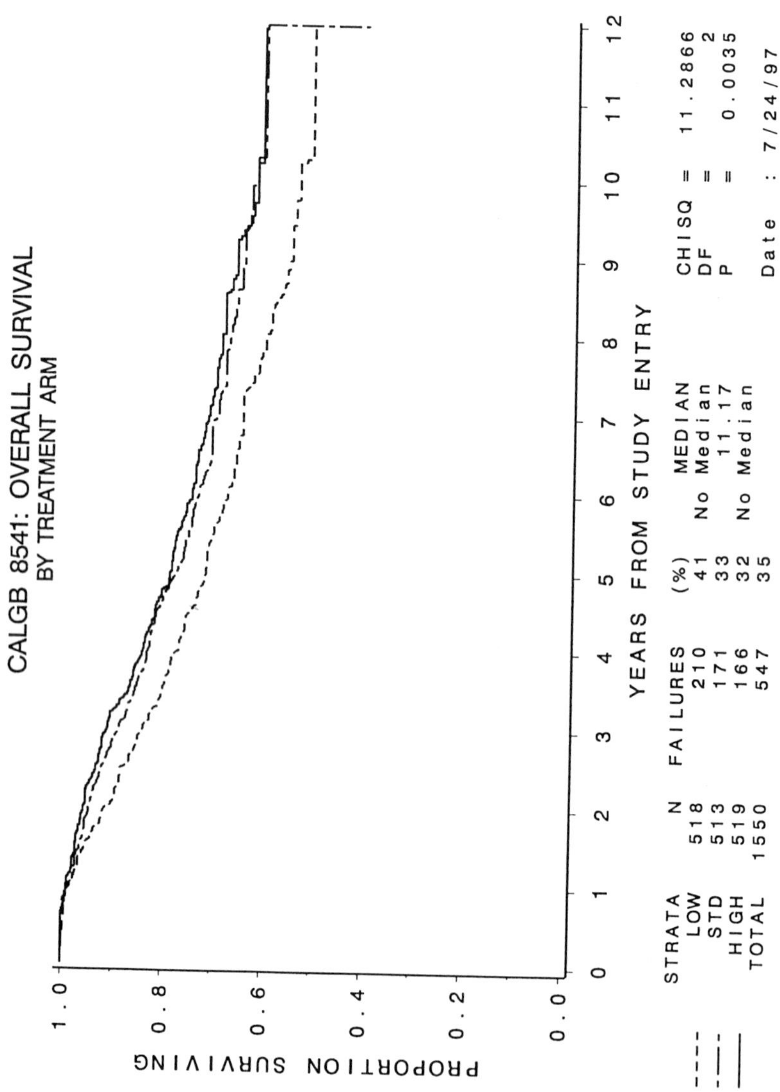
CALGB 8541: OVERALL SURVIVAL
BY TREATMENT ARM
PROPORTION SURVIVING
1.0
0.8
0.6
0.4
0.2
0.0
0 1 2 3 4 5 6 7 8 9 10 11 12
YEARS FROM STUDY ENTRY
STRATA N FAILURES (%) MEDIAN
LOW 518 210 41 No Median
STD 513 171 33 11.17
HIGH 519 166 32 No Median
TOTAL 1550 547 35
CHISQ = 11.2866
DF = 2
P = 0.0035
Date : 7/24/97

Fig. 1.

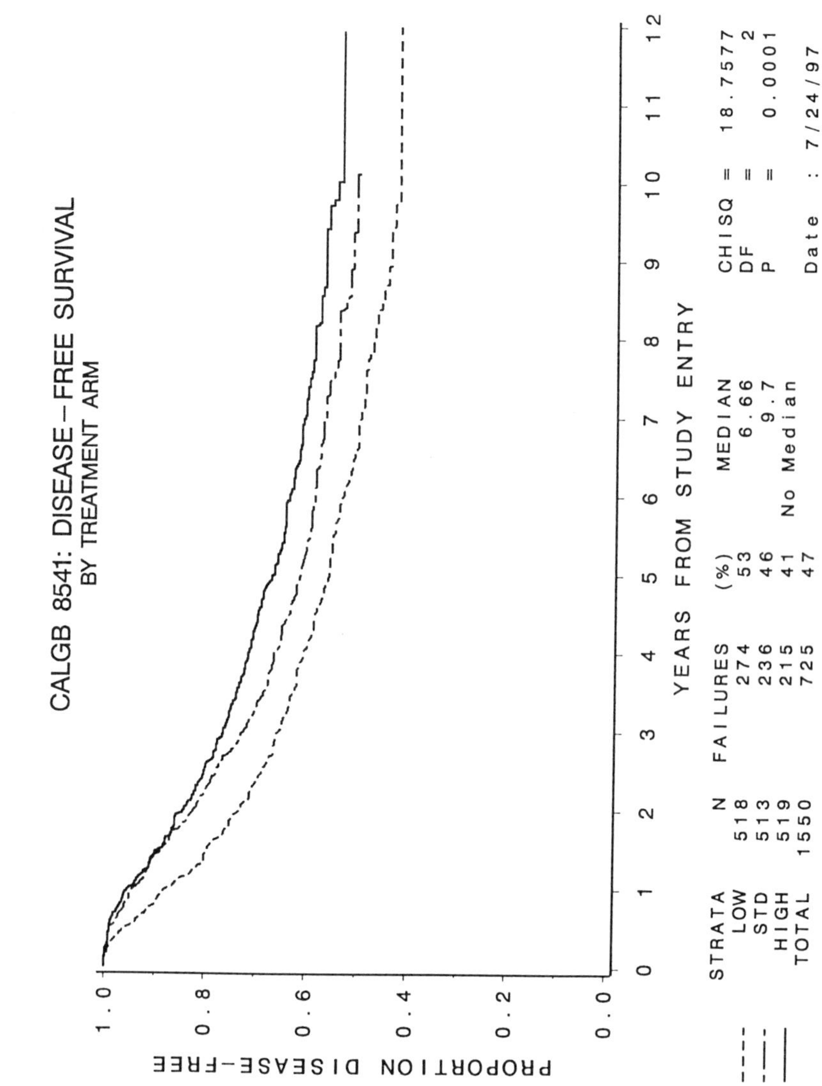
CALGB 8541: DISEASE – FREE SURVIVAL
BY TREATMENT ARM
PROPORTION DISEASE-FREE
1.0
0.8
0.6
0.4
0.2
0.0
0 1 2 3 4 5 6 7 8 9 10 11 12
YEARS FROM STUDY ENTRY
STRATA N FAILURES (%) MEDIAN
LOW 518 274 53 6.66
STD 513 236 46 9.7
HIGH 519 215 41 No Median
TOTAL 1550 725 47
CHISQ = 18.7577
DF = 2
P = 0.0001
Date : 7/24/97

Fig. 2.

TABLE 2

EXAMPLE 1: RECURRENT/METATASTIC HEAD AND NECK CANCER (Jacobs, et al, 1992)

RAND →	N	Response	MST
cisplatin	83	17%	5.0 mos
+ 5-FU	83	13%	6.1 mos
cisplatin + 5-FU	79	32%	5.5 mos
	245	20%	5.7 mos

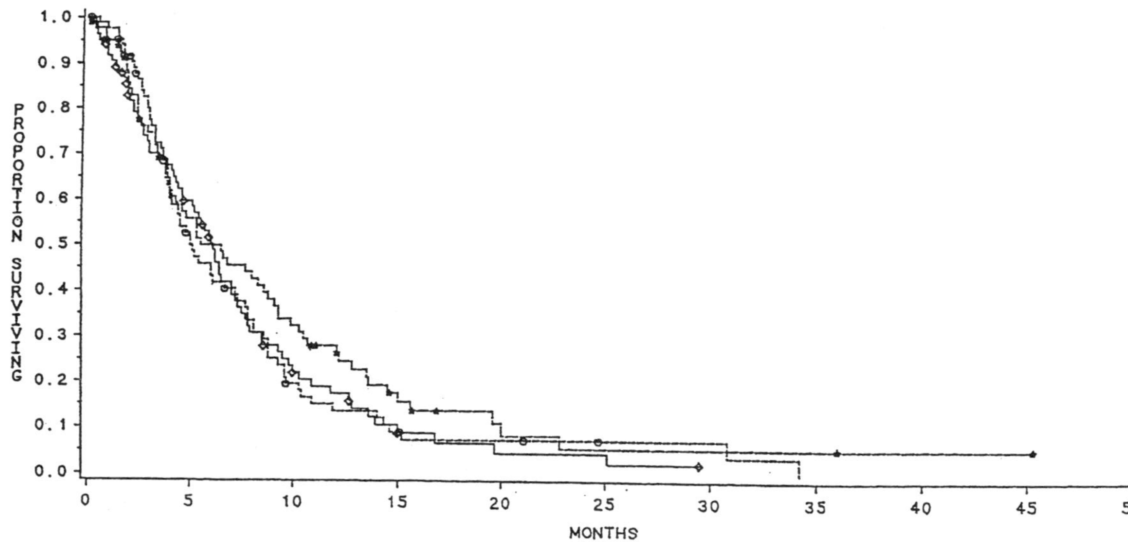

FIG. 3. *Overall survival by treatment arm. Cisplatin plus 5-FU* ($N = 79; *$)*: uncensored,* 62*, median,* 5.5 *months* (95% *Cl,* 4.0 *to* 8.8). *Cisplatin* ($N = 83; 0$)*: uncensored,* 71*; median,* 5.0 *months* (95% *Cl,* 4.1 *to* 7.2). 5-*FU* ($N = 83; \diamond$)*: uncensored,* 70*; median,* 6.1 *months* (95% *Cl,* 4.6 *to* 7.2). *By log-rank test, stratified by PS and prior radiation,* $P = .49$.

TABLE 3

EXAMPLE 2: RECURRENT/METASTATIC HEAD AND HECK CANCER (Forastiere, et al, 1992)

RAND	N	Response	MST
Mtx	88	10%	5.6 mos
carboplatin + 5-FU	86	21%	5.0 mos
cisplatin + 5-FU	87	32%	6.6 mos
	261	21%	5.7 mos

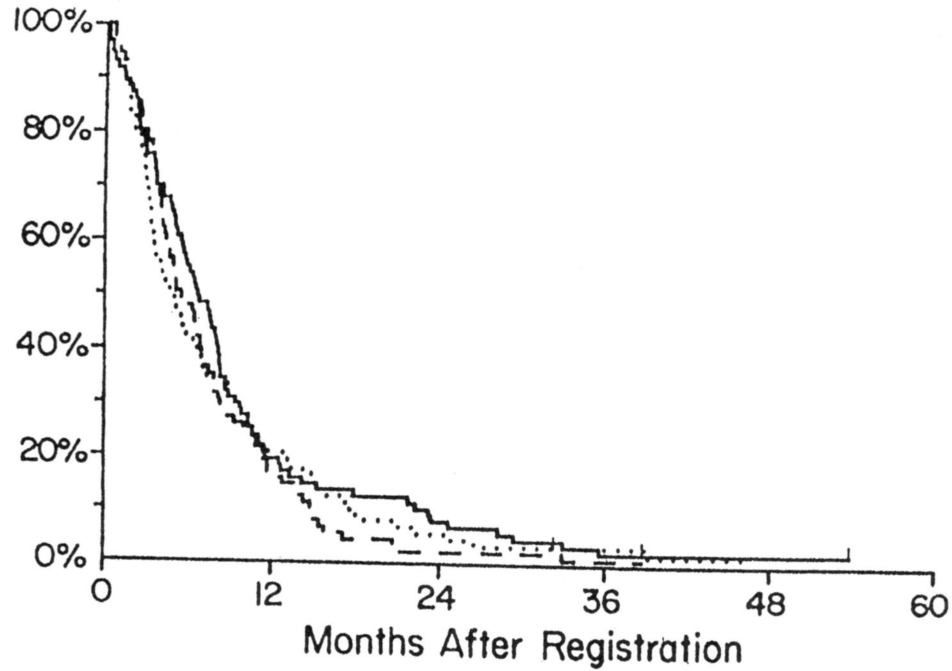

FIG. 4. *Overall survival by treatment arm of eligible patients with follow-up. —, cisplatin plus* 5-*FU, 87 patients at risk, 85 deaths, median survival time (MST)* 6.6 *months; ---, carboplatin plus 5-FU, 86 patients at risk, 85 deaths, MST 5.0 months; --, MTX, 88 patients at risk, 87 deaths, MST 5.6 months.*

REFERENCES

[1] PARKER, S.L., TONG, T., BOLDEN, S. AND WINGO, P.A., Cancer statistics, CA, 46:5–27, 1996.

[2] ELLENBERG, S.S., Surrogate endpoints in clinical trials (editorial), *British Medical Journal* 302:63–64, 1991.

[3] MACHADO, S.G., GAIL, M.H. AND ELLENBERG, S.S., On the use of laboratory markers as surrogates for clinical endpoints in the evaluation of treatment for HIV infection, *Journal of AIDS*, 3:1065–1073, 1990.

[4] TSIATIS, A.A., DAFNI, U., DEGRUTTOLA, V., PROPERT, K.J., STRAWDERMAN, R.L. AND WULFSOHN, M., *The relationship of CD4 counts over time to survival in patients with AIDS: Is CD4 a good surrogate marker? In: AIDS Epidemiology: Methodological Issues*, edited by Jewell, N.P., Dietz, K. and Farewell, V.T. Boston: Birkhauser, 1992, 245–274.

[5] DE GRUTTOLA, V., FLEMING, T., LIN, D.Y. AND COOMBS, R., Perspective: validating surrogate markers – are we being naive?, *J. Infect. Dis.*, 175:237–246, 1997.

[6] MILDVAN, D., LANDAY, A., DE GRUTTOLA, V., MACHADO, S.G. AND KAGAN, J., An approach to the validation of markers for use in AIDS clinical trials, *Clin. Infect. Dis.*, 24:764–774, 1997.

[7] FLEMING, T.R., Surrogate markers in AIDS and cancer trials, *Stat. Med.*, 13:1423–1435, 1994.

[8] ELLENBERG, S.S., Surrogate endpoints [editorial], *Br. J. Cancer*, 68:457–459, 1993.

[9] ELLENBERG, S.S. AND HAMILTON, J.M., Surrogate endpoints in clinical trials: Cancer., *Stat. Med.*, 8:405–413, 1989.

[10] TEMPLE, R.J., A regulatory authority's opinion about surrogate endpoints, In: *Clinical Measurement in Drug Evaluation*, edited by Nimmo, W.S. and Tucker, G.T., New York: John Wiley & Sons, 1995, 3–22.

[11] PRENTICE, R.L., Surrogate endpoints in clinical trials: definition and operational criteria, *Stat. Med.*, 8:431–440, 1989.

[12] ANONYMOUS, Effect of the antiarrhythmic agent moricizine on survival after myocardial infarction, The Cardiac Arrhythmia Suppression Trial II Investigators, *N. Engl J. Med.*, 327:227–233, 1992.

[13] ANONYMOUS, Preliminary report: effect of encainide and flecainide on mortality in a randomized trial of arrhythmia suppression after myocardial infarction, The Cardia Arrhythmia Suppression Trial (CAST) Investigators, *N. Engl. J. Med.*, 321:406–412, 1989.

[14] BYAR, D.P., Proceedings: The Veterans Administration Cooperative Urological Research Group's studies of cancer of the prostate, *Cancer*, 32:1126–1130, 1973.

[15] FLEMING, T.R. AND DEMETS, D.L., Surrogate end points in clinical trials: are we being misled? *Ann. Intern. Med.*, 125:605–613, 1996.

[16] FREEDMAN, L.S., GRAUBARD, B.I. AND SCHATZKIN, A., Statistical validation of intermediate endpoints for chronic diseases, *Stat. Med.*, 11:167–178, 1992.

[17] SCHATZKIN, A., FREEDMAN, L.S. AND SCHIFFMAN, M.H., Validation of intermediate end points in cancer research, *J. Natl. Can. Inst.*, 82:1746–1752, 1990.

[18] JEWELL, N.P. AND KALBFLEISCH, J.D., Marker models in survival analysis and applications to issues associated with AIDS. In: *AIDS epidemiology: Methodological Issues*, edited by Jewell, N.P., Dietz, K. and Farewell, V. Boston: Birkhauser, 1992, 211–230.

[19] FLEMING, T.R., PRENTICE, R.L., PEPE, M.S. AND GLIDDEN, D., Surrogate and auxiliary endpoints in clinical trials, with potential applications in cancer and AIDS research, *Stat. Med.*, 13:955–968, 1994.

[20] MEYSKENS, F.L., JR., Biomarker intermediate endpoints and cancer prevention, [Review], *Monogr. Natl. Cancer Inst.*, 177–181, 1992.

[21] SZARKA, C.E., GRANA, G. AND ENGSTROM, P.F., Chemoprevention of cancer, *Curr. Probl. Cancer*, 18:6–79, 1994.

[22] BOSTWICK, D.G. AND AQUILINA, J.W., Prostatic intraepithelial neoplasia (PIN) and other prostatic lesions as risk factors and surrogate endpoints for cancer chemoprevention trials, *J. Cell Biochem. Suppl.*, 25:156–164, 1996.

[23] GRIZZLE, W.E., MYERS, R.B. AND MANNE, U., The use of biomarker expression to characterize neoplastic process, *Biotech. Histochem*, 72:96–104, 1997.

[24] KELLOFF, G.J., HAWK, E.T., CROWELL, J.A., ET AL., Strategies for identification and clinical evaluation of promising chemopreventive agents, *Oncology*, 10:1471–1484, 1996.

[25] KELLOFF, G.J., BOONE, C.W., CROWELL, J.A., ET AL., Risk biomarkers and current strategies for cancer chemoprevention, *J. Cell Biochem. Suppl.*, 25:1–14, 1996.

[26] LA, D.K. AND SWENBERG, J.A., DNA adducts: biological markers of exposure and potential applications to risk assessment, *Mutat. Res.*, 365:129–146, 1996.

[27] GOHAGAN, J.K., KRAMER, B.S. AND GREENWALD, P., Screening for prostate cancer [editorial], *Am. J. Prev. Med.*, 10:245–246, 1994.

[28] BOSTWICK, D.G., BURKE, H.B., WHEELER, T.M., ET AL., The most promising surrogate endpoint biomarkers for screening candidate chemopreventive compounds for prostatic adenocarcinoma in short-term phase II clinical trials, *J. Cell Biochem. Suppl.*, 19:283–289, 1994.

[29] FEIGL, P., BLUMENSTEIN, B., THOMPSON, I., ET AL., Design of the Prostate Cancer Prevention Trial (PCPT), *Control. Clin. Trials*, 16:150–163, 1995.

[30] PITOT, H.C., The tamoxifen controversy–clinical chemopreventive agent and experimental carcinogen, *Proc. Soc. Exp. Biol. Med.*, 208:139–140, 1995.

[31] ANONYMOUS, The effect of vitamin E and beta carotene on the incidence of lung cancer and other cancers in male smokers, The Alpha-Tocopherol, Beta Carotene Cancer Prevention Study Group, *N. Engl. J. Med.*, 330:1029–1035, 1994.

[32] THORNQUIST, M.D., OMENN, G.S., GOODMAN, G.E., ET AL., Statistical design and monitoring of the Carotene and Retinol Efficacy Trial (CARET), *Control.Clin.Trials*, 14:308–324, 1993.

[33] GOHAGAN, J.K., PROROK, P.C., KRAMER, B.S. AND CORNETT, J.E., Prostate cancer screening in the prostate, lung, colorectal and ovarian cancer screening trial of the National Cancer Institute, *J. Urol*, 152:1905–1909, 1994.

[34] FLETCHER, S.W., BLACK, W., HARRIS, R., RIMER, B.K. AND SHAPIRO, S., Report of the International Workshop on Screening for Breast Cancer, *J. Natl. Cancer Inst.*, 85:1644–1656, 1993.

[35] HARRIS, R. AND LEININGER, L., Clinical strategies for breast cancer screening: weighing and using the evidence, *Ann. Intern. Med.*, 122:539–547, 1995.

[36] FONTANA, R.S., SANDERSON, D.R., WOOLNER, L.B., ET AL., Screening for lung cancer. A critique of the Mayo Lung Project, *Cancer*, 67:Suppl.:1155–64, 1991.

[37] STRAUSS, G.M., GLEASON, R.E. AND SUGARBAKER, D.J., Chest X-ray screening improves outcome in lung cancer. A reappraisal of randomized trials on lung cancer screening, *Chest*, 107:Suppl.:270S–279S, 1995.

[38] CARTER, S.K., Clinical research and drug development of antivirals in HIV: an industry perspective, J. Acquir. Immune. Defic. Syndr. Hum. Retrovirol., 10:Suppl 2:S107–S113, 1995.

[39] JOHNSON, J.R. AND TEMPLE, R., Food and Drug Administration requirements for approval of new anticancer drugs, *Cancer Treat. Rep.*, 69:1155–1159, 1985.

[40] SCHELLHAMMER, P., COCKETT, A., BOCCON-GIBOD, L., ET AL., Assessment of endpoints for clinical trials for localized prostate cancer, *Urology*, 49:27–38, 1997.

[41] SCHER, H.I., MAZUMDAR, M. AND KELLY, W.K., Clinical trials in relapsed prostate cancer: defining the target, *J. Natl. Can. Inst.*, 88:1623–1634, 1996.

[42] STEINECK, G., KELLY, W.K., MAZUMDAR, M., VLAMIS, V., SCHWARTZ, M. AND SCHER, H.I., Acid phosphatase: defining a role in androgen-independent prostate cancer, *Urology*, 47:719–726, 1996.

[43] Zietman, A.L., Dallow, K.C., McManus, P.A., Heney, N.M. and Shipley, W.U., Time to second prostate-specific antigen failure is a surrogate endpoint for prostate cancer death in a prospective trial of therapy for localized disease, Urology, 47:236–239, 1996.

[44] Dunn, J., Doxorubicin-induced cardiomyopathy, *J. Pediatr Oncol Nurs*, 11:152–160, 1994.

[45] de Forni, M. and Armand, J.P., Cardiotoxicity of chemotherapy, *Curr Opin Oncol*, 6:340–344, 1994.

[46] Lawley, P.D., Alkylation of DNA and its aftermath, *Bioessays*, 17:561–568, 1995.

[47] Wood, W.C., Budman, D.R., Korzun, A.H., et al., Dose and dose intensity of adjuvant chemotherapy for stage II, node-positive breast carcinoma, *N.Engl.J. Med.*, 330:1253–1259, 1994.

[48] Jacobs, C., Lyman, G., Velez-Garcia, E., et al., A phase III randomized study comparing cisplatin and fluorouracil as single agents and in combination for advanced squamous cell carcinoma of the head and neck, *J Clin. Oncol*, 10:257–263, 1992.

[49] Forastiere, A.A., Metch, B., Schuller, D.E., et al., Randomized comparison of cisplatin plus fluorouracil and carboplatin plus fluorouracil versus methotrexate in advanced squamous-cell carcinoma of the head and neck: a Southwest Oncology Group study, *J Clin.Oncol*, 10:1245–1251, 1992.

[50] Buyse, M. and Piedbois, P., On the relationship between response to treatment and survival time, *Stat. Med.*, 15:2797–2812, 1996.

Statistical Models in Epidemiology and Environment List of Participants

- Norman Breslow, Department of Biostatistics, University of Washington
- Bradley P. Carlin, Division of Biostatistics, University of Minnesota
- Raymond J. Carroll, Department of Statistics, Texas A&M University
- Nilanjan Chatterjee, Department of Biostatistics, University of Washington
- Li Chen, Division of Biostatistics, University of Minnesota
- Lin Chen, Department of Statistics, Purdue University
- Eric Ray Cohen, Center for Magnetic Resonance Research, University of Minnesota
- David Dorr, Biology and Biomedical Sciences, Washington University-St. Louis
- David B Dunson, Department of Biostatistics, Emory University
- Gregory Golm, Department of Biostatistics, Emory University
- M. Elizabeth Halloran, Department of Biostatistics, Emory University
- Andrew Lawson, Mathematical Sciences Division, University of Abertay Dundee
- George Maldonado, School of Public Health, University of Minnesota
- Carl Morris, Department of Statistics, Harvard University
- Gary W Oehlert, Department of Applied Statistics, University of Minnesota
- James M. Robins, Department of Epidemiology, Harvard University
- Joel Schwartz, Department of Environmental Health, Harvard School of Public Health
- Douglas Simpson, University of Illinois-Urbana
- Mark Van der Laan, Division of Biostatistics, University of California-Berkley
- Lance Waller, Division of Biostatistics, University of Minnesota
- Naisyin Wang, Statistics Department, Texas A&M University

Design and Analysis of Clinical Trials
List of Participants

- Don Berry Institute of Statistics, Duke University
- Gregory Campbell, Division of Biostatistics, Center for Devices and Radiological Health
- Kathryn Chaloner, School of Applied Statistics, University of Minnesota
- Li Chen, Division of Biostatistics, University of Minnesota
- Tim Church, University of Minnesota
- Eric Ray Cohen, Center for Magnetic Resonance Research, University of Minnesota
- Ori Davidov, Department of Biostatistics, Division of Public Health Science, Fred Hutchinson Cancer Research Center
- Dennis Dixon, Coordinating Centers Branch, National Institutes of Health
- David Dorr, Biology and Biomedical Sciences, Washington University-St. Louis
- Constantine Gatsonis, Department of Biostatistics, Brown University
- Steve George, Biometry-Medical Center, Duke University
- Chi Gu, Department of Biostatistics, Washington University
- M. Elizabeth Halloran, Department of Biostatistics, Emory University
- Ping Hu, Department of Biostatistics, Harvard School of Public Health
- Roger J. Lewis, Department of Emergency Medicine, UCLA
- Thomas Louis, Department of Biostatistics, University of Minnesota
- Barry Margolin, Department of Biostatistics, University of North Carolina-Chapel Hill
- Ross Prentice, Fred Hutchinson Cancer Research Center
- Amy Racine-Poone, Mathematical Applications, Novartis Pharma
- John Simes, NHMRC Clinical Trials Centre, University of Sydney
- Richard Simon, National Institutes of Health
- Dalene Stangl, Duke University
- Peter Thall, Department of Biomathematics, U of Texas M.D. Anderson Cancer Center
- L.J. Wei, Department of Biostatistics, Harvard University
- Stanley Young, Research Computing, Glaxo Wellcome, Inc.
- Marvin Zelen, Department of Biostatistics, Harvard School of Public Health

IMA SUMMER PROGRAMS

1987 Robotics
1988 Signal Processing
1989 Robust Statistics and Diagnostics
1990 Radar and Sonar (June 18 - June 29)
New Directions in Time Series Analysis (July 2 - July 27)
1991 Semiconductors
1992 Environmental Studies: Mathematical, Computational, and Statistical Analysis
1993 Modeling, Mesh Generation, and Adaptive Numerical Methods for Partial Differential Equations
1994 Molecular Biology
1995 Large Scale Optimizations with Applications to Inverse Problems, Optimal Control and Design, and Molecular and Structural Optimization
1996 Emerging Applications of Number Theory (July 15 – July 26)
Theory of Random Sets (August 22 – August 24)
1997 Statistics in the Health Sciences
1998 Coding and Cryptography (July 6 – July 18)
Mathematical Modeling in Industry (July 22 – July 31)
1999 Decision Making under Uncertainty: Energy and Environmental Models (July 20-24, 1999)
Codes, Systems and Graphical Models (August 2-13, 1999)

SPRINGER LECTURE NOTES FROM THE IMA:

The Mathematics and Physics of Disordered Media
Editors: Barry Hughes and Barry Ninham
(Lecture Notes in Math., Volume 1035, 1983)

Orienting Polymers
Editor: J.L. Ericksen
(Lecture Notes in Math., Volume 1063, 1984)

New Perspectives in Thermodynamics
Editor: James Serrin
(Springer-Verlag, 1986)

Models of Economic Dynamics
Editor: Hugo Sonnenschein
(Lecture Notes in Econ., Volume 264, 1986)

The IMA Volumes in Mathematics and its Applications

Current Volumes:

23 **Signal Processing Part II: Control Theory and Applications of Signal Processing** L. Auslander, F.A. Grünbaum, J.W. Helton, T. Kailath, P. Khargonekar, and S. Mitter (eds.)

24 **Mathematics in Industrial Problems, Part 2** A. Friedman

25 **Solitons in Physics, Mathematics, and Nonlinear Optics** P.J. Olver and D.H. Sattinger (eds.)

26 **Two Phase Flows and Waves** D.D. Joseph and D.G. Schaeffer (eds.)

27 **Nonlinear Evolution Equations that Change Type** B.L. Keyfitz and M. Shearer (eds.)

28 **Computer Aided Proofs in Analysis** K. Meyer and D. Schmidt (eds.)

29 **Multidimensional Hyperbolic Problems and Computations** A. Majda and J. Glimm (eds.)

30 **Microlocal Analysis and Nonlinear Waves** M. Beals, R. Melrose, and J. Rauch (eds.)

31 **Mathematics in Industrial Problems, Part 3** A. Friedman

32 **Radar and Sonar, Part I** R. Blahut, W. Miller, Jr., and C. Wilcox

33 **Directions in Robust Statistics and Diagnostics: Part I** W.A. Stahel and S. Weisberg (eds.)

34 **Directions in Robust Statistics and Diagnostics: Part II** W.A. Stahel and S. Weisberg (eds.)

35 **Dynamical Issues in Combustion Theory** P. Fife, A. Liñán, and F.A. Williams (eds.)

36 **Computing and Graphics in Statistics** A. Buja and P. Tukey (eds.)

37 **Patterns and Dynamics in Reactive Media** H. Swinney, G. Aris, and D. Aronson (eds.)

38 **Mathematics in Industrial Problems, Part 4** A. Friedman

39 **Radar and Sonar, Part II** F.A. Grünbaum, M. Bernfeld, and R.E. Blahut (eds.)

40 **Nonlinear Phenomena in Atmospheric and Oceanic Sciences** G.F. Carnevale and R.T. Pierrehumbert (eds.)

41 **Chaotic Processes in the Geological Sciences** D.A. Yuen (ed.)

42 **Partial Differential Equations with Minimal Smoothness and Applications** B. Dahlberg, E. Fabes, R. Fefferman, D. Jerison, C. Kenig, and J. Pipher (eds.)

43 **On the Evolution of Phase Boundaries** M.E. Gurtin and G.B. McFadden

44 **Twist Mappings and Their Applications** R. McGehee and K.R. Meyer (eds.)

45 **New Directions in Time Series Analysis, Part I** D. Brillinger, P. Caines, J. Geweke, E. Parzen, M. Rosenblatt, and M.S. Taqqu (eds.)

46 **New Directions in Time Series Analysis, Part II**
D. Brillinger, P. Caines, J. Geweke, E. Parzen, M. Rosenblatt, and M.S. Taqqu (eds.)

47 **Degenerate Diffusions**
W.-M. Ni, L.A. Peletier, and J.-L. Vazquez (eds.)

48 **Linear Algebra, Markov Chains, and Queueing Models**
C.D. Meyer and R.J. Plemmons (eds.)

49 **Mathematics in Industrial Problems, Part 5** A. Friedman

50 **Combinatorial and Graph-Theoretic Problems in Linear Algebra**
R.A. Brualdi, S. Friedland, and V. Klee (eds.)

51 **Statistical Thermodynamics and Differential Geometry of Microstructured Materials**
H.T. Davis and J.C.C. Nitsche (eds.)

52 **Shock Induced Transitions and Phase Structures in General Media** J.E. Dunn, R. Fosdick, and M. Slemrod (eds.)

53 **Variational and Free Boundary Problems**
A. Friedman and J. Spruck (eds.)

54 **Microstructure and Phase Transitions**
D. Kinderlehrer, R. James, M. Luskin, and J.L. Ericksen (eds.)

55 **Turbulence in Fluid Flows: A Dynamical Systems Approach**
G.R. Sell, C. Foias, and R. Temam (eds.)

56 **Graph Theory and Sparse Matrix Computation**
A. George, J.R. Gilbert, and J.W.H. Liu (eds.)

57 **Mathematics in Industrial Problems, Part 6** A. Friedman

58 **Semiconductors, Part I**
W.M. Coughran, Jr., J. Cole, P. Lloyd, and J. White (eds.)

59 **Semiconductors, Part II**
W.M. Coughran, Jr., J. Cole, P. Lloyd, and J. White (eds.)

60 **Recent Advances in Iterative Methods**
G. Golub, A. Greenbaum, and M. Luskin (eds.)

61 **Free Boundaries in Viscous Flows**
R.A. Brown and S.H. Davis (eds.)

62 **Linear Algebra for Control Theory**
P. Van Dooren and B. Wyman (eds.)

63 **Hamiltonian Dynamical Systems: History, Theory, and Applications**
H.S. Dumas, K.R. Meyer, and D.S. Schmidt (eds.)

64 **Systems and Control Theory for Power Systems**
J.H. Chow, P.V. Kokotovic, R.J. Thomas (eds.)

65 **Mathematical Finance**
M.H.A. Davis, D. Duffie, W.H. Fleming, and S.E. Shreve (eds.)

66 **Robust Control Theory** B.A. Francis and P.P. Khargonekar (eds.)

67 **Mathematics in Industrial Problems, Part 7** A. Friedman

68 **Flow Control** M.D. Gunzburger (ed.)

69 **Linear Algebra for Signal Processing**
A. Bojanczyk and G. Cybenko (eds.)
70 **Control and Optimal Design of Distributed Parameter Systems**
J.E. Lagnese, D.L. Russell, and L.W. White (eds.)
71 **Stochastic Networks** F.P. Kelly and R.J. Williams (eds.)
72 **Discrete Probability and Algorithms**
D. Aldous, P. Diaconis, J. Spencer, and J.M. Steele (eds.)
73 **Discrete Event Systems, Manufacturing Systems, and Communication Networks**
P.R. Kumar and P.P. Varaiya (eds.)
74 **Adaptive Control, Filtering, and Signal Processing**
K.J. Åström, G.C. Goodwin, and P.R. Kumar (eds.)
75 **Modeling, Mesh Generation, and Adaptive Numerical Methods for Partial Differential Equations** I. Babuska, J.E. Flaherty, W.D. Henshaw, J.E. Hopcroft, J.E. Oliger, and T. Tezduyar (eds.)
76 **Random Discrete Structures** D. Aldous and R. Pemantle (eds.)
77 **Nonlinear Stochastic PDEs: Hydrodynamic Limit and Burgers' Turbulence** T. Funaki and W.A. Woyczynski (eds.)
78 **Nonsmooth Analysis and Geometric Methods in Deterministic Optimal Control** B.S. Mordukhovich and H.J. Sussmann (eds.)
79 **Environmental Studies: Mathematical, Computational, and Statistical Analysis** M.F. Wheeler (ed.)
80 **Image Models (and their Speech Model Cousins)**
S.E. Levinson and L. Shepp (eds.)
81 **Genetic Mapping and DNA Sequencing**
T. Speed and M.S. Waterman (eds.)
82 **Mathematical Approaches to Biomolecular Structure and Dynamics**
J.P. Mesirov, K. Schulten, and D. Sumners (eds.)
83 **Mathematics in Industrial Problems, Part 8** A. Friedman
84 **Classical and Modern Branching Processes**
K.B. Athreya and P. Jagers (eds.)
85 **Stochastic Models in Geosystems**
S.A. Molchanov and W.A. Woyczynski (eds.)
86 **Computational Wave Propagation**
B. Engquist and G.A. Kriegsmann (eds.)
87 **Progress in Population Genetics and Human Evolution**
P. Donnelly and S. Tavaré (eds.)
88 **Mathematics in Industrial Problems, Part 9** A. Friedman
89 **Multiparticle Quantum Scattering With Applications to Nuclear, Atomic and Molecular Physics** D.G. Truhlar and B. Simon (eds.)
90 **Inverse Problems in Wave Propagation** G. Chavent, G. Papanicolau, P. Sacks, and W.W. Symes (eds.)
91 **Singularities and Oscillations** J. Rauch and M. Taylor (eds.)

92 **Large-Scale Optimization with Applications, Part I: Optimization in Inverse Problems and Design** L.T. Biegler, T.F. Coleman, A.R. Conn, and F. Santosa (eds.)

93 **Large-Scale Optimization with Applications, Part II: Optimal Design and Control** L.T. Biegler, T.F. Coleman, A.R. Conn, and F. Santosa (eds.)

94 **Large-Scale Optimization with Applications, Part III: Molecular Structure and Optimization** L.T. Biegler, T.F. Coleman, A.R. Conn, and F. Santosa (eds.)

95 **Quasiclassical Methods** J. Rauch and B. Simon (eds.)

96 **Wave Propagation in Complex Media** G. Papanicolaou (ed.)

97 **Random Sets: Theory and Applications** J. Goutsias, R.P.S. Mahler, and H.T. Nguyen (eds.)

98 **Particulate Flows: Processing and Rheology** D.A. Drew, D.D. Joseph, and S.L. Passman (eds.)

99 **Mathematics of Multiscale Materials** K.M. Golden, G.R. Grimmett, R.D. James, G.W. Milton, and P.N. Sen (eds.)

100 **Mathematics in Industrial Problems, Part 10** A. Friedman

101 **Nonlinear Optical Materials** J.V. Moloney (ed.)

102 **Numerical Methods for Polymeric Systems** S.G. Whittington (ed.)

103 **Topology and Geometry in Polymer Science** S.G. Whittington, D. Sumners, and T. Lodge (eds.)

104 **Essays on Mathematical Robotics** J. Baillieul, S.S. Sastry, and H.J. Sussmann (eds.)

105 **Algorithms For Parallel Processing** M.T. Heath, A. Ranade, and R.S. Schreiber (eds.)

106 **Parallel Processing of Discrete Problems** P.M. Pardalos (ed.)

107 **The Mathematics of Information Coding, Extraction, and Distribution** G. Cybenko, D.P. O'Leary, and J. Rissanen (eds.)

108 **Rational Drug Design** D.G. Truhlar, W. Howe, A.J. Hopfinger, J. Blaney, and R.A. Dammkoehler (eds.)

109 **Emerging Applications of Number Theory** D.A. Hejhal, J. Friedman, M.C. Gutzwiller, and A.M. Odlyzko (eds.)

110 **Computational Radiology and Imaging: Therapy and Diagnostics** C. Börgers and F. Natterer (eds.)

111 **Evolutionary Algorithms** L.D. Davis, K. De Jong, M.D. Vose, and L.D. Whitley (eds.)

112 **Statistics in Genetics** M.E. Halloran and S. Geisser (eds.)

113 **Grid Generation and Adaptive Algorithms** M.W. Bern, J.E. Flaherty, and M. Luskin (eds.)

114 **Diagnosis and Prediction** S. Geisser (ed.)

115 **Pattern Formation in Continuous and Coupled Systems: A Survey Volume**
M. Golubitsky, D. Luss, and S.H. Strogatz (eds.)

116 **Statistical Models in Epidemiology, the Environment, and Clinical Trials**
M.E. Halloran and D. Berry (eds.)

117 **Structured Adaptive Mesh Refinement (SAMR) Grid Methods**
S.B. Baden, N.P. Chrisochoides, D.B. Gannon, and M.L. Norman (eds.)

118 **Dynamics of Algorithms**
R. de la Llave, L.R. Petzold, and J. Lorenz (eds.)

FORTHCOMING VOLUMES

1992–1992: *Control Theory*

Robotics

1996 Summer Program: *Emerging Applications of Number Theory*

1996–1997: *Mathematics in High Performance Computing*

Algorithms for Parallel Processing
Evolutionary Algorithms
The Mathematics of Information Coding, Extraction and Distribution
Structured Adaptive Mesh Refinement Grid Methods
Computational Radiology and Imaging: Therapy and Diagnostics
Mathematical and Computational Issues in Drug Design
Rational Drug Design
Grid Generation and Adaptive Algorithms
Parallel Solution of Partial Differential Equations

1997 Summer Program: *Statistics in the Health Sciences*

Week 1: Genetics
Week 2: Imaging
Week 3: Diagnosis and Prediction
Weeks 4 and 5: Design and Analysis of Clinical Trials
Week 6: Statistics and Epidemiology: Environment and Health

1997–1998: *Emerging Applications for Dynamical Systems*

Numerical Methods for Bifurcation Problems
Multiple-time-scale Dynamical Systems
Dynamics of Algorithms